Proceedings of the Vth World Congress on Cardiac Rehabilitation

Proceedings of the Vth World Congress on Cardiac Rehabilitation

held in Bordeaux, France, July 5–8 1992

edited by

J. P. BROUSTET

Hôpital Cardiologique du Haut-Lévêque, Pessac, France

Intercept Ltd

Andover

British Library CIP Data available
ISBN 0 946707 67 7

Published by Intercept Limited, P.O. Box 716, Andover, Hampshire SP10 1YG, England

Typeset in Times by Techset Ltd., Salisbury, Wilts.
Printed in Great Britain by Athenaeum Press, Newcastle upon Tyne

List of Contributors

S. Adamopoulos
Department of Cardiac Medicine
National Heart and Lung Institute
Dovehouse Street
London SW3 6LY
UK and
Department of Cardiovascular Medicine
John Radcliffe Hospital
Oxford OX3 9DU
UK

J. W. Allen
Hospital of the Good Samaritan and University of Southern California
Los Angeles, California
USA

M. M. Al-Nozha
World Health Organization
Geneva
Switzerland

R. Aurisch
Kardiologische Abteilung
Klinik für Innere Medizin der Medizinische Fakultät (Charité) und Klinik für Nuklearmedizin
Humboldt-Universität zu Berlin
Luisentrasse 11-13
0-1040 Berlin
Germany

M. V. del Barrio
Cardiac Rehabilitation Unit
University General Hospital
GV Marquès del Turia 7
46005 Valencia
Spain

A. Bayès de Luna
Departamento de Cardiologia y Cirugia Cardiovascular
Hospital de Sant Pau
Avd S. Antonio Mª Claret 167
08025 Barcelona
Spain

G. Bennett
Medical Branch
Civil Aviation Authority
Gatwick Airport
South Area, Gatwick
West Sussex RH6 0YR
UK

W. E. Berger
Kaiser Permanente Medical Center
1150 Veterans Boulevard
Redwood City
CA 94063
USA

K. Berra
Stanford Center for Research in Disease Prevention
Stanford University
730 Welch Road
Palo Alto
CA 94304
USA

A. Bertrand
Department of Nuclear Medicine
CHU Nancy-Brabois
54500 Vandoeuvre-les-Nancy
France

P. Besse
Hôpital Cardiologique du Haut-Lévêque
Avenue de Magellan
33604 Pessac
France

H. Blackburn
School of Public Health
University of Minnesota
1300 South 2nd Street
Minneapolis
MN 55454
USA

C. Blaquière
Hôpital Cardiologique du Haut-Lévêque
Avenue de Magellan
33604 Pessac
France

J.-P. Broustet
Department of Clinical Cardiology A and Department of Exercise Testing
Hôpital Cardiologique du Haut-Lévêque
Avenue de Magellan
33604 Pessac
France

L. M. Buja
Division of Cardiology
University of Texas Southwestern Medical Center
Dallas, Texas
USA

F. Burkart
Division of Cardiology
Department of Internal Medicine
University Hospital
CH-4031 Basel
Switzerland

J. D. Cantwell
Cardiac Rehabilitation and the Internal Medicine Residency Programme
Georgia Baptist Medical Center
300 Boulevard NE
Atlanta
GA 30312
USA

A. Cavalli
Ospedale G. Fornaroli
Divisione di Cardiologia
Magenta (Milano)
Italy

E. L. Cay
Astley Ainslie Hospital
Grange Loan
Edinburgh EH9 2HL
UK

F. Cherrier
Department of Cardiology
CHU Nancy-Brabois
54500 Vandoeuvre-les-Nancy
France

A. J. S. Coats
Department of Cardiac Medicine
National Heart and Lung Institute
Dovehouse Street
London SW3 6LY
UK and
Department of Cardiovascular Medicine
John Radcliffe Hospital
Oxford OX3 9DU
UK

C. Coustry-Degré
Médico-Surgical and Rehabilitation Divisions
CUB Hôpital Erasme
808 Route de Lennik
B-1070 Brussels
Belgium

T. A. Cox
Hospital of the Good Samaritan and University of Southern California
Los Angeles, California
USA

N. Danchin
Department of Cardiology
CHU Nancy-Brabois
54500 Vandoeuvre-les-Nancy
France

J.-F. Dartigues
Laboratoire de Statistiques Médicales
Unité Inserm 330
Université de Bordeaux II
Rue Léo Saignat
33000 Bordeaux
France

P. Davey
Department of Cardiovascular Medicine
John Radcliffe Hospital
Oxford OX3 9DU
UK

R. F. DeBusk
Stanford Cardiac Rehabilitation Program
Stanford University School of Medicine
780 Welch Road, Suite 106
Palo Alto
CA 94304-1517
USA

S. G. L. G. Degré
Médico-Surgical and Rehabilitation Divisions
CUB Hôpital Erasme
808 Route de Lennik
B-1070 Brussels
Belgium

H. Denolin
Ave Winston Churchill
1180 Brussels
Belgium

M. Dorado
Departamento de Cardiologia y Cirugia Cardiovascular
Hospital de Sant Pau
Avd S. Antonio Mª Claret 167
08025 Barcelona
Spain

H. Douard
Hôpital Cardiologique du Haut-Lévêque
Avenue de Magellan
33604 Pessac
France

H. Drexler
Falk C. V. Research Center
Standford University
300 Pasteur Drive
Stanford
CA 94305
USA

R. Eckels
Division of Cardiology
University of Texas Southwestern Medical Center
Dallas, Texas
USA

M. H. Ellestad
Memorial Heart Institute
Long Beach Memorial Medical Center
Long Beach
CA 90901-1428
USA

A. O. Falase
World Health Organization
Geneva
Switzerland

A. Förster
Kardiologische Abteilung
Klinik für Innere Medizin der Medizinische Fakultät (Charité) und Klinik
für Nuklearmedizin
Humboldt-Universität zu Berlin
Luisentrasse 11-13
0-1040 Berlin
Germany

N. Frasure-Smith
McGill University and Montreal Heart Institute
5000 Belanger East
Montreal
Quebec H1T 1C8
Canada

E. S. Froelicher
Department of Physiological Nursing
School of Nursing and Department of Epidemiology and Biostatistics
School of Medicine
University of California
San Francisco
CA 94143-0610
USA

V. F. Froelicher
Division of Cardiology
111C Palo Alto VA Medical Center
3801 Miranda Avenue
Palo Alto
CA 94304
USA

M. Galvao
Department of Medicine
Division of Cardiology
Albert Einstein College of Medicine
1300 Morris Park Avenue
Forchheimer G-42
Bronx, New York
NY 10461
USA

A. J. Goble
National Heart Foundation Centre for Social and Preventive Research
Suite 1A 333 Drummond Street
Carlton
Melbourne
Victoria 3053
Australia

P. Golino
Division of Cardiology
University of Texas Southwestern Medical Center
Dallas, Texas
USA

F. L. Goss
Human Energy Research Laboratory
Health and Physical Education
School of Education
University of Pittsburgh
Pittsburgh
PA 15261
USA

J. Guindo
Departamento de Cardiologia y Cirugia Cardiovascular
Hospital de Sant Pau
Avd S. Antonio Mª Claret 167
08025 Barcelona
Spain

I. Gyarfas
World Health Organization
Geneva
Switzerland

O. M. Hess
Department of Internal Medicine, Cardiology
Institute of Pathology and Clinic of Cardiovascular Surgery
University Hospital
CH-8091 Zurich
Switzerland

E. Homs
Departamento de Cardiologia y Cirugia Cardiovascular
Hospital de Sant Pau
Avd S. Antonio Mª Claret 167
08025 Barcelona
Spain

D. R. Jacobs
School of Public Health
University of Minnesota
1300 South 2nd Street
Minneapolis
MN 55454
USA

M. Jakob
Department of Internal Medicine, Cardiology
Institute of Pathology and Clinic of Cardiovascular Surgery
University Hospital
CH-8091 Zurich
Switzerland

F. W. James
Division of Cardiology
Children's Hospital Medical Center
Cincinatti
Ohio 45229-2899
USA

M. Jelinek
Cardiac Investigation Unit
St Vincent's Hospital
Melbourne
Victoria 3065
Australia

G. Jondeau
Department of Medicine
Division of Cardiology
Albert Einstein College of Medicine
1300 Morris Park Avenue
Forchheimer G-42
Bronx, New York
NY 10461
USA

M. Joy
Medical Branch
Civil Aviation Authority
Gatwick Airport
South Area, Gatwick
West Sussex RH6 0YR
UK

Y. Juillière
Department of Cardiology
CHU Nancy-Brabois
54500 Vandoeuvre-les-Nancy
France

G. Karcher 83,179
Department of Nuclear Medicine
CHU Nancy-Brabois
54500 Vandoeuvre-les-Nancy
France

S. D. Katz
Department of Medicine
Division of Cardiology
Albert Einstein College of Medicine
1300 Morris Park Avenue
Forchheimer G-42
Bronx, New York
NY 10461
USA

T. Kavanagh
Toronto Rehabilitation Centre
345 Rumsey Road,
Toronto
Ontario M4G 1R7
Canada

J. J. Kellermann
Chaim Sheba Medical Centre
Tel Hashomer
Israel

M. Klapholz
Department of Medicine
Division of Cardiology
Albert Einstein College of Medicine
1300 Morris Park Avenue
Forchheimer G-42
Bronx, New York
NY 10461
USA

R. A. Kloner
Hospital of the Good Samaritan and University of Southern California
Los Angeles, California
USA

M. Koch
Department of Clinical Cardiology A and Department of Exercise Testing
Hôpital Cardiologique du Haut-Lévêque
Avenue de Magellan
33604 Pessac
France

K. Kothe
Kardiologische Abteilung
Klinik für Innere Medizin der Medizinische Fakultät (Charité) und Klinik für Nuklearmedizin
Humboldt-Universität zu Berlin
Luisentrasse 11-13
0-1040 Berlin
Germany

H. P. Krayenbuehl
Department of Internal Medicine, Cardiology
Institute of Pathology and Cardiovascular Surgery
University Hospital
CH-8091 Zurich
Switzerland

O. N. Krogmann
Department of Internal Medicine, Cardiology
Institute of Pathology and Clinic of Cardiovascular Surgery
University Hospital
CH-8091 Zurich
Switzerland

J. Larrue
Unité de Recherche Cardiovasculaire
U8 INSERM
Groupe Hospitalier Haut-Lévêque
33600 Pessac
France

T. H. LeJemtel
Department of Medicine
Division of Cardiology
Albert Einstein College of Medicine
1300 Morris Park Avenue
Bronx, New York
NY 10461
USA

P. Levato
Department of Medicine
Division of Cardiology
Albert Einstein College of Medicine
1300 Morris Park Avenue
Bronx, New York
NY 10461
USA

B. Lewis
4 Sutcliffe Close
London NW11 6NT
UK

P. R. Lichtlen
Department of Internal Medicine
Division of Cardiology
Hannover Medical School
Konstanty-Gutschow-Str 8
D-3000 Hannover 61
Germany

P.-Y. Marie
Department of Cardiology and
Department of Nuclear Medicine
Hôpital de Brabois
Rue du Morvan
54500 Vandoeuvre-les-Nancy
France

A. Martin
Department of Public Health
University of Sydney
Sydney
New South Wales 2006
Australia

I. Martin
World Health Organization
Geneva
Switzerland

T. Marwick
Service de Cardiologie
Cliniques Universitaires St Luc
Université Catholique de Louvain
Avenue Hippocrate 10
1200 Brussels
Belgium

E. Mazaudier
Hôpital Cardiologique du Haut-Lévêque
Avenue de Magellan
33604 Pessac
France

D. Mertens
Toronto Rehabilitation Centre
University of Toronto
320 Huron Street
Toronto
Ontario M5S 1A1
Canada

M. V. Mestre
Cardiac Rehabilitation Unit
University General Hospital
GV Marquès del Turia 7
46005 Valencia
Spain

K. F. Metz
Human Energy Research Laboratory
Health and Physical Education
School of Education
University of Pittsburgh
Pittsburgh
PA 15261
USA

T. E. Meyer
Department of Cardiovascular Medicine
John Radcliffe Hospital
Oxford OX3 9DU
UK

N. Houston Miller
Stanford Cardiac Rehabilitation Program
Stanford University School of Medicine
780 Welch Road
Suite 106
Palo Alto
CA 94304-1517
USA

R. Mulcahy
Department of Preventive Cardiology
St Vincent's Hospital
Dublin 4
Ireland

L. F. Nikolaeva
World Health Organization
Geneva
Switzerland

G. Niset
Médico-surgical and Rehabilitation Divisions
CUB Hôpital Erasme
808 Route de Lennik
B-1070 Brussels
Belgium

B. Oldenburg
Department of Public Health
University of Sydney
Sydney
New South Wales 2006
Australia

N. Oldridge
Department of Health Sciences
University of Wisconsin
Milwaukee
WI 53201
USA

C. H. Oon
Singapore General Hospital
Outram Road
Singapore

D. Ornish
Preventive Medicine Research Institute
1001 Bridgeway
Suite 305
Sausalito
CA 94965
USA

N. Oysel
Hôpital Cardiologique du Haut-Lévêque
Avenue de Magellan
33604 Pessac
France

C. Panchaud
World Health Organization
Geneva
Switzerland

F. J. Pashkow
Department of Cardiology
Cleveland Clinic Foundation
9500 Euclid Avenue
Cleveland
OH 44195-5064
USA

P. Pastor
Division of Cardiology
University of Texas Southwestern Medical Center
Dallas, Texas
USA

C. Penas
Cardiac Rehabilitation Unit
University General Hospital
GV Marquès del Turia 7
46005 Valencia
Spain

M. Pfisterer
Division of Cardiology
Department of Internal Medicine
University Hospital
CH-4031 Basel
Switzerland

M. Piepoli
Department of Cardiac Medicine
National Heart and Lung Institute
Dovehouse Street
London SW3 6LY
UK and
Department of Cardiovascular Medicine
John Radcliffe Hospital
Oxford OX3 9DU
UK

F. Platieau
Médico-Surgical and Rehabilitation Divisions
CUB Hôpital Erasme
808 Route de Lennik
B-1070 Brussels
Belgium

P. A. Poole-Wilson
Department of Cardiology
National Heart and Lung Institute
Dovehouse Street
London SW3 6LY
UK

J. A. Queiroz
Memorial Heart Institute
Long Beach Memorial Medical Center
Long Beach
CA 90801-1428
USA

S. Qureshi
Toronto Rehabilitation Centre
University of Toronto
320 Huron Street
Toronto
Ontario M5S 1A1
Canada

A. Radaelli
Department of Cardiovascular Medicine
John Radcliffe Hospital
Oxford OX3 9DU
UK and
Department of Internal Medicine
First Medical Clinic
University of Pavia
Pavia
Italy

F. Ridocci
Cardiac Rehabilitation Unit
University General Hospital
GV Marquès del Turia 7
46005 Valencia
Spain

R. J. Robertson
Human Energy Research Laboratory
Health and Physical Education
School of Education
University of Pittsburgh
Pittsburgh
PA 15261
USA

H. Roskamm
Rehabilitationszentrum für Herz- und Kreislaufkranke
Südring 15
D-7812 Bad Krozingen
Germany

P. Rougier
Hôpital Cardiologique du Haut-Lévêque
Avenue de Magellan
33604 Pessac
France

C. E. Ruiz
Hospital of the Good Samaritan and University of Southern California
Los Angeles, California
USA

P.-A. Salamin
Division of Mathematical Applications
Central Research Laboratories
Ciba-Geigy Ltd
Basel
Switzerland

L. Samek
Rehabilitationszentrum für Herz- und Kreislaufkranke
Südring 15
D-7812 Bad Krozingen
Germany

J. Schneider
Department of Internal Medicine, Cardiology
Institute of Pathology and Clinic of Cardiovascular Surgery
University Hospital
CH-8091 Zurich
Switzerland

A. H. Shandling
Memorial Heart Institute
Long Beach Memorial Medical Center
Long Beach, California
USA

R. J. Shephard
Toronto Rehabilitation Centre and School of Physical and Health Education
University of Toronto
320 Huron Street
Toronto
Ontario M5S 1A1
Canada

P. Sleight
Department of Cardiovascular Medicine
John Radcliffe Hospital
Oxford OX3 9DU
UK

H. van der Sluys
Department of Cardiology
Building 1/C5-P
University Hospital
PO Box 9600
2300 RC Leiden
Netherlands

S. Solomon
Department of Medicine
Division of Cardiology
Albert Einstein College of Medicine
1300 Morris Park Avenue
Bronx, New York
NY 10461
USA

R. H. Startt-Selvester
Memorial Heart Institute
Long Beach Memorial Medical Center
Long Beach
CA
USA

T. Strasser
World Health Organization
Geneva
Switzerland

M. J. Sullivan
Department of Medicine
Division of Cardiology and Center for Living
Duke University VA Medical Center
Durham
NC 27710
USA

R. H. Superko
Alta Bates—Herrick Hospital
3030 Telegraph Avenue
Berkeley
CA 94705
USA

L. Tavazzi
Fondazione Clinica del Lavoro
Centro Medico di Riabilitazione
Divisione di Cardiologia
Via S. Boezio 26
27100 Pavia
Italy

A. L. Taylor
Associate Professor of Medicine
Division of Cardiology
Department of Medicine
University Hospital of Cleveland
2074 Abington Road
Cleveland
OH 44106
USA

C. B. Taylor
Department of Psychiatry
Stanford University School of Medicine
Stanford
CA 94305
USA

J. Traber
Department of Internal Medicine, Cardiology
Institute of Pathology and Clinic of
Cardiovascular Surgery
University Hospital
CH-8091 Zurich
Switzerland

M. Turina
Department of Internal Medicine, Cardiology
Institute of Pathology and Clinic of
Cardiovascular Surgery
University Hospital
CH-8091 Zurich
Switzerland

J. A. Velasco
Cardiac Rehabilitation Unit
University General Hospital
GV Marquès del Turia 7
46005 Valencia
Spain

X. Viňolas
Departamento de Cardiologia y Cirugia
Cardiovascular
Hospital de Sant Pau
Avd S. Antonio Mª Claret 167
08025 Barcelona
Spain

A. Volpi
Ospedale G. Fornaroli
Divisione di Cardiologia
Magenta (Milano)
Italy

C. Vongprateep
Children's Hospital
420/8 Rajvitee Road
Payatai
Bangkok 10400
Thailand

H. W. H. Weeda
Department of Cardiology
Building 1/C5-P
University Hospital
PO Box 9600
2300 RC Leiden
The Netherlands

N. K. Wenger
Department of Medicine
Division of Cardiology
Emory University School of Medicine
69 Butler Street SE
Atlanta
GA 30303
USA

T. Willerson
University of Texas Southwestern Medical Center
Dallas, Texas
USA

M. C. Worcester
National Heart Foundation Centre for Social and Preventive Research
Suite 1a 333 Drummond Street
Carlton
Melbourne
Victoria 3053
Australia

M. H. Yacoub
Department of Cardiothoracic Surgery
National Heart and Lung Institute
Harefield Hospital
Harefield, Middlesex
UK

Preface

Following on from Hamburg in 1977, Jerusalem in 1981, Caracas in 1984, and Broadbeach near Brisbane in 1988, the Vth World Congress of Cardiac Rehabilitation was held in Bordeaux, France from July 5–8 1992. More than 900 delegates attended; seven conference halls and two areas for posters were available. Through lectures, conferences, round tables, workshops, oral and poster communications 370 speakers were able to air their opinions and transmit information on all aspects of comprehensive rehabilitation.

Rehabilitation touches on all the many and varied aspects of the management of cardiac patients: the state of patients must first of all be assessed cardiologically – the haemodynamic repercussions, risks of arrhythmia, the quantity of viable myocardium, hibernating or creeping ischaemia and very often the coronary network are increasingly identified and measured using methods and equipment which are in themselves more and more sophisticated and which must be used judiciously: isotropy, ultrasonics, x-rays, electrocardiography leave little to chance after an infarction, a bypass or cardiac failure.

But assessment also covers the respiratory system, the muscular and osteo-articular state of the patient since the cardiovascular system is fed by the lungs and is there to service the muscles.

Beyond this and often to the fore are the psychological and socio-professional repercussions. A reaction of mourning after such a heavy blow and loss of health, or news of continuing progression, or another onset of the disease all provoke various types of reactions: depression, anxiety, negation. Recognition and psychotherapy can often do much more for the future welfare of the patient than any specific treatment of the cardiac disease itself.

Retraining for exercise under stress, both long- and short-term, has benefited considerably from progress in the knowledge of metabolism thanks to magnetic resonance imaging. We now understand that it is neither dangerous nor a waste of time to offer graded physical exercise to patients with chronic heart disease. The necessity of retraining appeared with the problems of weakness of muscle in cardiac transplant patients.

While the patient pursued his rehabilitation from Phase I and Phase II, if he has returned to work, there remained the development of the relationship with and between the rehabilitation team, those of the medical services and the representatives of occupational medicine. There remains a lot to be done in many countries to see that information circulates correctly and rapidly, and that the preparation for return to work is carried out effectively.

Progress in therapeutic treatment means that life expectancy is increasing all the time. More and more coronary patients and those suffering from cardiac failure are over the age of 75. Those who have undergone coronary revascularization between the ages of 60 and 70 present specific problems of strategy and care when 10 or 15 years later they come back with angina pectoris or an infarction, more often than not complicated by heart failure. If there is any improvement at all everything must be done to give them back as much autonomy as possible to enable them, if such is their desire, to continue to live at home, even if some assistance is required.

In short, the rehabilitation of cardiac patients means applying a full range of medical techniques, with Hippocratic and humanistic approaches to the fore. It is differentiated from other approaches by concentrating in particular on the physiology and physiopathology of an individual patient and his or her tolerance to exercise and training by not restricting cardiology to the acute phases of cardiac disease or to exploration by sophisticated technical means, which are marvellous in their technicity but are extremely costly and deal with the patient's heart as an organ rather than with the patient as a whole. These techniques are also mostly inaccessible to most developing countries. The Scientific Council of the Section on Cardiac Rehabilitation of the International Society and Federation of Cardiology and the World Health Organization have both given much consideration to modes of rehabilitation.

It is all this that the papers which follow and which were given by the invited speakers at the Vth World Congress on Cardiac Rehabilitation have tried to express. Inevitably the reader will get the impression of dispersal or, according to his own specialization within the subject, he might only feel a scant interest. But is it not the true duty of all those who work in the field of cardiac rehabilitation to have a wide knowledge? To be competent in all the diagnostic and therapeutic fields linking the first sensation of pain or suffocation to a successful return to work and long-term absence of development of symptoms. What other field of medicine enables the practitioner to take such a total approach, one of such unceasing and sustained effort, and so prolonged in time as that of the rehabilitation of cardiac patients? Those who practise rehabilitation conscientiously refuse to be considered as specialists who know a lot about a little, or generalists who know a little about a lot. They have the ambition of knowing a lot about everything concerning the diagnosis, treatment and psychology of cardiac patients. The object of the World Congress and this volume of Proceedings is to assist them.

I would like to address our thanks to all concerned with the publication of this volume:

First and foremost the authors who kindly agreed to supply the text of their papers within a short time and who have accepted editorial constraints to which they are not accustomed.

Next I would like to thank all those who worked to make the Vth World Congress on Cardiac Rehabilitation a success: Doctors Douard, Monpère, Goepfert, Sellier and our friends on the Scientific Council of the Section on Cardiac Rehabilitation of the International Society and Federation of Cardiology. Their advice, example and experience were of great assistance.

Marianne de Figueiredo, the indefatigible and devoted Secretary of the International Society and Federation of Cardiology who gave us constant support during the preparation of the Congress and who circulated information about it throughout the world in their magazine *Heartbeat*.

Our gratitude must also go to Jane Coulter who has done much to harmonize the style of the texts and who stimulated the authors with perseverance and determination in reminding them of the deadlines to be met.

Our thanks also to Intercept and its very forward-looking system of computer-aided publication which has enabled us to bring you these Proceedings so rapidly.

Finally, but not least, we are indebted to the pharmaceutical companies and manufacturers of medical equipment who have given us their unstinting backing, in some cases several years in advance. Without them and their assistance, and that too of the Aquitaine Regional Council, none of this would have been possible.

Our final wish would be that the readers of this volume will be pursuaded to attend the VIth World Congress on Cardiac Rehabilitation to be held in Buenos Aires in 1996 under the chairmanship of Professor Bernardo Boskis.

January 1993 J.P. Broustet

Contents

PART VII REHABILITATION IN CHRONIC HEART FAILURE

PART VIII REHABILITATION IN CARDIAC TRANSPLANTATION

PART XI REGRESSION OF ATHEROSCLEROSIS

PART XII SECONDARY PREVENTION

PART XIII RETURN TO WORK

PART XIV IMPLEMENTATION OF CARDIAC REHABILITATION THROUGHOUT THE WORLD

I Stratification of Risk After Myocardial Infarction

1 Risk Assessment after Myocardial Infarction: Role of Clinical and Electrocardiographic Information

Matthias Pfisterer[1]*, Paul-André Salamin[2], Felix Burkart[1]

[1] *Division of Cardiology, Department of Internal Medicine, University Hospital, CH-4031 Basel* and [2] *Division of Mathematical Applications, Central Research Laboratories, Ciba-Geigy Ltd, Basel, Switzerland*

Introduction

Myocardial necrosis, viable myocardium remaining at jeopardy, and ventricular arrhythmias are the main determinants of prognosis after myocardial infarction. Clinical and non-invasive testing after myocardial infarction aims, therefore, at evaluation of infarct size as well as detection of ischaemia and severe ventricular arrhythmias. There is a multitude of non-invasive tests available for this purpose. However, in view of the cost constraints in medicine today, multiple non-invasive testing for risk assessment in the large group of patients with recent myocardial infarction has to be restricted. A decision protocol should be available which would allow risk assessment based on relevant clinical data combined if necessary with non-invasive tests. Accordingly, the aim of our study was to determine prospectively markers of infarct size, ischaemia and ventricular arrhythmias based on clinical and electrocardiographic findings in a large consecutive group of patients surviving their first acute coronary event and to follow these patients for 2.5–5 years. In view of the limitations of standard prediction models [1] and in order to simulate clinical practice, a recursive partitioning algorithm was used to define a decision tree for risk assessment based on data collected at hospital discharge.

* To whom all correspondence should be addressed.

Proceedings of the Vth World Congress on Cardiac Rehabilitation

Methods

Subjects

A consecutive series of 744 patients below the age of 71 years admitted to our coronary care unit with acute myocardial infarction between July 1981 and June 1984 were screened for this study. Those patients who were excluded included 219 with a history or ECG signs of a previous infarct, 60 who died in the hospital, 19 with severe secondary disease (carcinoma, cerebrovascular disability, renal or liver insufficiency), 15 with urgent coronary artery bypass graft surgery during hospitalization, 9 who did not consent and 56 patients who lived so far away that no follow-up was possible. Thus, 366 patients were included, but 5 were later lost for follow-up (moved to a foreign country), leaving a final study population of 361 survivors of a first myocardial infarction.

The 290 men and 71 women were aged 23–70 years (median 59 years). Of these, 204 had a Q-wave, 113 a non-Q-wave and 44 an impending infarction ($>$30 min ischaemic chest pain at rest with only transient ST-T wave changes and without enzyme rise above normal limits). Since the patients were entered consecutively into the study at hospital admission, this latter group remained in the analysis, although their acute coronary event did not lead to a definite infarction. The location of the electrocardiographic infarct was anterior in 114 (32%) patients, inferior in 175 (48%) and elsewhere in 72 (20%). No patient had thrombolytic therapy. Treatment at hospital discharge was by β-blocking drugs in 120 patients, nitrates in 60, calcium channel blockers in 178, anti-arrhythmics in 60 and diuretics in 97, while 41 patients had coronary artery bypass graft surgery during the first year after their infarct, 8 of them without symptoms (i.e. for prophylactic reasons). Anti-anginal and other drug therapy as well as coronary artery bypass graft surgery was left to the discretion of the physician responsible and registered as in an observational study.

Study protocol

During the acute phase of infarction, the usual clinical parameters were recorded including a 12-lead ECG, an upright chest X-ray and serial determinations of creatine kinase activity. At hospital discharge, the same clinical, ECG and chest X-ray measurements were obtained. In addition, all patients had a 24 h Holter ECG recording (Instruments for Cardiac Research Inc., Syracuse, NY, model 6004C Holter electrocardio-scanner; playback at 60 times real-time speed and printed condensed on fibre optic paper for visual control) after discontinuation of all anti-arrhythmic therapy. Three to four weeks after the acute event, a symptom-limited upright bicycle ergometer test was performed for evaluation of physical work capacity and exercise ECG.

In order to compare the clinical data with non-invasive test results, planar thallium-201 myocardial perfusion scintigraphy was performed according to standard protocols. Thallium-201 scintigraphy defect size was semi-quantitatively scored as previously described [2]. Usually on the same day, the patients also had equilibrium radionuclide angiocardiography at rest and during symptom-limited supine bicycle ergometry for determination of left ventricular ejection fraction. All non-invasive tests were evaluated immediately, i.e. long before follow-up information was available, and independently of clinical data. Heart failure was diagnosed clinically if more than one of the following four signs were present: (1) chest X-ray: cardiothoracic ratio >0.5 and/or pulmonary congestion; (2) third heart sound and/or clinically enlarged left ventricle; (3) dyspnoea New York Heart Association class $\geq$ II; (4) use of diuretics. The patients were then followed at our out-patient clinic after 3, 6 and 12 months, including a full clinical examination and 12-lead ECG after 1 year. Thereafter, all patients and/or their doctors were contacted by questionnaire and if necessary by telephone for a final survival assessment 2.5–5 years (median 3.4 years) after their index infarction.

The critical events were cardiac death and non-fatal ischaemic events, i.e. documented non-fatal reinfarction and unstable angina pectoris (= angina at rest or increase ≥ 2 classes in Canadian Heart Association classification) as assessed during the follow-up visits.

This study protocol was approved by the Ethical Committee of the University Hospital of Basel, Switzerland on 29 January 1981.

Statistical analysis

The data are presented as the mean ± 1 standard deviation (SD). There were initially 52 clinical variables (including exercise ECG). For analysis, each was subdivided into three sub-groups based on patient distribution (highest and lowest quartiles) and clinical judgement. The prognostic power of each variable was assessed by calculating the relative risk, together with a 95% confidence interval, using the method suggested by Koopman [3]. The confidence interval is asymmetric about the estimate of the relative risk and is consistent with Pearson's chi-square test for testing the hypothesis that the relative risk is equal to 1. Logistic regression, based on the variables for which the relative risk was significantly larger than 1 with a P-value <0.02, was used to identify independent risk factors for death and ischaemic events separately.

In view of the large number of variables (some continuous and others categorical), a small amount of missing data, the three separate endpoints (death, non-fatal ischaemic events and no events) and the aim of arriving at a simple decision tree useful for clinical practice, a recursive partitioning algorithm (CART software) was applied [4]. A family of decision trees was constructed to find an optimal risk prediction for the death, non-fatal ischaemic event and no-event patient groups. To compensate for the large differences (76 *vs* 20 *vs* 4%) in the observed frequency of no events, non-fatal events and death, the misclassification "costs" were chosen proportional to the inverse of the observed frequency of the outcomes. The "costs" were then in the relation 1:4:20, meaning that a non-fatal event was weighted four times as much as no event and death five times as much as a non-fatal event. It can be shown that this choice of "cost" is equivalent to assuming unit misclassification "cost" and equal probability of the outcomes.

Since there were few deaths and ischaemic events after the first year and since information during late follow-up was reliable for myocardial infarction and death only, the predictive power of all variables was calculated for first-year events only.

Results

Occurrence of cardiac events

Critical events occurred mainly in the first 6 months after the acute event and there were very few additional deaths after the first year (Fig. 1). One year mortality in hospital survivors of a first myocardial infarction below age 71 years was 4.2%. In this time period, five patients died of severe congestive heart failure, six died suddenly (defined as within 1 h of symptoms, two of whom had cardiac rupture at autopsy) and three were found dead without prior symptoms or alarm, whereas only one patient died after reinfarction in cardiogenic shock. Non-fatal ischaemic events were five times more frequent than fatal events during the first year (20%); thereafter, these data were reliable only for reinfarction, since they were obtained by questionnaire and/or telephone interview (Fig. 1).

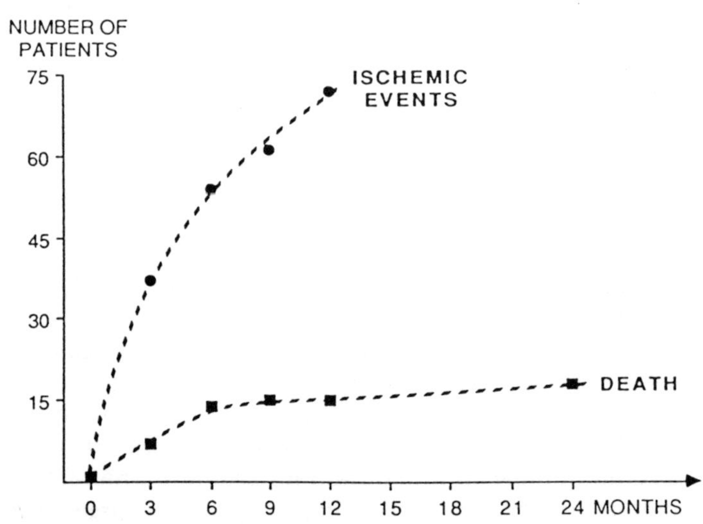

Fig. 1. Cumulative cardiac event rate over time, separated for death (■) and non-fatal ischaemic events (●) for the first 12 months and for death up to 48 months (actual data points, fitted curve). Note that most of the deaths occurred during the first 6 months after the acute event.

Predictors of death and non-fatal ischaemic events

According to univariate analysis, there were 11 clinical or electrocardiographic predictors of death with a relative risk increase of 4.7-fold to 20.7-fold, mainly related to age, infarct size and arrhythmias (Table 1). In addition, there were nine predictors of non-fatal ischaemic events related to risk factors, history of

Table 1

Predictors of death and ischaemic events according to univariate analysis[a]

Variable	Comparison	Relative risk	95% confidence interval	*P*
Predictors of death				
Age (years)	≥65 *vs* 52	13.2	1.6–∞	0.0117
Heart rate (beats/min)	≥81 *vs* 60–80	6.6	2.4–20.9	0.0001
LV palpation	abnormal *vs* normal	5.2	1.9–12.7	0.0007
Third heart sound	present *vs* absent	4.8	1.7–11.8	0.0015
Heart failure	≥2 signs *vs* no sign	10.0	2.4–86.1	0.0006
Diuretics	yes *vs* no	7.1	2.7–22.2	0.0001
Chest X-ray	oedema *vs* normal	9.2	1.9–33.9	0.0021
ST segment at rest	depressed *vs* normal	7.9	1.0–26.3	0.0155
Max. CK (IU/l)	>2500 *vs* <750	4.7	1.3–18.8	0.0177
VPB/h average	>9 *vs* 0	20.7	2.6–∞	0.0012
Lown class	>III *vs* 0	15.9	2.0–∞	0.0046
TL score at rest	≥12 *vs* ≤2	4.9	1.2–42.6	0.0309
LVEF at rest	≤30 *vs* ≥52	6.4	1.4–33.5	0.0118
LVEF exercise	≤30 *vs* ≥52	12.3	2.8–107.3	0.0005
WMA	>1 segment *vs* no	5.5	1.3–47.2	0.0199
Predictors of ischaemic events				
Sex	female *vs* male	1.7	1.1–2.6	0.0098
Angina history	yes *vs* no	1.7	1.1–2.6	0.0072
Diabetes history	yes *vs* no	2.0	1.2–3.1	0.0083
Risk factors	≥3 *vs* ≤1	2.6	1.2–7.6	0.0180
Systolic blood pressure (mmHg)	≥125 *vs* ≤105	3.0	1.7–5.9	0.0001
Diastolic blood pressure (mmHg)	≥80 *vs* ≤65	2.1	1.2–3.8	0.0067
ECG	non-Q *vs* Q	1.8	1.2–2.8	0.0089
Exercise ST segment[b]	sign. depression *vs* no	1.9	1.0–3.2	0.0349
Max. CK (IU/l)	<750 *vs* >2500	3.5	1.3–15.9	0.0109
ΔLVEF rest–exercise	≤−5% *vs* >0%	2.2	1.3–3.6	0.0024
WMA	0 *vs* ≥1 segment	2.0	1.2–3.5	0.0054
ΔTL score rest–exercise	0 *vs* >1	1.6	1.3–4.3	0.0059

[a] Risk increase for sub-groups as indicated. All parameters assessed at hospital discharge.
[b] For patients without beta-blocking drugs.
Abbreviations: IU/l = international units per litre; LVEF = left ventricular ejection fraction; Max. CK = maximal creatine kinase level; VPB/h = ventricular premature beats per hour; WMA = wall motion abnormalities; Δ = change.

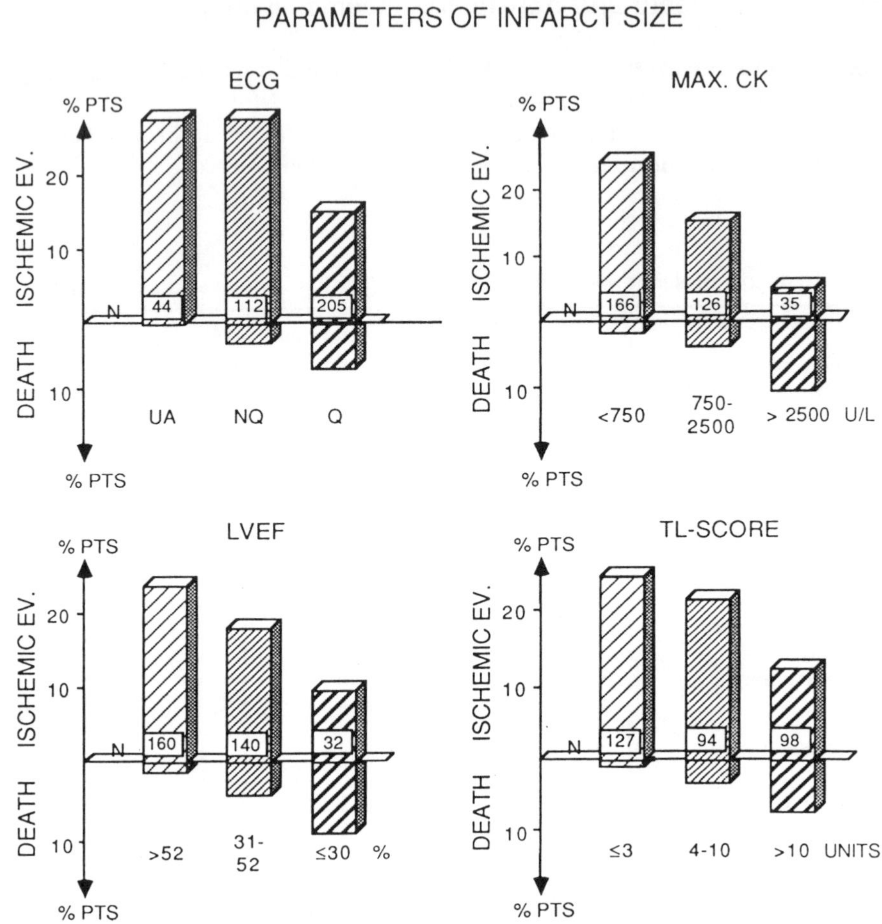

Fig. 2. Parameters of infarct size and left ventricular function at rest (a) arrhythmias and heart failure (b) each subdivided into three groups in relation to their power to predict death (downwards) and non-fatal ischaemic events (upwards) over the 1-year follow-up. *Note*: for all these parameters, there is a direct relation to fatal and an inverse relation to non-fatal events, the sum remaining relatively constant.

angina and persistent ischaemia, with a risk increase between 1.6-fold and 3.0-fold. In Table 1, the relative risk increase for different clinical variables is given and compared to that of non-invasive test results.

The parameters infarct size, left ventricular function at rest and ventricular arrhythmias (Fig. 2) were directly related to fatal and inversely related to non-fatal ischaemic events during the 1-year follow-up. This means that the lower the left ventricular ejection fraction, the higher the rate of subsequent death, but the lower the rate of later non-fatal ischaemic events. This was true for all univariate predictors of death. Thus, Q-wave infarct had a 1-year

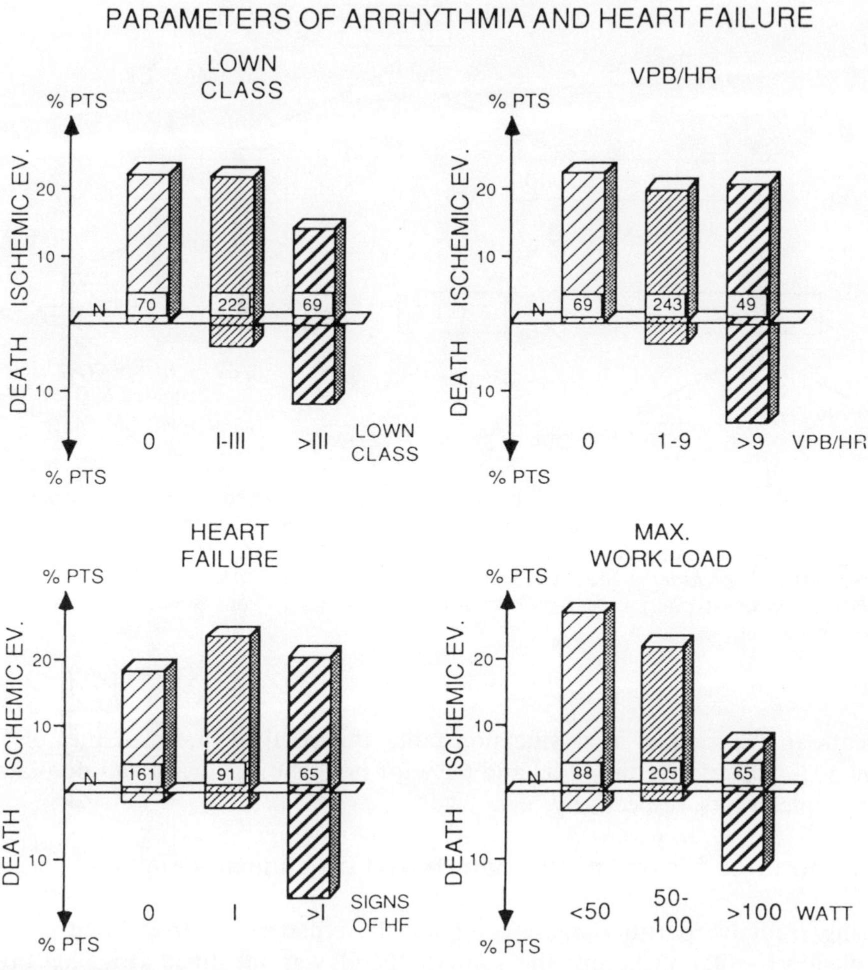

Fig. 2 (*continued*)

mortality rate double that of non-Q-wave infarcts (5.9 *vs* 2.7%; $P < 0.01$); however, non-fatal ischaemic events were almost twice as frequent in non-Q-wave as compared to Q-wave infarcts (27 *vs* 15%; $P < 0.05$). On the other hand, such a relation was not present for non-invasive signs of ischaemia which predicted ischaemic events only.

Logistic regression analysis performed separately for the two main endpoints identified ventricular arrhythmias (maximal Lown grade) ($P = 0.013$) and heart rate at rest ($P = 0.032$) as independent clinical predictors of death, and systolic blood pressure at rest ($P = 0.001$), maximally tolerated workload ($P = 0.014$) and diabetes mellitus ($P = 0.034$) as independent clinical predictors of non-fatal ischaemic events. In addition, wall motion abnormalities detected by radionuclide ventriculography strongly predicted death as well as non-fatal ischaemic

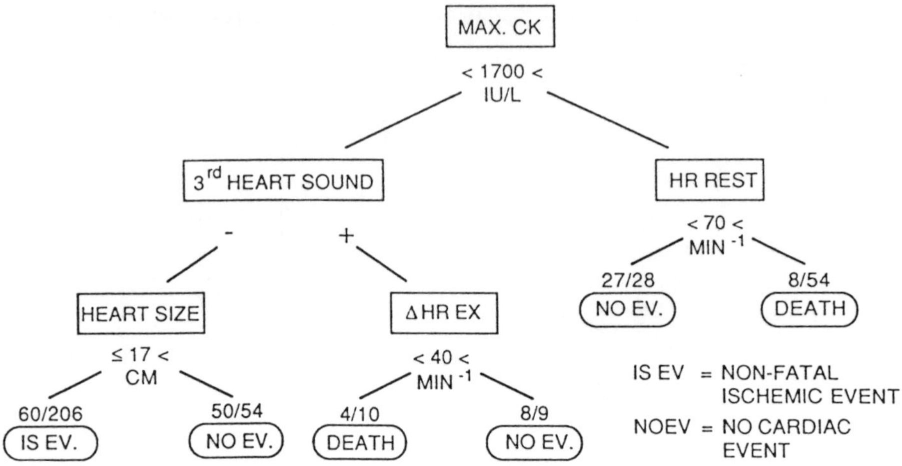

Fig. 3. Risk assessment after first myocardial infarction based on clinical variables. Prediction of death, ischaemic events and no events. The quotients with each final sub-group indicate number of patients with event/total number of patients in that sub-group. *Abbreviations*: Max. CK = maximal creatine kinase level; HR = heart rate; Δ HR EX = heart rate increase with exercise; IS EV = non-fatal ischaemic event; NO EV = no event.

events. In the form of a classification table, this resulted in sensitivities of 53 and 59% and specificities of 89 and 62% for prediction of death and non-fatal ischaemic events, respectively.

Decision tree for risk assessment based on clinical variables

Using recursive partitioning, a computer-derived decision tree based on 52 clinical variables including the exercise ECG was identified (Fig. 3). Five parameters were selected by the computer algorithm to differentiate between patients with fatal, non-fatal and no events: maximal creatine kinase above or below 1700 IU per litre; the presence or absence of a third heart sound, resting heart rate above or below 70 beats/min, heart size in the chest X-ray of above or below 17 cm and a heart rate increase with upright exercise of above or below 40 beats/min, all at hospital discharge. This decision tree resulted in an excellent prediction of death (80%) and non-fatal events (82%), but only a poor prediction of the low-risk group with no events (31%, Table 2).

Table 2 compares the predictive power based on such decision trees using either clinical variables, radionuclide angiocardiography, thallium-201 scintigraphy, including exercise parameters in each, or Holter-ECG, each for itself. Those patients who died during follow-up were particularly well identified by radionuclide angiocardiography and Holter-ECG, whereas patients with no further events were best predicted by thallium-201 scintigraphy.

Table 2
Risk assessment (%) after first myocardial infarction based on clinical and non-invasive testing: Classification matrix (predicted *vs* true class)

	True class		
Predicted class	Death	Ischaemic event	No event
Clinical variables			
Death	80	10	16
Ischaemic event	20	82	53
No event	0	8	31
Holter ECG			
Death	93	32	41
Ischaemic event	0	59	48
No event	7	10	11
RNA			
Death	93	26	27
Ischaemic event	0	64	24
No event	7	10	49
Thallium			
Death	67	19	20
Ischaemic event	7	40	18
No event	26	41	62

Discussion

The computer-derived decision tree defined in this report stresses the importance of simple clinical variables for risk assessment after a first myocardial infarction. High-risk patients could be identified based on clinical data alone without further testing. However, this approach included too many low-risk patients who would also undergo catheterization if this were the next step in this "high-risk" group. Therefore, additional non-invasive testing is necessary. Several aspects of this study have to be discussed, however, especially the selection of patients with a first myocardial infarction only and the relevance of such a decision tree.

Selection of first myocardial infarction patients

Published studies of risk stratification after myocardial infarction have paid remarkably little attention to patients having their first myocardial infarction [5–9], despite the fact that their early and late survival is significantly better than in patients who have had previous infarctions [9,10]. Still, they constitute the main sub-group of 60–80% of all patients with acute infarctions.

Generally, they have a relatively preserved left ventricular function, but the uninvolved myocardium is the Achilles heel for subsequent infarctions. This is shown in the present study by a low 1-year mortality rate but a high incidence of recurrent non-fatal ischaemic events, especially in non-Q-wave infarctions. This is in accordance with previous reports by Krone *et al.* [11], who showed a similarly high survival rate in these patients, and by Benhorin *et al.* [12], who identified non-fatal reinfarction as the most important mortality risk after the first myocardial infarction. Thus, prevention of a second infarction has high priority in survivors of a first myocardial infarction. This implies that identification of patients at risk for future events is particularly important in this population.

Q *vs* non-Q infarctions

Previous reports have shown that patients with non-Q-wave infarctions have a higher incidence of previous infarction than patients with Q-wave infarctions [9,13] and thus the prognostic implications of Q-wave and non-Q-wave infarctions are similar. However, several reports have identified previous infarctions as a separate and powerful prognostic factor [9,14,15]. If this factor is omitted as in the present study where only first myocardial infarctions were included, this results in a prognostic difference between Q-wave and non-Q-wave infarctions regarding mortality but not regarding all cardiac events. Again this calls for careful evaluation of patients after first myocardial infarction, especially after a first non-Q-wave myocardial infarction; on the other hand, this is probably also applicable to patients with a first myocardial infarction after successful thrombolysis.

Differentiation between fatal and non-fatal events

Finally, this patient population allowed us to differentiate death from non-fatal ischaemic events during follow-up. At first glance, it may not seem pathophysiologically logical to separate predictors of fatal from non-fatal events [16]. However, the present findings may lead to a different interpretation: markers of infarct size predict death due to congestive heart failure similar to the observation that ventricular ectopy predicts death due to ventricular fibrillation, whereas recurrent ischaemic events seem not to be lethal in the great majority of patients. This is supported by the findings of the present study where only one cardiac death was due to documented recurrent infarction and all the others were either due to congestive heart failure or occurred suddenly. The observed non-invasive test results indicate clearly that there is an inverse relationship between many of the most powerful risk predictors and fatal or non-fatal events. A given predictive factor may, therefore, lose its predictive power if an analysis on "all cardiac events" is carried out. This should be appreciated not only for the present analysis but also for other studies on risk assessment after myocardial infarction.

Role of exercise testing after myocardial infarction

Since the activity of coronary artery disease is variable and unpredictable after myocardial infarction and angiographic assessment of the severity of coronary stenoses proved to be inadequate to predict time or location of a subsequent occlusion [17], it is important to detect jeopardized myocardium in order to identify patients at high risk who may benefit from coronary angiography and possible revascularization. Here exercise testing, including an exercise ECG, has a central role as shown in several studies [18]. Accordingly, this test was analysed together with clinical variables in the present study. The question as to which and how many additional and more expensive non-invasive tests would have to be added to optimize risk prediction will have to be analysed separately.

Recursive partitioning for multivariate analysis

Standard multivariate logistic regression analysis identified several independent predictors of death and ischaemic events. For risk assessment in daily clinical practice, a simple classification rule as provided by recursive partitioning seems preferable: it is designed to identify synergistic interactions among factors as applied in clinical practice; it may identify non-linear relationships between different endpoints as observed for exercise ejection fraction in this study; it provides a simple format for constructing homogeneous risk strata; it is relatively insensitive for missing values and it considers prior probabilities and penalties for misclassification in its variable selection process [19]. Thus, for the present analysis, the cost of a false negative (e.g. missing a patient who later died) was five times as high as the cost of a patient who experienced a non-fatal cardiac event and 20 times as high as the cost of a false positive (e.g. including a patient with no future events), whereas commonly available parametric models search for factors that separate two groups under the assumption that costs for a false positive and a false negative are equal – which, in the setting of risk assessment, does not reflect clinical judgement. Still, the present study may serve as a clinical example to evaluate the relative merits of the two statistical methods, which identified very similar variables as being most important but grouped them differently, thereby underlining some of the practical advantages of recursive partitioning in a complex clinical situation.

Relevance of the decision tree/implications

The aim of this study was to find a simple, clinically useful decision tree based on clinical data. Of course, such a decision protocol warrants further large-scale prospective testing and is therefore not ready for routine clinical use. A similar type of analysis, however, has been used for patients with acute chest pain in an emergency room situation and the protocol proved to be valid during subsequent testing [20]. Some of the branch points of the present decision tree were reached on the basis of a relatively small number of patients and the protocol may need modification and improvement on the basis of experience with a larger number of patients. Still, it provides a practical guideline for risk assessment in the large sub-group of patients with a first myocardial infarction where it is most important to prevent further myocardial damage in order to improve prognosis.

Acknowledgements

We are indebted to all of the nurses and doctors for enrolling, examining and following the patients. We also thank Jan Müller-Brand for performing the scintigraphic studies and Mrs Hanka Jordi for the analysis of the Holter tracings. Special thanks go to Luzia Glaus for her help with statistical analysis. Finally, we appreciate the secretarial skills of Cathy Faes and the help of Gaby Frey in preparing the figures.

This study was supported by Grant No. 3.966-080 of the Swiss National Foundation for Scientific Research, Berne, Switzerland. A detailed report of this study has been published in *Chest* 1992; **102**: 1499–1504.

References

1. Diamond GA. Future imperfect: The limitations of clinical prediction models and the limits of clinical prediciton. *J Am Coll Cardiol* 1989; **14**: 12A–22A.
2. Sieber R, Pfisterer M, Emmenegger H, Müller-Brand J. Enzymatisch und szintigraphisch bestimmte Infarktgrösse: Bedeutung für die linksventrikuläre Funktion nach Infarkt. *Z Kardiol* 1984; **73**: 748–755.
3. Koopman PAR. Confidence limits for the reration of two binominal proportions. *Biometrics* 1984; **40**: 513–517.
4. Breiman L, Friedman J, Olshen R, Stone C. *Classification and Regression Trees.* Wadsworth Intl. Group: Belmont, CA, USA, 1984.
5. Henning H, Gilpin EA, Covell JW, Swan EA, O'Rourke RA, Ross J. Prognosis after acute myocardial infarction: A multivariate analysis of mortality and survival. *Circulation* 1979; **59**: 1124–1134.
6. Sanz G, Castaner A, Betriu A, Magrina J, Roig E, Coll S, Parc JC, Navarro-Lopez F. Determinants of prognosis in survivors of myocardial infarction. *N Engl J Med* 1982; **306**: 1065–1070.
7. The Multicenter Postinfarction Research Group. Risk stratification and survival after myocardial infarction. *N Engl J Med* 1983; **309**: 331–336.
8. Mukharji J, Rude RE, Poole WK, Gustafson N, Thomas LJ, Strauss HW, Jaffe AS, Muller JE, Roberts R, Raabe DS, Croft CH, Passamani E, Braunwald E, Willerson JT. Risk factors for sudden death after acute myocardial infarction: Two-year follow-up. *Am J Cardiol* 1984; **54**: 31–36.
9. Ahnve S, Gilpin E, Dittrich H, Nicod P, Henning H, Carlisle J, Ross J. First myocardial infarction: Age and ejection fraction identify a low-risk group. *Am Heart J* 1988; **116**: 925–932.
10. Kannel WB, Sorlie P, McNamara PM. Prognosis after initial myocardial infarction: The Framingham study. *Am J Cardiol* 1979; **44**: 53–59.
11. Krone RJ, Friedmann E, Thanavaro S, Miller JP, Kleiger RE, Oliver GC. Long-term prognosis after first Q-wave (transmural) or non-Q-wave (non-transmural) myocardial infarction: Analysis of 593 patients. *Am J Cardiol* 1983; **52**: 234–239.

12. Benhorin J, Moss AJ, Oakes D, Multicenter Diltiazem Post-infarction Trial Research Group. The prognostic significance of non-fatal reinfarction. *J Am Coll Cardiol* 1990; **15**: 23–28.
13. Gibson RS, Watson DD, Craddock GB, Crampton RS, Kaiser DL, Denny MJ, Beller GA. Prediction of cardiac events after uncomplicated myocardial infarction: A prospective study comparing predischarge exercise thallium-201 scintigraphy and coronary angiography. *Circulation* 1983; **68**: 321–336.
14. Nicod P, Gilpin E, Dittrich H, Polikar R, Hjalmarson A, Blacky AR, Henning H, Ross J. Short- and long-term clinical outcome after Q wave and non-Q wave myocardial infarction in a large patient population. *Circulation* 1989; **79**: 528–536.
15. Fioretti P, Brower RW, Simoons ML, ten Katen H, Beelen A, Baardman T, Lubsen J, Hugenholtz PG. Relative value of clinical variables, bicycle ergometry, rest radionuclide ventriculography and 24 hours ambulatory electrocardiographic monitoring at discharge to predict one-year survival after myocardial infarction. *J Am Coll Cardio* 1986; **8**: 40–49.
16. Fleiss JL, Bigger JT, McDermott M, Miller JP, Moon T, Moss AJ, Oakes D, Rolnitzky LM, Therneau TM. Nonfatal myocardial infarction is, by itself, an inappropriate endpoint in clinical trials. *Circulation* 1990; **81**: 684–685.
17. Little WC, Constantinescu M, Applegate RJ, Kutcher MA, Burrows MT, Kahl FR, Santamore WP. Can coronary angiography predict the site of a subsequent myocardial infarction in patients with mild-to-moderate coronary artery disease? *Circulation* 1988; **78**: 1157–1166.
18. DeBusk RF. Specialized testing after recent acute myocardial infarction. *Ann Intern Med* 1989; **110**: 470–481.
19. Cook EF, Goldman L. Empiric comparison of multivariate analytic techniques: Advantages and disadvantages of recursive partitioning analysis. *J Chron Dis* 1984; **37**: 721–731.
20. Goldman L, Weinberg M, Weisberg M, Olshen, R, Cook EF, Sargent RK, Lamos GA, Dennis C, Wilson C, Deckelbaum L, Fineberg H, Stiratelli R. A computer-derived protocol to aid in the diagnosis of emergency room patients with acute chest pain. *N Engl J Med* 1982; **307**: 588–596.

2 Risk Stratification in Post-infarction Patients: Special Reference to Multi-vessel Disease

Helmut Roskamm, L. Samek

Rehabilitationszentrum für Herz- und Kreislaufkranke, Südring 15, D-7812 Bad Krozingen, Germany

Introduction

Multi-vessel involvement in post-infarction patients influences short- and, in particular, long-term prognosis, short- and long-term management (PTCA, ACBS), and probably the intensity of risk factor corrections. It is generally accepted, though, that vessel involvement is not everything when it comes to prognosis or management, which has clearly been shown, for instance, by the CAS-Study [1]. Even patients with triple vessel disease had a good prognosis and did not profit from surgery if they were asymptomatic or only mildly symptomatic, and if they had fairly good ventricular function.

The view is different, however, depending on whether we look for bad prognosis or look for multi-vessel disease. Short-term survival will predominantly be impaired as a result of bad ventricular function, and there is little that can be done to prevent this. Multi-vessel disease, on the other hand, is important as regards long-term prognosis. For post-infarction patients with multi-vessel disease, we do have something to offer, especially bypass surgery. Thus, independent of survival it seems to be worthwhile to predict multi-vessel disease.

Proceedings of the Vth World Congress on Cardiac Rehabilitation

Prediction of multi-vessel disease by clinical parameters

The most important clinical factors influencing the prevalence of multi-vessel disease in a post-infarction patient are age and post-infarction angina pectoris. Thus Chaitman *et al.* [2] correlated clinical variables with the angiographic findings of multi-vessel disease in 108 men with previous inferior myocardial infarction. Of 71 men in angina class 2–3, 42 had triple vessel disease; of the 37 who were either asymptomatic or in angina class 1, only 7 had triple-vessel disease (Canadian Cardiovascular Society Classification). Multi-vessel disease was present in 35 of the 36 patients with anterior ST/T abnormalities at rest, and 16 of the 17 with cardiomegaly. Among the men at age 55 and older, the incidence of multi-vessel disease was 94%, compared to 70% in patients younger than 55 years [2]. This and other clinical parameters have to be considered in addition to exercise testing results.

Prediction of multi-vessel disease by exercise testing

In a recent study, Miranda *et al.* [3] found that the positive predictive value of exercise testing for the identification of multi-vessel disease was 71% on average, which has been shown in 15 studies. This is valid for Q-wave as well as for non-Q-wave infarction.

In our own study, 261 post-infarction patients (mean age 46 years, range 29–62 years) were investigated to find out whether the involvement of a second or third vessel could be predicted on the basis of angina pectoris and/or ST-segment depression during exercise [4]. The main findings were:

> Severe lesions (≥75%) of a second or third vessel were found in 61.7% of patients with *inferior* myocardial infarction who developed angina pectoris and ST-segment depression in the anterior leads during exercise.
> In patients with neither angina pectoris nor ST-segment depression during exercise, only 3.4% had multi-vessel disease.

In patients with *anteroseptal* infarction, the correlations were not so clear. However, in this group, patients with neither angina pectoris nor ST-segment depression during exercise rarely had multi-vessel disease. A minor sensitivity to exercise testing in patients with anterior wall infarction has also been shown by Tubau *et al.* [5].

The consequences of these results are:

1. Critical stenosis of a second or third vessel is rare, if neither angina pectoris nor ST-segment depression occurs during maximal exercise testing.
2. Patients with transmural inferior infarction who develop angina and ST-segment depression during exercise testing 8 weeks post-infarction, have a high incidence of critical stenosis in a second or third vessel.

The most important problem is, indeed, further vessel involvement in patients after inferior wall infarction. In inferior myocardial infarction, the main question is whether the left anterior descending (LAD) coronary artery is also involved, because this will also influence prognosis in patients with double vessel disease [6].

Prediction of multi-vessel disease by the combination of clinical parameters and exercise testing

Tubau *et al.* [5] found that the maximal diagnostic value of exercise testing after infarction was for patients in angina class 0 or 1. A positive test in this subset increased the likelihood of multi-vessel disease from 50–55% to 80–100%, and a negative test reduced the risk of triple vessel disease to less than 10%.

But how many patients with multi-vessel disease will be missed if one relies on angina pectoris in daily life and on exercise testing? Cross *et al.* [7] investigated 200 consecutive patients below the age of 60 years who had undergone coronary angiography. They found that if only those 174 patients with a positive exercise test or angina in daily life had been catheterized, 5 patients with triple-vessel disease and none with left main stem disease would have been missed; but none of these 5 patients were referred for surgery.

In our own series of rather young patients ($n = 296$, age < 40 years) with transmural myocardial infarction in whom coronary angiography was performed more or less systematically, more than 20% of the patients with ST-segment depression and angina pectoris went to surgery, whereas only 1% of those patients with neither ST-segment depression nor angina pectoris during exercise testing did.

The question of percutaneous transluminal coronary angioplasty (PTCA) is of less importance in this context, as patients after transmural infarction and with critical involvement of a further important vessel are more likely candidates for surgery than for PTCA.

Prediction of left main stem stenosis

Basing selection for angiography on the presence of angina and exercise test results, Cross *et al.* [7] did not miss patients with critical (>50%) left main stem disease.

In our own retrospective study, we investigated the exercise tolerance of 133 patients with left main stem disease who had undergone surgery [8]. The majority of patients had an angina-free exercise tolerance below 50 W as well as ST-segment depression of 0.2 mV–0.5 mV. Thus the majority showed very pronounced signs and symptoms of ischaemia during exercise. However, 16 patients had a rather high angina pectoris-free exercise tolerance of 75 W or more; 31 had an ST-segment depression of below 0.2 mV or none at all; 16 patients had no angina during exercise. The combination of high exercise tolerance and only slight ST-segment depression during exercise is rare, however. Only 5 patients (i.e. 4%) were able to exercise at 75 W or more with only slight ST-segment depression below 0.2 mV. Thus moderately limited exercise tolerance in patients with left main stem stenosis is possible, though rare.

If the results of exercise testing are unclear, we additionally use floating catheterization. Scintigraphy or stress echo may also be used.

Are there sub-groups with different prognoses among post-infarction patients with multi-vessel disease?

In patients with double or triple vessel disease, prognosis is influenced by several factors. Left ventricular dysfunction is generally accepted; arrhythmias may also be. But the results of simple exercise testing are also of importance. Gohlke *et al.* [9] found that patients with double or triple vessel disease and a moderately impaired left ventricle had a 72% 5-year survival if they reached exercise values in the lower half, but survival was significantly better with 88% if they reached exercise values in the upper half.

In summary, the prognostic relevance of multi-vessel disease can only be specified within the framework of anatomic and functional parameters.

Should knowledge of multi-vessel disease influence the intensity of risk factor modification?

In the past, the identification of patients with multi-vessel disease would have had immediate consequences, such as invasive therapy. Our diagnostic approach was primarily oriented at severe stenosis. Today, it is important to know whether a patient, in addition to his infarction-related severe stenosis, has other small stenoses, (e.g. several stenoses below 50%). These patients do not, by definition, have double or triple vessel disease, but multivessel involvement. And because of the only slightly stenosed additional vessels, this will not be reflected in the exercise test results.

However, multi-vessel involvement influences the further progression of coronary heart disease. In our own study of young post-infarction patients [10], progression was 10 times as frequent in the sub-group of patients with multilocular disease in the first angiogram than in the group with initial unilocular disease (34.3 *vs* 3.6%). We also know from a number of studies that further myocardial infarction develops from slight or medium stenoses, rather than from an originally severe stenosis, and this cannot be detected by exercise testing [11,12].

Very aggressive lipid lowering, for example to low density lipoprotein (LDL)-values of below 100 mg/dl, can be especially justified if we know that a patient who already has multi-vessel involvement has a high probability of future progression of the disease. This means that the search for multi-vessel involvement should be widened, especially among young patients.

References

1. Coronary Artery Surgery Study (CASS). A randomized trial of coronary artery bypass surgery. Survival data. CASS Principal Investigators and their associates. *Circulation* 1983; **68**: 939.
2. Chaitman BR, Waters DD, Corbara F, Bourassa MG. Prediction of multivessel disease after inferior myocardial infarction. *Circulation* 1978; **57:** 1085.
3. Miranda CP, Herbert WG, Dubach P, Lehmann KG, Froehlicher VF. Post-myocardial infarction exercise testing. Non-Q wave versus Q-wave correlation with coronary angiography and long-term prognosis. *Circulation* 1991; **84**: 2357.
4. Samek L, Roskamm H, Rentrop P, Kaiser P, Stürzenhofecker P, Schober B, Görnandt L, Velden R. Belastungsprüfungen und Koronarangiogramm im chronischen Infarktstadium. *Z Kardiol* 1975; **64:** 809.
5. Tubau JF, Chaitman BR, Bourassa MG, Waters DD. Detection of multivessel disease after myocardial infarction using exercise stress testing and multiple ECG lead systems. *Circulation* 1980; **61:** 44.
6. European Coronary Surgery Study Group. Prospective randomized study of coronary artery bypass surgery in stable angina pectoris: A progress report on survival. *Lancet* 1980; **ii:** 491.
7. Cross S, Lee HS, Kenmure A *et al.*: Should every patient under 60 with acute myocardial infarction undergo cardiac catheterization? Experience with a consecutive series of patients. *J Am Coll Cardiol* 1992; **19:** 81A.
8. Roskamm H, Samek L. Comparison of exercise ECG and coronary angiography. In: Loogen F, Seipel L (eds), *Detection of Ischemic Myocardium with Exercise.* Springer: Berlin, 1982, p.113.
9. Gohlke H, Samek L, Betz P, Roskamm H. Exercise testing provides additional prognostic information in angiographically defined subgroups of patients with coronary artery disease. *Circulation* 1983; **68:** 979–985.
10. Roskamm H, Gohlke H, Stürzenhofecker P, Droste C, Thomas H, Samek L, Schnellbacher K, Betz P: Der Herzinfarkt im jugendlichen Alter (unter 40 Jahren): Koronarmorphologie, Risikofaktoren, Langzeitprognose der Erkrankung und Progression der Koronargefäßsklerose. *Z Kardiol* 1983; **72:** 1.
11. Little WC, Constantinescu M, Applegate RJ, Kutcher MA, Borrows MT, Kahl FR, Santamore WP. Can coronary angiography predict the site of a subsequent myocardial infarction in patients with mild-to-moderate coronary artery disease? *Circulation* 1988; **78:** 1157–1166.
12. Ellis S, Alderman E, Cain K, Fisher L, Sanders W, Bourassa M and the CASS Investigators. Prediction of risk of anterior myocardial infarction by lesion severity and measurement of stenosis in the left anterior descending coronary distribution: A CASS registry study. *J Am Coll Cardiol* 1988; **11:** 908–916.

3 Can Follow-up Studies Yield Accurate Clinical Prediction Rules for Managing Patients with Coronary Artery Disease?

Victor F. Froelicher[1], Erika Sivarajan Froelicher[2]

[1] *Division of Cardiology, 111C, Palo Alto VA Medical Center, 3801 Miranda Avenue, Palo Alto, CA 94304* and [2] *Department of Physiological Nursing, N611Y, University of California, San Francisco, CA 94143-0610, USA*

Introduction

Maintaining quality medical care is dependent upon the constant assessment of technological efficiency and patient outcomes. Though databases exist for the formulation of clinical prediction rules, population and procedure peculiarities require confirmation of these rules. Clinical evaluation, exercise testing and coronary angiography are routinely used by physicians to decide whether or not interventions are needed in patients with coronary artery disease. The purpose of this review is to determine if rules can be developed from available studies to optimize this decision.

Statistical methods

To develop and demonstrate clinical prediction rules, follow-up studies must be performed and special statistical methods called survival analysis applied. Survival analysis consists of a group of univariate and multivariate mathematical techniques that consider time of observation as a continuous variable or censored observation called person-time of exposure, and use it to calculate a hazards ratio or risk ratio. The key difference between survival analysis and other statistical methods is censoring, which is the removal of the subject from observation before the outcome of interest is observed. Censoring is carried out

Proceedings of the Vth World Congress on Cardiac Rehabilitation

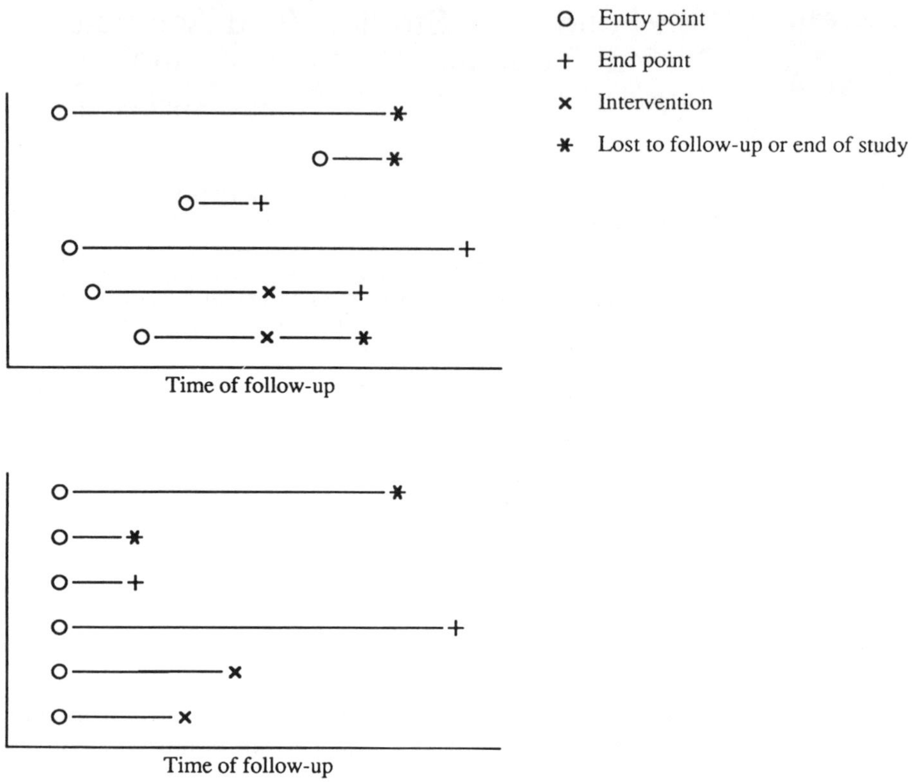

Fig. 1. The basic concepts of survival analysis. The top graph shows that patients can enter and leave the study at various times and thus have differing exposure time periods. As shown in the bottom graph, entry time must be set to zero and patients censored appropriately so that exposure times can be compared.

at time of "lost to follow-up", at completion of medical procedures that should alter risk (i.e. CABS, PTCA), or termination of the study. The key principles of survival analysis are illustrated in Fig. 1.

The two most commonly used survival techniques are the Kaplan-Meier survival curves for univariate analysis and the Cox-Hazard model for multivariate analysis. Multivariate analysis is necessary because of the multifactorial nature of many chronic diseases, because of the interrelationships or multicolinearity among variables. Univariately, variables can be associated with the outcome measure (i.e. cardiovascular death), but the association may be through other variables (i.e. digoxin use through a history of congestive heart failure, exercise-induced ST elevation through Q-waves on the resting ECG). Univariate analysis is confused both by confounding and proxy variables. The following is a review of the studies that have applied these techniques in patients with stable coronary disease and they are summarized in Table 1.

Literature review

Since the pioneering studies at the University of Alabama [1,2], numerous investigators have utilized clinical, exercise test and catheterization data to predict prognosis in patients with coronary artery disease. Implicit in these studies has been the question of which variables are predictive, and whether exercise test variables and coronary angiography data improve prediction sufficiently to merit their use despite their expense and risk. It must be remembered, however, that selection for cardiac catheterization on clinical grounds results in a sub-population quite different from the unselected clinical population in whom decision rules should be used. Making conclusions from these studies is also complicated by the fact that the variables were not standardized by consistent definitions. For instance, congestive heart failure was defined quite differently from study to study. In addition, very often, variables of interest were not reported. To perform our review, we had to contact all of the investigators to obtain many of the data listed in Table 1, since they were missing in their publications. It is surprising how often it is not even stated what percentage of study patients were women. Further complicating comparison, very often the variables included in the Cox-Hazard function model are not listed. This makes comparison of these studies very difficult.

Oberman *et al.* [1] found cardiac enlargement on chest X-ray and a history of congestive heart failure to be the two most predictive independent clinical variables and that angiography improved prediction of death. They did not consider exercise test results because of incomplete data but found that those unable to perform the test had a poorer prognosis. Ellestad and co-workers [3] reported the predictive implications of maximal exercise testing in 2700 individuals followed from 6 months to 9 years. ST-segment depression and prior myocardial infarction were both associated with mortality. This study did not require coronary angiography and so selection bias is lessened.

From the Seattle Heart Watch, Hammermeister *et al.* [4] assessed 733 medically treated patients using a stepwise regression an analysis of clinical markers and then the exercise test markers. Cox's regression analysis showed ejection fraction, older age, number of diseased vessels and resting ventricular arrhythmias in that order to be most predictive. A prospective study by Gohlke *et al.* [5] of 1034 patients with coronary artery disease showed that exercise-induced ST-segment depression was only independently predictive in the subgroup with triple vessel disease and normal ventricular function.

From the Italian Multicentre Study, Brunelli *et al.* [6] reported their findings in 1083 patients less than 65 years of age followed for a mean of $5\frac{1}{2}$ years. They found clinical markers to stratify risk and that coronary angiography added prognostic information only in patients with moderately severe disease. Q-wave presence and a history of infarction were the most important clinical predictors (congestive heart failure was not considered). Exercise-induced ST-segment depression was not considered independently but rather was combined with angina and exercise capacity in order to create a score associated with cardiovascular death.

Table 1
Summary of all studies found using Med-Line that required clinical assessment, exercise testing and coronary angiography to evaluate patients with stable coronary artery disease[a]

	LBVAMC (no cath.)	LBVAMC	VACABS	CASS	Duke
Clinical					
Years entered	1984–90	1984–90	1970–74	1974–79	1969–81
Population size	2546	588	245	4083	2842
Age (years)	59	59 (mean)	51 (mean)	50	49 (median)
Males (%)	100	100%	100%	80%	70%
Congestive heart failure	5%	8%	9%	8%	4%
Myocardial infarction	23%	45%	54%	40%	29%
Q-waves (at least one)	21%	37%	38%	22%	22%
Digoxin	8%	8%	NA	14%	11%
Beta blockers	22%	35%	14%	40%	54%
Typical angina	21%	52%	100%	50%	47%
Exercise test					
% with 1 mm ST-dep.	22%	58%	72%	44%	35%
% Angina	4%	35%	66%	80%	50%
Maximal heart rate (beats/min)	137	124	125	138	134
Maximal SBP (mmHg)	175	159	156	171	160
METs	8.4	6.6	5.7	NA	7
PVCs	5%	12%	19%	12%	6%
Cardiac catheterization findings					
Triple vessel disease (%)	NA	14%	55%	23%	22%
Left main (%)	NA	7%	13%	7%	5%
No significant lesion (%)	NA	26%	0%	34%	40%
Ejection fraction (mean)	NA	60 (mean)		57%	60 (median)
Significant lesion criteria	NA	70%	50%	70%	75%
Follow-up					
Years	5	5	7	5	5
CABS(%)	2%	20%	24%	35%	24%
Annual cv mortality	1.5%	2.7%	NA	1.0%	1.6%
Annual total mortality	2.8%	3.5%	4.0%	1.6%	1.8%
Independent predictors of mortality by priority					
	CHF/DIG	CHF	E-I PVCs	CHF	ST-dep.
	METs	SBP drop	MHR > 140	Treadmill stage	Angina index
	Max. SBP	Rest ST-dep.	Ex. ST-dep. >2 mm	Ex. ST-dep.	Treadmill time
	Ex. ST-dep.				

[a] All studies included a follow-up for cardiovascular or total deaths and used the Cox-Hazard model. Variables chosen are ordered by their relative weight.

Italy	Belgium	Belgium (no PMI)	Germany	Seattle	Buenos Aires
1976–79	1972–77	1978–85	1975–78	1971–74	1972–82
1083	372	470	1238	733	180
49 (mean)	48	52	50 (mean)	52 (mean)	51 (mean)
90%	100%	100%	90%	80%	96%
Exclude	1%		Exclude	13%	Exclude
42%	39%	Exclude	> 50%	40%	64%
37%	39%	Exclude	50%	45%	
	0%	Exclude	8%	18%	
	0%				
95%	67%	75%	95%	86%	71%
42%	27%	54%	56%		65%
60%	49%	44%	61%		60%
130	148	140	118	145	128
171	NA	186	182	160	151
5.4	9	8	5	6.5	5.2
15%	2%	NA		18%	21%
15%	34%	26%	33%	12%	44%
5%	8%	8%	0%		8
26%	18%	22%	0%	39%	0%
60	NA	65	60	60	
75%	50%	50%	50%	70%	75%
5.5	5	5	5	3.5	6
15%	28%	29%			9%
1.5%	1.8%	2.0		2.6%	4.6%
2.0%	2.4%		2.4%	1%	
Q-wave	Age	Age	Ex. capacity	CHF	Max. SBP < 130
Prior MI	Ex. capacity	Max. EX score (−2 to +2)	Angina	Max. DP	ST-elevation
Effort ischaemia		(MHR, ST_{60}, AP, WATTS, ST-slope)	MHR	Max. SBP	<4 Mets
Ex. capacity				Angina frequency Resting ST-dep.	Inappropriate dyspnea

In the Coronary Artery Surgery Study (CASS), Weiner *et al.* [7] analysed exercise test, coronary angiographic and clinical variables in 4083 patients to identify predictors of mortality in medically treated patients with symptomatic coronary artery disease. This study was based on analysis of 16% of the registry of patients with no previous coronary artery byass surgery who were able to undergo a standard or modified Bruce protocol within 1 month of their catheterization. During the mean follow-up of 4 years, 212 or 5% died. Approximately 40% of the patients had a prior myocardial infarction and 36% underwent coronary artery bypass surgery. Standard clinical variables including chest pain, congestive heart failure, physical examination, family history, risk factor index, drugs and cardiac catheterization findings were considered. Regression analysis demonstrated that 7 of 30 variables tested were independent predictors of survival. A high-risk sub-group (annual mortality about 5%) was identified consisting of patients with either congestive heart failure or ST-segment depression and a final exercise stage in the Bruce protocol of one or less (5 METs or less). When all 30 variables were analysed jointly, the left ventricular contraction pattern and the number of diseased vessels were the best predictors of survival. In a sub-group of 572 patients with triple vessel disease and good left ventricular function, the probability of survival at 4 years ranged from 53% for patients only able to achieve stage 1 or 2 to 100% for patients able to exercise into stage 5 (10 METs).

Mark *et al.* [8] studied 2842 consecutive patients who underwent cardiac catheterization and exercise testing and whose data were entered into the Duke computerized medical information system. The median follow-up for the study population was 5 years and follow-up was 98% complete. All patients underwent a Bruce protocol exercise test and had standard ECG measurements recorded. A treadmill angina index was assigned a value of zero if angina was absent, 1 if typical angina occurred during exercise and 2 if angina was the reason the patient stopped exercising. Before the test, 54% of the patients had taken propranolol and 11% had taken digoxin. The ST measurements considered were sum of the largest net ST depression and elevation, sum of the ST displacements in all 12 leads, the number of leads showing ST displacement of 0.1 mV or more, and the product of the number of leads showing ST displacement and the largest single ST displacement in any lead. To make the score apply to other treadmill protocols, it is necessary to convert minutes in the Bruce protocol to METs with the equation: METs equals 1.3 (min) – 2.2 or minutes in the Bruce protocol equals METs + 2.2 divided by 1.3. Patients with ST-segment elevation in ECG leads with pathological Q-waves were excluded because this ST-segment response has a different meaning than ST depression.

The largest net ST deviation recorded during exercise in any one of the 12 leads proved to be the single most important variable for predicting prognosis. After adjusting for maximum net ST deviation using the Cox proportional hazards model, only two other variables contained additional prognostic information: the treadmill angina index and exercise time. The results did not change substantially when patients taking β-blockers or digoxin were excluded. The results also remained unchanged when patients treated surgically were excluded from the study. The authors did not offer any explanation for these observations. Regarding the latter, either the prevalence of surgical treatment was very low or other variables were highly intercorrelated with the choice of surgical treatment so that the information was contained in those variables, or residual confounding exists. A score was calculated as exercise time minus ($5 \times$ ST maximum net deviation) minus ($4 \times$ angina index), where exercise time is measured in minutes and ST deviation in millimetres [8]. Patients at high risk with a score of -11 or lower had a 5-year survival of 72%. Patients at moderate risk with a score of -10 to $+4$, had a 5-year survival of 91%, and patients with a low risk score of $+5$ or greater had a 5-year survival risk of 97%. The treadmill score contained important prognostic information even after the information provided by clinical and catheterization data was considered. The prognostic stratifying power of the treadmill score was greatest in patients with triple vessel disease and lowest in those with single vessel disease.

From the Veterans Administration randomized trial of coronary artery bypass surgery, Peduzzi *et al.* [9] reported on the 7-year follow-up of 245 patients randomized to medical management who had a baseline treadmill test. Univariately and using Cox proportional hazards modelling, ST depression (≥ 2 mm), exercise-induced PVC's, and final heart rate greater than 140 beats/min were significant predictors. As mentioned earlier, caution must be exerted when comparing studies that the identical variables are used in the same numbers and combination in each study analysis and that the measurements and classifications are comparable. These results are in marked contrast with other studies, since PVCs have not had independent predictive power and high heart rates have been protective rather than associated with risk. These unusual results might be explained by their failure to censor on interventions; 24% had coronary artery bypass surgery and the possible confounding effects of this intervention may in part explain these differences.

Lerman *et al.* [10] reported on 190 patients with exercise test and coronary angiograms who were followed for 6 years. Their study began in 1978. Patients had a high annual mortality and a small proportion (9%) had interventions, yet exercise-induced ST-segment depression failed to predict prognosis. Maximal systolic blood pressure of less than 130 mmHg was the strongest predictor. This study did not apply survival analysis techniques and must be viewed with caution. This study is only mentioned because one hypothesis is that exercise-induced ST-segment depression is not consistently selected as a prognostic marker because of interventions. This study has the lowest intervention rate, yet ST-segment depression was not associated with mortality.

Wyns *et al.* [11] evaluated independent prognostic information provided by exercise testing by calculating survival rates with the life-table method in 372 men referred for coronary arteriography. A previous myocardial infarction (MI) was noted in 39% and 66% had typical angina. During a mean follow-up of 29 months, 32 patients (8%) died and 27 patients (7%) had non-fatal events.

Both typical angina pectoris and/or an old MI and an abnormal exercise test (angina and/or the presence of ST-segment shifts) had a significant prognostic value. In patients with an MI and/or angina, the 5-year cumulative survival rate was 76% if the exercise test was abnormal *vs* 94% if it was normal. Proportional hazards analysis was performed. By univariate analysis, age and maximal workload were the only non-invasive variables associated with cardiac events. Cox proportional hazards analysis was performed and exercise capacity was found to provide prognostic information which was not available either from the clinical history or from cardiac catheterization. Because the ST-segment response was coded combining elevation and depression with angina, it can be assumed that the ST-segment depression was not an independent risk predictor in this study.

A second study from Saint-Luc Hospital in Brussels is worthy of discussion because patients with a prior MI were excluded [12]. From 1978 to 1985, 470 consecutive male patients with complaints of chest pain underwent a maximal exercise test with a thallium scan and coronary angiography. During follow-up (1–8 years), 32 of the patients (6.8%) died of cardiovascular causes and another 30 (6.3%) had a non-fatal MI. The average annual cardiovascular death rate was 2%. Of the historical variables, only age was statistically chosen as significant in multivariate analysis, whereas angina and pre-test likelihood were significant univariately. A maximal exercise test score based on maximal heart rate, ST_{60} at maximal exercise, angina during the test, maximal workload and ST slope in the lateral X lead was predictive. This combined score is similar to the ischaemic index used in the Italian study, which made a test abnormal if one or more of the following occurred: angina, ST depression, poor exercise capacity. Such combined scores make it impossible to calculate the weight of individual variables, such as ST-segment depression or exercise capacity, from the data provided in the papers.

At the Long Beach Veterans Administration Medical Center, 588 male patients with an average follow-up of 3 years were examined to determine whether coronary artery disease outcomes could be predicted by clinical and exercise test data. Over the follow-up period, there were 39 cardiovascular deaths and 45 non-fatal myocardial infarctions. The Cox proportional hazards model demonstrated the following characteristics to have a significant independent hazards ratio: history of congestive heart failure (4 ×), resting ST depression (3 ×), and a drop in systolic blood pressure during exercise below standing pre-exercise (5 ×). Exercise-induced ST depression was not associated with either outcome. Out of the cardiac catheterization variables, only ejection fraction added independent information to the model. A simple score based on three factors – a history of congestive heart failure, ST depression on a resting electrocardiogram and exertional hypotension – stratified patients from low risk (annual cardiac mortality of 1% for 4 years after testing) to high risk (annual cardiac mortality of 12%).

In a study that did not consider exercise test results, Califf *et al.* [13] applied clinical measures of ischaemia to predict infarct-free survival in 5896 patients with angina and angiographic (>75% lesions) coronary artery disease. The Cox proportional hazards model chose the following variables in descending order: more than 1 mm of resting ST depression or T-wave inversion, frequency of angina, unstable angina, typical angina and duration of symptoms. An angina score was derived from the Cox coefficients and, when entered into a model with catheterization data, the following variables were chosen in descending order to predict survival: ejection fraction, number of diseased vessels, left main stenosis, angina score, age and sex. This score helped predict prognosis independent of catheterization data.

In another study that did not consider exercise testing, Detre *et al.* [14] developed a multivariate risk function from 508 patients randomized to medical treatment in the Veterans Administration (VA) randomized study of coronary bypass surgery. The variables, in order of importance, were ST-segment depression on resting ECG, history of myocardial infarction, history of hypertension and New York Heart Association functional classification III or IV. Investigation of treatment effects in approximate terciles obtained by collapsing the probability distribution into low-, middle- and high-risk groups showed that surgery was beneficial for patients in the high-risk tercile even after removal of patients with left main coronary artery disease (17% surgical *vs* 34% medical mortality at 5 years; $P < 0.01$). This finding was accentuated when patients in the 10 hospitals with the lowest operative mortality (3.3%) were compared. Mortality results in the low-risk tercile favoured medical treatment (medical *vs* surgical mortality 7% *vs* 17%; $P < 0.05$). The risk function predicted mortality well not only for the VA medical group, but also for an independent symptomatic coronary heart disease population from the University of Alabama arteriographic registry.

Why do these excellent studies fail to agree?

A. The analytical, theoretical, statistical answer is that you cannot expect them to agree for the following reasons. In order to allow for a comparison of results between and among the studies, the following three conditions must be met:

1. The same variables and the same number of variables (i.e. combination) must be included in each analysis.
2. Even when condition 1 has been met, each variable must be measured and classified in the same way to allow for comparison between studies.
3. Population characteristics between studies need to be delineated sufficiently to be sure that there are no other major confounders with a different distribution.

B. From a practical point of view, four universal problems in performing these studies explain the lack of consistent findings:

1. The wide spectrum of the pathophysiology resulting in cardiovascular death.

2. The impact of invasive interventions that alter the natural history of coronary disease (percutaneous transluminal coronary angioplasty and coronary artery bypass surgery).
3. The effect of selection bias.
4. The effect of misclassification.

These practical points will be discussed in the following paragraphs:

Spectrum of cardiovascular death

Cardiac patients die in a pathophysiological spectrum ranging from those that die due to congestive heart failure with relatively little myocardium remaining to those who die from an event related to ischaemia with ample myocardium intact. The clinical and exercise test variables most likely associated with congestive heart failure death include a history or symptoms of congestive heart failure, prior myocardial infarction, Q-waves, and other indicators of left ventricular dysfunction. The variables most likely associated with ischaemic death are angina and both rest and exercise-induced ST-segment depression. Some variables are associated with either type of cardiovascular death – exercise capacity, maximal heart rate and maximal systolic blood pressure – which explains why they are reported most consistently among the available studies. It appears that ischaemic deaths occur later in follow-up and are more likely to occur in those lost to follow-up, whereas congestive heart failure deaths are more likely to occur early (within 2 years) and are more likely to be identified. The impact of this problem is further illustrated in Table 2.

Interventions

Most available studies of stable coronary artery disease patients included a 5-year follow-up and, during that time, 25% of their populations underwent coronary artery bypass surgery. Only since 1980 has percutaneous transluminal coronary angioplasty (PTCA) influenced studies and its impact will only increase in the future. Patients with ischaemic markers are certainly favoured for these interventions and many argue that risk can no longer be associated. Most statisticians advocate that censoring on these interventions (i.e. removing patients who undergo PTCA or coronary artery bypass surgery from the study at the point they undergo them) is appropriate. Some clinicians argue that including these interventions as endpoints is appropriate, particularly if there is a lag time between testing and the procedure. Certainly, using interventions as endpoints is not appropriate since ischaemic test results lead physicians to perform interventions, even if there is a time delay. We feel that censoring is appropriate, but one of the assumptions of the Cox proportional hazards model is still not met (i.e. censoring should be random). Populations with low intervention rates should be studied whenever possible to validate the findings in other populations with high censoring rates due to intervention. An alterna-

Table 2
The population features and follow-up or study conditions that favour either of the two far ends of the cardiovascular pathophysiological spectrum

Factors favouring ischaemic endpoints
Lower prevalence of prior myocardial infarctions
Lower prevalence of Q-waves or ECG abnormalities on resting ECG
Shorter course of symptoms
Better long-term follow-up
Lower prevalence of congestive heart failure confounders (i.e. alcoholism, diabetes, hypertension)
Longer complete follow-up
Younger mean age
Fewer interventions during follow-up
Higher prevalence of angina
Less digoxin administration
Factors favouring congestive heart failure endpoints
Higher prevalence of prior myocardial infarctions
Higher prevalence of Q-waves and LVH with strain on resting ECG
Chronicity of disease
Better short-term follow-up than long term follow-up
Short follow-up
Higher prevalence of congestive heart failure confounders (i.e. alcoholism, diabetes, hypertension)
More patients taking digoxin
Older mean age
More interventions during follow-up
Lower prevalence of angina

tive to the dilemma of how to handle interventions in the analysis would be to analyse the data with coronary artery bypass grafts or PTCA censored, and then conduct a repeat analysis in which they are not censored and compare the results, keeping all other variables constant. This can provide revealing information.

Selection bias

The studies presented are based on selected populations seen at research centres in university-affiliated hospitals, and are unlike the patients a clinician encounters in community hospitals. Since cardiac catheterization is a prerequisite to enter the studies, clinical judgement led to this inclusion. This is often referred to as "work-up bias" by clinicians, but is more correctly called "selection bias" by epidemiologists. What we would really like to know is, what should be used to select patients to undergo catheterization? If they have already been selected, then the developed rules cannot apply. Several attempts have been made to lessen work-up bias – one is to have patients agree to both procedures prior

Prognostic Scores

- DUKE SCORE

  (METs - 5 * [mm E-I ST Depression] - 4 * [TM AP Index])

- VA SCORE

  (5 * [CHF/Dig] + mm E-I ST Depression + change in SBP score - METs)

E-I = exercise-induced

Fig. 2. The Duke and Veterans Administration prognostic scores.

to testing and another is to test or develop the models in populations not selected for cardiac catheterization. Using the Veterans Administration database, when analysis was performed in a larger population not selected for cardiac catheterization, exercise test-induced ST-segment depression was selected by the Cox proportional hazards model, whereas it was not selected in the sub-group selected for catheterization. However, the Duke group obtained similar results in both an in-patient population (selected for catheterization) and an outpatient population (not selected for catheterization) [15]. These two scores are listed in Fig. 2 and their performance in the VA population illustrated in Fig. 3.

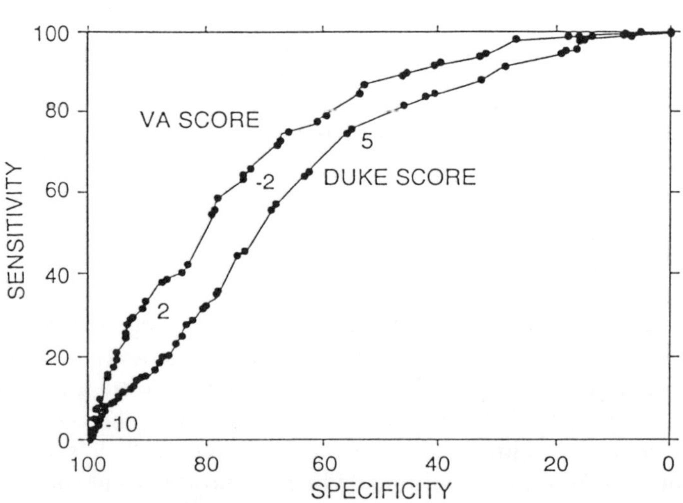

Fig. 3. ROC curves comparing the performance of the Duke score to the Veterans Administration score in the VA population.

Misclassification

This can occur with either the prediction or outcome variables and merely means that a mistake was made in their identification. For instance, exercise-induced ST-segment depression was actually due to digoxin use or left ventricular hypertrophy rather than exercise-induced ischaemia, or a non-cardiac death was considered a cardiac death, or a diagnosis of congestive heart failure was actually pneumonia. Careful record review rather than reliance on death certificates alone and prospective collection of clinical and test variables with well-defined criteria and forms can lessen misclassification. In all circumstances, the observer should be "blinded" to the outcome variable.

Conclusion

Are there solutions to these problems? One could study populations with patients that have a low intervention rate. Scheduling follow-up visits at a sufficient frequency to capture all clinical changes to allow more accurate classification is recommended. Censoring on interventions should be done. Classification of deaths as being due to either ischaemia or congestive heart failure should be attempted and non-cardiac deaths should be so classified. Obtaining autopsy certification of death can be planned into the study design. Since routinely only a very small number of deaths receive autopsy confirmation (<20%), this should be budgeted in prospective studies. Using a multi-centre design permits a larger sample size and standardized protocols can improve classification.

For current practice given the problems discussed, can we answer the question of who needs to undergo cardiac catheterization among patients with stable coronary artery disease? This is easy to decide when symptoms cannot be controlled, but otherwise it is often difficult to decide who should be considered for intervention to prolong life.

Can we identify low-risk patients who do not need catheterization and high-risk patients who may benefit? Risk can be assessed by considering simple clinical variables – more than 5 METs exercise capacity, no evidence or history of congestive heart failure or ventricular damage (Q-waves or cardiomegaly), a normal systolic blood pressure response to exercise and no ST-segment depression are all associated with a very low risk. These patients are at a low risk for complications in exercise programmes and need not be considered for intervention solely to prolong their lives. High-risk patients can be identified by the presence of multiple clinical or exercise test markers (i.e. the presence of two or more abnormal findings or responses). The identification of high risk implies that exercise training should have lesser goals and should be monitored. Such patients should be considered for coronary artery bypass surgery to improve their survival. While intervention should be considered, it may not be feasible for clinical or personal reasons. Ischaemic markers are associated with a later and lesser risk, whereas congestive heart failure or left ventricular dysfunction markers are associated with an earlier and greater risk of death. Of the reported scores, only the Duke score has been appropriately validated and shown to function in other populations. Until the limitations in the reviewed studies are overcome, this pragmatic approach can be used to make clinical decisions.

Acknowledgement

This study was supported in part by the Veterans Administration Cooperative Studies Program.

References

1. Oberman, A., Jones, WB, Riley, CP, Reeves TJ, Sheffield LT. Natural history of coronary artery disease. *Bull NY Acad Med* 1972; **48:** 1109–1125.
2. Reeves TJ, Oberman A, Jones WB, Sheffield LT. Natural history of angina pectoris. *Am J Cardiol* 1974; **33:** 423–430.
3. Ellestad M, Wan M. Prediction implications of stress testing. *Circulation* 1975; **51:** 363–369.
4. Hammermeister KE, DeRouen TA, Dodge HT. Variables prodictive of survival in patients with coronary disease: Selection by univariate and multivariate analyses from the clinical, electrocardiographic, exercise, arteriographic, and quantitative angiographic evaluation. *Circulation* 1979; **59:** 421–430.
5. Gohlke H, Samek L, Betz P, Roskamm H. Exercise testing provides additional prognostic information in angiographically defined subgroups of patients with coronary artery disease. *Circulation* 1983; **68:** 979–985.
6. Brunelli C, Cristofani R, L'Abbate A, for the ODI Study Group. Long-term survival in medically treated patients with ischemic heart disease and prognostic importance of clinical and electrocardiographic data. (The Italian CNR Multicenter Prospective Study.) *Eur Heart J* 1989; **10:** 292–303.
7. Weiner DA, Ryan T, McCabe CH, Chaitman BR, Sheffield T, Ferguson JC, Fisher LD, Tristani F. Prognostic importance of a clinical profile and exercise test in medically treated patients with coronary heart disease. *J Am Coll Cardiol* 1984; **3:** 772–779.
8. Mark DB, Hlatky MA, Harrell FE, Lee KL, Califf RM, Pryor DB. Exercise treadmill score for predicting prognosis in coronary heart disease. *Ann Intern Med* 1987; **106:** 793–800.
9. Peduzzi P, Hultgren H, Thomsen J, Angell W. Prognostic value of baseline exercise tests. *Prog Cardiovasc Dis* 1986; **28:** 285–292.
10. Lerman J, Svetlize H, Capris T, Perosia A. Follow-up of patients after exercise test and catheterization. *Medicina (Buenos Aires)* 1986; **46:** 210–211.
11. Wyns W, Musschaert-Beauthier E, Van Domburg R, Lubsen J, Rousseau MF, Cosyns J, Detry JMR. Prognostic value of symptom limited exercise testing in men with a high prevalence of coronary artery disease. *Eur Heart J* 1985; **6:** 939–945.
12. Detry JM, Luwaert RJ, Melin JA, Brohet CR, Rousseau MF, Ponlot R, D'Hondt AM, Vanbutsele R, Robert A. Non-invasive data provide independent prognostic information in patients with chest pain without previous myocardial infarction:

Findings in male patients who have had cardiac catheterization. *Eur Heart J* 1988; **9:** 418–426.

13. Califf RM, Mark DB, Harrell FE, Hlatky MA, Lee KL, Rosati RA, Pryor DB. Importance of clinical measures of ischemia in the prognosis of patients with documented coronary heart disease. *J Am Coll Cardiol* 1988; **11:** 20–26.
14. Detre K, Peduzzi R, Murphy M, Hultgren H, Thomsen J, Oberman A, Takaro T. Effect of bypass surgery on survival in patients in low- and high-risk subgroups delineated by the use of simple clinical variables. *Circulation* 1981; **63:** 1329–1338.
15. Mark DB, Shaw L, Harrell FE, Hlatky MA, Lee KL, Bengtson JR, McCants CB, Califf RM, Pryor DB. Prognostic value of a treadmill exercise score in outpatients with suspected coronary artery disease. *N Engl J Med* 1991; **325:** 849–853.

4 Routine Coronary Angiography After Each Major Coronary Event

Michael Jelinek

Cardiac Investigation Unit, St Vincent's Hospital, Melbourne, Victoria 3065, Australia

Acute coronary occlusion and acute coronary insufficiency

In the 1930s, the first generation of cardiologists to confront the waxing epidemic of coronary heart disease sought to differentiate clinically between the entities of coronary thrombosis and coronary insufficiency. Based on the findings of (hospitalized) patients, coronary thrombosis was characterized by acute severe chest pain, features of shock or heart failure, and evidence of fever and leucocytosis. Such patients frequently died in shock or heart failure or suddenly early in their hospital stay, and at autopsy had at least one coronary artery totally occluded with fresh thrombus. On the other hand, patients with coronary insufficiency were characterized by a history of angina often with recent deterioration prior to admission. The attack of pain which brought them to hospital was usually not as severe or as prolonged as in patients with coronary thrombosis. They were often quite well on admission to hospital and did not develop fever or leucocytosis; and frequently they went on to develop a coronary thrombosis either later than admission or not long after discharge from hospital. It was postulated that coronary insufficiency was characterized by coronary artery narrowing, not total occlusion, with a high risk of subsequent coronary thrombosis and death [1].

Proceedings of the Vth World Congress on Cardiac Rehabilitation

Myocardial infarction, Q-waves and myocardial ischaemia

The term coronary thrombosis was replaced by myocardial infarction due to persisting controversy lasting decades as to whether coronary thrombosis was consequent on reduced coronary flow from other causes, particularly coronary artery spasm. The pathogenic role of coronary artery thrombosis was finally proven by coronary angiography and thrombolysis in acute myocardial infarction. However, the term myocardial infarction has persisted. It is known that Q-wave myocardial infarctions (coronary thrombosis) have a relatively high mortality in hospital but a low mortality thereafter. On the other hand, patients with non-Q-wave infarctions (coronary insufficiency) have a low hospital mortality but increased death rate after hospital discharge due to recurrent myocardial infarction [2]. However, coronary angiography has shown that some patients with acute Q-wave myocardial infarctions do not have acute 100% occlusions, whereas some patients with acute non-Q-wave infarctions do have 100% occlusions [3,4].

Although tests for myocardial ischaemia after myocardial infarction have shown a correlation with the severity of coronary artery disease at angiography, they have not consistently predicted deaths within 1 year after discharge from hospital [5,6]. Thus, the presence of a narrowed but patent coronary artery, vulnerable to coronary thrombosis and fatal myocardial infarction, is only imprecisely assessed by clinical features, the presence or absence of Q-waves on the ECG and tests of myocardial ischaemia. The only way to assess whether or not a coronary artery is patent, narrowed or occluded in a patient with chest pain syndrome is by coronary angiography.

The prognostic significance of coronary angiography

It has been known for almost 20 years that the more vessels that are narrowed by more than 50% in diameter at coronary angiography, the worse is the prognosis over the next 5 years [7]. However, the major determinant of prognosis in patients in patients studied by angiography is the left ventricular systolic function, which can be assessed non-invasively by ejection fraction and end-systolic volume [8]. There is a statistical relationship in ischaemic heart disease between the number of major vessels narrowed and the ejection fraction, but a close relationship exists between the number of major occlusions (coronary thromboses) and reduced left ventricular ejection fraction. It is not possible clinically to be sure which patients have two mainstem occlusions and one residual, patent artery and which patients have there narrowed but patent main vessels with a better prognosis. Only coronary angiography can establish just how vulnerable a patient is to coronary occlusion.

In recent years, other features on the coronary angiogram have been shown to have prognostic significance. The 3-year risk of myocardial infarction in any vessel depends on the severity of its maximum stenosis varying from 2% risk with <50% diameter narrowing to 15% risk with >90% narrowing [9]. Thus a tightly narrowed coronary artery segment may be eight times as likely to occlude than a minimally narrowed segment. Occlusion is more likely if the lesion is long, eccentric in the lumen, or irregular in shape [10]. The latter two characteristics have been shown by coronary angioscopy to be the appearance of coronary thrombus without total occlusion. Thus there are a number of independent prognostic indicators with therapeutic implications which can be derived from the coronary angiogram.

Improved survival with coronary artery bypass surgery

There have been three large trials of coronary artery surgery for angina. Taken individually, the European Cardiac Surgery Study showed that a policy of routine coronary artery bypass surgery for severe narrowing of two or three main coronary arteries was superior to a policy of medical treatment in such cases [11]. This was not confirmed by either the Veterans Administrative Trial or the Coronary Artery Surgery Study [12,13]. However, retrospective analysis of these trials has shown consistently the surgery for patients with left main coronary artery stenosis >50% or patients with three mainstem vessel narrowings – particularly if associated with reduced ejection fraction consequent on total occlusion of one or more mainstream vessels – have improved survival with surgery [14].

The potential impact of coronary bypass surgery in prolonging life can best be shown by data bank experiences which combine large numbers of patients treated together with the frequency of triple vessel and left main coronary disease in practice. In recent years, these have shown uniformly that patients undergoing coronary bypass surgery for triple vessel disease and left main stenosis have better survival over 5 years than did similar patients treated medically [15–17].

Non-invasive predictors of improved surgical survival

Retrospective analyses from the large trials of coronary artery surgery have suggested that improved survival in patients randomly assigned to surgical therapy should be confined to patients with >1 mm of ST-segment depression on exercise testing [11,18,19]. This suggested that patients with <1 mm of ST-segment shift on exercise testing might not require coronary angiography in order to define the role of surgery in improving prognosis. However, wider experience of exercise testing in predicting survival of patients with angina has not shown a consistent role for ST shifts but has emphasized more consistently that low measured exercise tolerance – itself well predicted by history-taking – is the major determinant of poor survival in such patients [20,21].

Routine coronary angiography for effort angina

My views on the need for routine coronary angiography for effort have been created by a retrospective study of 434 patients who were regarded as having angina at the time of an exercise test in the years 1975–79, which resulted in reproduction of anginal pain and/or ST-segment depression on exercise. In those days, coronary angiography was offered only to patients limited by angina on ordinary effort and bypass surgery to patients with more severe disease an angiography. Thus 208 (48%) of the patients underwent coronary angiography and 125 (60%) of these had coronary artery bypass surgery. Despite being more limited symptomatically, patients who underwent coronary angiography had a 96% survival at 5 years compared with 86% survival in those patients "not sick enough" to investigate by angiography ($P < 0.001$). The patients who died averaged 1.80 mm of ST-segment depression compared with the 1.29 mm in survivors ($P < 0.01$). There were eight deaths among 59 patients (13.5%) without ST-segment changes treated medically without angiography in the following period averaging 6 years. Acknowledging the various potential biases in this retrospective study, we concluded that "coronary angiography is a superior technique to exercise testing for detecting patients with effort angina who are at high risk of premature mortality". We also noted"such a hypothesis should be tested by a randomized trial of angiography in patients thought to have angina. However, such a trial is not likely to be performed" [22].

The natural history of coronary heart disease

Although lipid deposition in arteries is a linear process over many decades, the natural history of coronary heart disease (CHD) reflects thrombosis episodes and represents stepwise necrosis of heart muscle, deterioration of health and eventual death. Two-thirds of these deaths occur outside a hospital setting and can be regarded as sudden [23].

If we combine sudden death and first episodes of myocardial infarction, then 35% of first coronary events are fatal [24]. If we include angina as a first manifestation of CHD, then the case fatality rate of first coronary events is 16% in men and much less in women. While the incidence of first and fatal events is age-dependent, the risk of coronary death as the first event of 1.5 per 1000 per year in middle-aged men and one-third of that in women [25]. Primary prevention is the only way to reduce the toll of sudden death as the first coronary event; better hospital care, especially with thrombolytic therapy, has almost certainly lowered hospital death rates from first myocardial infarctions [26].

Survivors of acute myocardial infarction have an excess mortality risk for the first six months after the event and then a stable mortality risk of 4% per annum [27,28]. However, the mortality risk depends on severity of left ventricular damage from heart attacks and is assessed clinically by the presence and severity of heart failure and life-threatening arrhythmias during and subsequent to the initial phase of the heart attack. Patients presenting with non-Q-wave myocardial infarction, unstable angina and progressive effort angina have a low initial mortality but an increased risk of recurring coronary events requiring hospitalization and a higher mortality risk after hospitalization. While the mortality risk of stable coronary heart disease in the absence of complications may be 1–2% per annum, the mortality risk of patients discharged from hospital with acute coronary syndrome without evidence of heart failure may be 2–5% within the next six months [29].

As indicated earlier, there are no completely reliable ways of distinguishing between patients with occluded arteries (coronary thrombosis, completed events) and patients with severe narrowings (coronary insufficiency) capable of subsequent complete occlusion and potential death of the patient. Although the mortality risk of coronary insufficiency is much higher in patients presenting in hospital with this syndrome as a *second* or subsequent clinical event in the course of CHD [30], preventable mortality may occur in patients surviving a first uncomplicated coronary event. Since coronary bypass surgery has been shown to delay early death in patients with multi-vessel disease, it follows that *all patients should have coronary angiography if they survive the first coronary event*. Furthermore, they should have this procedure as part of assessment early after their subsequent coronary event.

References

1. Master AM, Dacu S, Freed LE, Horn H. Diagnosis and treatment of acute coronary diseases. *JAMA* 1949; **14:** 887–891.
2. Marmor A, Geltman EM, Schetman K, Sobel BE, Roberts, R. Recurrent myocardial infarction: Clinical predictors and prognostic implications. *Circulation* 1982; **66:** 415–421.
3. Dewood MA, Spores J, Notske R, Mouser LT, Burroughs R, Golden MS, Lang HT. Prevalence of total coronary occlusions during the early hours of transmural myocardial infarction. *N Engl J Med* 1980; **303:** 897–902.
4. Dewood MA, Stiffer WF, Simpson CS, Spores J, Eugster GS, Judge TOP, Hinnen ML. Coronary anteriographic findings soon after non-Q-wave myocardial infarction. *N Engl J Med* 1986; **315:** 417–423.
5. Jelinek VM. Exercise testing after myocardial infarction. *Aust NZ J Med* 1985; **15:** 392–395.
6. Froelicher VF, Perdue S, Pewen W, Risch M. Application to meta-analysis using an electronic spread sheet to exercise testing in patients after myocardial infarction. *Am J Med* 1987; **83:** 1045–1054.
7. Bruscke AVG, Proudfit WL, Sones FM Jr. Progress study of 590 consecutive non-surgical cases of coronary disease followed 5–9 years. 1. Arteriographic correlation. *Circulation* 1973; **47:** 1147–1153.
8. Whitelock RML, Wild CJ. Left ventricular end-systolic volume as the major determinant of survival after recovery from myocardial infarction. *Circulation* 1987; **76:** 44–51.
9. Ellis S, Alderman E, Cain K, Fisher L, Sanders W, Bourassa M, and the CASS Investigations. Predicition of risk of anterior myocardial infarction by lesion severity and measurement method of stenoses in the left anterior descending distribution: A CASS registry study. *J Am Coll Cardiol* 1988; **11:** 908–916.

10. Ellis S, Alderman EL, Cain K, Wright A, Bourassa M. Fischer L, and the participants of the Coronary Artery Surgery Study (CASS). Morphology of left anterior descending coronary territory lesions as a predictor of anterior myocardial infarction: A CASS registry study. *J Am Coll Cardiol* 1989; **13:** 1481–1491.
11. European Coronary Surgery Study Group. Long term results of prospective randomized study of coronary artery bypass surgery in stable angina pectoris. *Lancet* 1982; **ii:** 1173–1180.
12. The Veterans Administration Coronary Artery Bypass Surgery Cooperative Study Group. Eleven year survival in the Veterans Administration randomized trial of coronary bypass surgery for stable angina. *N Engl J Med* 1984; **311:** 1333–1339.
13. Alderman EL, Bourassa MG, Cohen LS, Davis KB, Kaiser GG, Killip T, Mock MS, Pettinger M, Robertson TL, for the CASS Investigators. Ten-year follow-up of survival and myocardial infarction in the randomized coronary artery surgery study. *Circulation* 1990; **82:** 1629–1646.
14. Surgery in the treatment of coronary artery disease. *Circulation* 1985; **72** (Suppl. V): 1–168.
15. Vigilante GL, Weintraub WS, Klein LW. Medical and surgical survival in coronary disease in the 1980s. *Am J Cardiol* 1986; **58:** 926–931.
16. Pryor DB, Harrell FJ Jr, Rankin JS *et al.* The changing benefits of coronary revascularisation over time. *Circulation* 1987; **76** (Suppl. V): 13–21.
17. Proudfit WL, Kramer JR, Goormastic M, Loop FD. Survival of patients with mild angina or myocardial infarction without angina: A comparison of medical and surgical treatment. *Br Heart J* 1988; **59:** 641–647.
18. Ryan TJ, Weiner DA, McCabe CH *et al.* Exercise testing in the Coronary Artery Surgery Study randomized population. *Circulation* 1985; **72** (Suppl. V): 31–38.
19. Peduzzi P, Hultgren H, Thomsen J, Angell W. Prognostic value of baseline exercise tests. *Prog Cardiovasc Dis* 1986; **28:** 285–292.
20. Bruce RA, Derouen T, Peterson DR *et al.* Non-invasive predictors of sudden cardiac death in men with coronary heart disease: Predictive value of maximal stress testing. *Am J Cardiol* 1977; **39:** 833–840.
21. Jelinek VM, McDonald IG. History, exercise test, and prognosis of chest pain. *Med J Aust* 1980; **2:** 25–27.
22. Jelinek MV, Becker NG, Ryan WF, Clemens A. Routine coronary angiography for effort angina. *Med J Aust* 1991: **1:** 808–814.
23. Gordon T, Kannel WB. Premature mortality from coronary heart disease: The Framingham Study. *JAMA* 1971; **215:** 1617–1625.
24. Frank CW. The course of coronary heart disease: Factors relating to prognosis. *Bull NY Acad Med* 1968; **44:** 900–915.
25. Schatzkin A, Cupples LA, Heeren T, Morelock S, Kannel WB. Sudden death in the Framingham Heart Study: Differences in incidence and risk factors by sex and coronary disease status. *Am J Epidemiol* 1984; **120:** 888–899.
26. McGovern PG, Folson AR, Sprafka JM, Burke GL, Doliszny KM, Demirovic J, Naylor JD, Blackburn H. Trends in survival of hospitalized myocardial infarction patients between 1970 and 1985: The Minnesota Heart Survey. *Circulation* 1992; **85:** 172–179.
27. Gilpin EA, Koziol JA, Madsen EB, Henning H, Ross J Jr. Periods of differing mortality distribution during the first year after acute myocardial infarction. *Am J Cardiol* 1983; **52:** 240–244.
28. Schlant RC, Forman, S, Stamler J, Canner PL. The natural history of coronary heart disease: Prognostic factors after recovery from myocardial infarction in 2789 men. The 5-year findings of the Coronary Drug Project. *Circulation* 1982; **66:** 410–414.
29. Jelinek M, Powell A, Becker N, McDonald I. Uncomplicated acute myocardial infarction: A five year follow-up. *J Cardiopulmonary Rehab* 1988; **8:** 149–154.
30. Bayley N, Hunt D, Penington C, Sloman JG. Subendocardial myocardial infarction. *Aust NZ J Med* 1982; **12:** 166–169.

5 After a First Coronary Event, Clinical Assessment is Sufficient to Define the Need for Coronary Angiography

Risteard Mulcahy

Department of Preventive Cardiology, St Vincent's Hospital, Dublin 4, Ireland

Disagreements about many aspects of coronary heart disease (CHD) management can be attributed to conflicting or to equivocal or absent trial evidence, and such disagreements are compounded by wide variations in professional attitudes, experience, training and circumstances, and by differences in patient attitudes and circumstances.

The subject of risk stratification after myocardial infarction (MI) exemplifies the difficulties we encounter in reaching a consensus about the best approach. History-taking and clinical examination, the nature of the attack, and the residual symptoms and cardiac status, are obviously important components of risk stratification analysis. Investigations, including ECG, the exercise and thallium tests, echocardiography, radionucleotide studies and angiography are now widely used soon after MI to identify risk status, to assist in establishing prognosis and to provide guidelines about subsequent management. However, the widely varying practices in the use of these tests, and the varying opinions about their value in risk stratification reported in the literature, is a measure of their unsatisfactory sensitivity and specificity.

Because of the lack of consensus about the value of these investigations, it is important to take a balanced view of their place in establishing prognosis and in outlining guidelines about management. It is too easy to polarize a discussion of this sort, but I shall avoid doing so, particularly by avoiding the temptation of quoting selectively from the literature.

Proceedings of the Vth World Congress on Cardiac Rehabilitation

Let us look at the proposition of performing routine angiography early after the first MI. An angiogram might be deemed useful at this stage for three reasons.

1. To further research.
2. To establish prognosis.
3. To provide guidelines about treatment, including coronary artery bypass surgery (CABS) and angioplasty.

There are, however, alternative clinical and non-invasive investigations available to assess prognosis and to establish useful guidelines about intervention. Assessment is based on identifying and quantifying the factors which contribute to the patients' risk of further complications and of premature death. These factors are as follows:

1. Age.
2. The degree of left ventricular damage.
3. The extent, location and severity of disease in the coronary vessels.
4. The presence of post-infarction ischaemia, whether it is silent, or of the unstable or stable variety.
5. The presence of atrial fibrillation, ventricular arrhythmias and conduction defects.
6. The presence of concomitant disease.
7. The risk factor status and the potential for risk factor modification, and hence non-progression or regression of atheroma.

In the early stages after MI, left ventricular damage is the principal determinant of prognosis, at least during the first year after the event. Silent and symptomatic ischaemia, whether unstable or stable, are also relevant factors, and, in addition, affect quality of life. In the absence of left ventricular damage and in the absence of persistent ischaemia, it is doubtful if angiography is justified, at least in the early phase following MI, nor is it likely to be cost-effective because of its low yield in terms of identifying patients who are best treated by CABS or angioplasty. Neither is angiography justified in patients with severe left ventricular damage and pump failure.

What are the disadvantages of angiography after MI?

1. It alters what is and should be a functional assessment to a strictly anatomical one.
2. It is expensive, not without complications, and not always easily available. Hence, to be cost-effective, it should only be prescribed for patients who are likely to benefit by delineating the coronary anatomy, such as those requiring surgical intervention or angioplasty.

Left ventricular damage can be accurately measured by history-taking, clinical examination and non-invasive tests, including echocardiography. We are aware that patients with severe left ventricular damage, and those with atrial fibrillation or persistent ventricular arrhythmias, without residual ischaemia or ventricular damage, are unlikely to be helped by surgical intervention. We are also aware that patients with little or no heart muscle damage who are asymptomatic following MI, and who respond to risk factor modification and an exercise training programme, have an excellent prognosis. Models have been described, based on independent clinical, ECG and exercise testing variables, to identify low-risk cases not requiring angiography [1]. Nor do we have any evidence from trials or other means that, in high-risk cases, surgery or angioplasty reduce morbidity or mortality in the early post-infarction phase, so that there seems every reason to postpone angiography until the patient's response to risk factor intervention and routine rehabilitation measures, including aspirin and beta-blockers when indicated, has been measured.

A report from the Irish Cardiac Surgical Register [2] records that there was an early mortality of 13.2% among 53 patients submitted to CABS less than 6 weeks after MI, whereas the early mortality in 1467 patients operated at a later date was 3.09%. Since the early 1980s surgical mortality among patients submitted to early operation in Ireland has been substantially higher than mortality among those who are operated on at a later date, although the latest 1990 report from the Irish register [3] does not record this differential.

Angiography after MI should be reserved for those who have a high probability of benefiting from the procedure. If it is practised routinely or in a haphazard and less precise way, it may result in a number of undesirable consequences, over and above the expense of the procedure, its possible complications, the inconvenience to patients, and the waste of professional time and expertise. These consequences are principally the result of assessing prognosis on the strictly anatomical findings, and of ignoring the relevant functional features. Also ignored may be the potential benefits of conservative treatment, including risk factor modification, exercise programmes and appropriate medication. The widespread use of angiography encourages surgery in asymptomatic patients and in those who have single, two-vessel, or non-threatening three-vessel disease, and who have not been given the benefits of adequate medical treatment. It may also encourage surgery or angioplasty immediately after unstable angina or MI when it may be best left until a later date. The benefits of immediate surgery remain controversial, and immediate angioplasty may be harmful [4].

If we are to adhere strictly to guidelines indicating surgical benefit, we should confine operation to patients with left main stem, three-vessel or three-vessel equivalent disease, and particularly those with some left ventricular damage. We should also consider patients with persistent unstable or intractable chronic angina of effort. However, reference to the literature and our own experience would suggest that many patients with single- or two-vessel disease are submitted to surgery, as well as patients who are asymptomatic or who have non-disabling angina of effort.

In my experience, most patients with chronic angina will show considerable symptomatic improvement or resolution of symptoms on a graduated exercise programme combined with routine rehabilitation and secondary preventive measures. So-called intractable angina is rare in patients who are given adequate medical treatment, unless the ischaemia is unstable in nature.

The haphazard approach to surgery and to angioplasty can be partly attributed to the haphazard criteria which so frequently determine the indications for angiography. What are the circumstances that encourage this uncritical approach to employing angiography? They include the physician's training, the local medical culture, the preferences and prejudices of one's colleagues, the availability of facilities and equipment, personal and institutional financial interests, an uncritical approach to the literature, the absence of audit or evaluation of results and, finally, medico-legal considerations.

The modern training of cardiologists puts considerable emphasis on invasive expertise. Appointments to consultant posts are likely to favour the candidate highly trained in laboratory and angioplasty techniques. There is less emphasis today on the role of a cardiologist as a doctor treating and counselling the patient at the bedside. We exaggerate the value and relevance of our complex investigations and we now undervalue information that we can acquire from history-taking and physical examination. As doctors, we are distancing ourselves from our patients.

The local medical culture and the attitudes and practices of our colleagues consciously or unconsciously determine our own activities and beliefs. As a team, we like to reach a consensus when making clinical decisions. It makes us more comfortable and secure to agree or seem to agree. Nowhere is this more obvious than at the angiology conference.

The availability of equipment, staff and facilities plays a major role in encouraging angiography. When facilities are scarce, only the high-risk cases are likely to be referred and, indeed, under these circumstances we may err in underusing desirable investigations. When the facilities are adequate or unlimited, we not infrequently find Murphy's law in operation, the law which ordains that nature abhors a vacuum. Another important factor that encourages the overuse of angiography is the financial interests of the investigator and/or the institutions providing this service. This is a more important influence than we would care to admit.

Our response to the literature can be ambivalent. We are aware of the trials confirming the benefits of CABS in patients with a defined coronary anatomy, with moderate left ventricular damage or with persistent symptomatic ischaemia. We are aware also of the absence of evidence of benefit in patients without these presentations. Yet we prescribe surgery in many patients who, when assessed from the trial and epidemiological information available, do not qualify for intervention. And there is generally little attempt to evaluate our results in terms of a better quality of life, reduced morbidity and mortality, and health service exigencies by audit or peer review. Up to one-third of our proceedures have been shown to be inappropriate [5].

We must, however, be realistic about the pressures which are imposed on us to undertake active intervention when we are dealing with coronary patients. The diagnosis of CHD, whether angina or infarction, has important life-threatening implications for the patient and the family. As doctors, too, we are aware of the unpredictability of the condition in terms of further infarction or life-threatening arrhythmias. It is natural to abreact under these circumstances in response to patients' anxiety and our own forebodings. What easier way to abreact than to refer our patients to the laboratory and, with the evidence of the anatomical lesions in the coronary arteries, to prescribe urgent angioplasty or surgery. If the patient recovers and remains asymptomatic, as most patients do, great credit redounds to the medical attendants. If the patient dies or suffers some serious complication, at least we will have been perceived to have done everything in our power to bring benefit to our patient. How much easier it is to do an angiogram and to follow this up with active intervention than to prescribe a rehabilitation programme, to provide repeated counselling sessions, to emphasize that the mainstay of recovery and survival may require difficult changes in lifestyle, and to prescribe appropriate medication. The surgical patient requires the same rehabilitation programme, although this is not always made clear to the patient, nor is it made clear that surgery is merely a palliative procedure.

In this critique of modern cardiological practice, I hope that I shall not be misunderstood. There are important and compelling guidelines supporting the need for angiography and for surgical intervention. I merely make a plea that, despite the fact that valid management guidelines do exist, our diagnostic and therapeutic practices are frequently based on less well-defined criteria. Clear advantages in terms of reduced morbidity and mortality and/or a better quality of life should be adduced before angiography should be considered appropriate. Unfortunately, in the case of coronary angiography, the unnecessary performance of the test may lead to interventions which may not be justified on the grounds of current guidelines. As a profession responsible for its own standards, I believe we have a responsibility to be critical of all our actions on such issues as routine coronary angiography after a first MI. I must confess that I cannot therefore agree with Dr Jelinek's thesis.

References

1. Wilcox I, Freedman B, Allman KC *et al.* Prognostic significance of a predischarge exercise test in risk stratification after unstable angina. *J Am Coll Cardiol* 1991; **18:** 677–683.
2. Lonergan M, Daly L, Graham I. Mortality in the first year after coronary artery bypass surgery. *Ir J Med Soc* 1990; **159:** 289–291.
3. Personal report.
4. Baim DS. Angioplasty as a treatment for coronary artery disease (Editorial). *N Engl J Med* 1992; **326:** 56–58.
5. Ryan TJ, Baker CD, Abelmann WH *et al.* The Cardiology Working Group, Harvard: Cardiology and the quality of medical practice. *JAMA* 1991; **265:** 482–485.

6 Comparative Study of Two Populations Medically and Surgically Treated: A Ten-year Follow-up of 791 Patients

N.Oysel, P. Rougier, M. Koch, H. Douard, P. Besse, J.-P. Broustet*

Hôpital Cardiologique du Haut-Lévêque, 33604 Pessac, FRANCE

Introduction

The indications and long-term benefits of myocardial revascularization by coronary artery bypass surgery (CABG) in patients with stable angina pectoris are now well known after the results of three randomized multi-centre studies [1–3]. Mortality and morbidity are only improved in selected groups of patients, such as those with left main coronary artery disease, triple-vessel disease with impaired left ventricular function, or proximal stenosis in left anterior descending artery with multi-vessel disease.

In other cases, the assignment to medical or surgical treatment generally depends on an individually tailored approach to the information collected (medical history, exercise test and coronary angiography) [4]. In a retrospective study, we compared the long-term follow-up of two groups of patients: (1) patients with operable coronary lesions whose vital and functional prognosis appeared good enough in the short term to be maintained by medical treatment, and who were therefore treated medically as a first choice; (2) patients treated surgically as a first choice because of the severity of their symptoms and coronary lesions.

* To whom all correspondence should be addressed.

Proceedings of the Vth World Congress on Cardiac Rehabilitation

Patients and methods

The decision as to type of treatment was determined by data collected from the patient's medical history (symptoms, age, job and leisure demands), by the results of an exercise stress test free of anti-anginal medication, and by data from coronary angiography. The decision to carry out surgery as a first choice was designed to (a) improve symptoms and functional status and (b) to preserve the myocardium. There were four categories of choice (Fig. 1): First, not to operate but patients were operable. These were the medically treated patients of the study. This choice was called "deliberate abstention from coronary artery bypass graft (CABG)". Secondly, not to operate and patients were non-operable. These patients had usually had a myocardial infarction, or had mild symptoms, and coronary angiography showed only one occluded vessel or that the vessel could not be bypassed. Thirdly, to operate and patients were operable. These were the surgically treated patients of the study. Fourthly, to operate but patients were non-operable. These patients had severe and diffuse coronary lesions for whom surgery was impossible or extremely limited.

Follow-up information was obtained from a survey of medical records, by mail or by telephone. Comparison of the two groups was done on the basis of

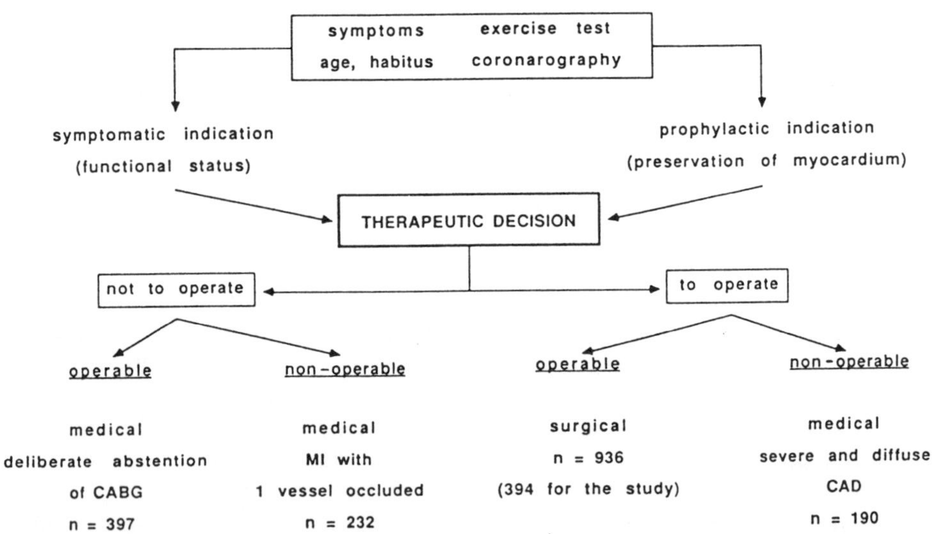

Fig. 1. Therapeutic decisions in coronary artery disease. Two indications lead to the therapeutic decision: a symptomatic indication and a prophylactic indication. Thus, four therapeutic schema appear. Between 1979 and 1985, of 1755 patients, 397 were medically treated but eligible for surgery (medical group of the study), 232 were medically treated because angiography showed one vessel occluded in the territory of myocardial infarction, 936 were immediately operated upon (394 were randomized for the study) and 190 were medically treated because of severe and diffuse coronary disease.

"intention to treat". Survival and morbidity were estimated by the actuarial method and the log-rank test was used to compare rates between the groups.

Results

Patients

Between 1979 and 1985, 397 patients with significant coronary artery disease (stenosis > 70%) were medically treated and 936 patients were surgically treated as a first choice. Among the 936 surgical patients, 394 were randomized for the purpose of the study. Comparison of clinical characteristics between the two groups (Table 1) showed a small difference for age, no difference for sex and previous myocardial infarction. Stable angina pectoris was more frequently observed in the medical group, while aggravated and unstable angina occurred more often in the surgical group. All patients underwent a symptom-limited exercise test free of anti-anginal medication. The results of the two groups were dramatically different (Table 2). In the surgical patients, the exercise test was terminated more frequently due to chest pain at a lower speed (3221 ± 2299 *vs* 5175 ± 3300 kilogram metres, $P < 0.001$) workload (90 watts 3 min *vs* 120 watts 3 min), maximal heart rate (121 ± 20 *vs* 133 ± 21 beats/min, $P < 0.001$), maximal ST segment depression in the CM_5 lead (-2.5 ± 1.6 *vs* -1.9 ± 1.6 mm, $P < 0.001$). An exercise test score developed in our laboratory [5], taking into account many parameters in a multivariate analysis, was more severe in the surgical group (12.1 ± 3.9 *vs* 7.9 ± 4.2, $P \pm 0.001$). Coronary angiography data showed a higher severity of coronary lesions in the surgical group compared to the medical group (Table 3). Three-vessel disease was more frequent in the surgical patients (245 *vs* 55, $P < 0.001$), whereas one-vessel disease was dominant in the medical patients (188 *vs* 31, $P < 0.001$). Proximal stenosis in the left anterior descending artery was present in 106 medical patients

Table 1
Clinical characteristics of medically and surgically treated patients at entry into the study

	Medical ($n = 397$)	Surgical ($n = 394$)	P
Age (years)	55.7 ± 9.0	57.0 ± 8.0	0.04
Male	347 (87.5%)	363 (92%)	NS
Previous MI	179 (45%)	176 (45%)	NS
Angina:			
stable	160 (40%)	33 (8.5%)	<0.01
aggravated	117 (29.5%)	149 (38.5%)	
unstable	120 (30.5%)	205 (53%)	

Table 2
Exercise test data of the medically and surgically treated patients at entry into the study

	Medical ($n = 397$)	Surgical ($n = 394$)	P
Pain at exercise test	38%	72%	<0.001
Total work (Kgm)	5157 ± 3300	3221 ± 2299	<0.001
HR_{max} (beats/min)	133 ± 21	121 ± 20	<0.001
ST_{max} (CM5, mm)	−1.9 ± 1.6	−2.5 ± 1.6	<0.001
Exercise test score	7.9 ± 4.2	12.1 ± 3.9	<0.001

Abbreviations: HR_{max}, maximal heart rate; ST_{max}, maximal ST-depression in CM5 lead; Kgm, kilogram metres.
Exercise test scores obtained by multivariate analysis.

and in 214 surgical patients ($P < 0.001$). The Friesinger score [6] was significantly increased in the surgical group (9.8 ± 2.5 *vs* 5.7 ± 2.7, $P < 0.001$).

Follow-up data

In the medical group (Fig. 2), with a mean follow-up of 78 ± 21 months, 46 patients died, 22 from cardiac causes. Of the 351 patients still living, 11 had been lost from sight but were alive according to the information provided by the Registry Office, 24 had suffered a myocardial infarction, 83 had undergone CABG and 11 coronary angioplasty (PTCA). Finally, 265 patients who had been eligible for surgery had had no cardiac event. In the surgical group (Fig. 3), with a longer mean follow-up (90 ± 27 months), 63 patients had died, 38 from cardiac causes. Out of the 331 patients still living, 10 had been lost from sight during the follow-up, 22 had had repeat CABG, 12 had undergone PTCA, 24 had suffered a myocardial infarction and 306 patients had had no cardiac event.

Table 3
Coronary angiography data of medically and surgically treated patients at entry into the study

	Medical ($n = 397$)	Surgical ($n = 394$)	P
One-vessel disease	188 (47.3%)	31 (7.9%)	<0.001
Two-vessel disease	154 (38.8%)	118 (29.9%)	NS
Triple-vessel disease	55 (13.9%)	245 (62.2%)	<0.001
Ejection fraction (%)	61 ± 12	63 ± 12	<0.05
Prox. LAD	106 (26.7%)	214 (54.8%)	<0.001
Friesinger score	5.7 ± 2.7	9.8 ± 2.5	<0.001

Abbreviation: Prox. LAD, presence of proximal stenosis in the left anterior descending artery.

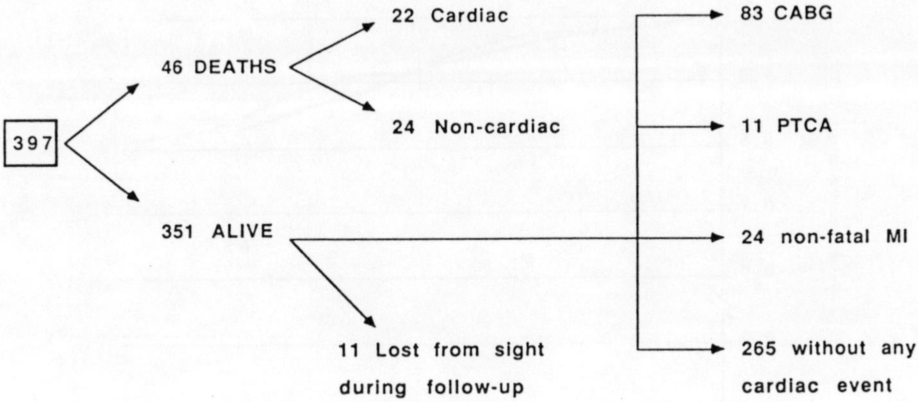

Fig. 2. Follow-up of medically treated patients (78 ± 21 months).

Survival

Cumulative survival rates (Fig. 4) after assignment to treatment were the same for both groups, i.e. 82 and 81% at 5 and 10 years. There was no significant difference between the two groups in terms of actuarial cardiac mortality: about 5% at 5 years and 10% at 10 years. When the patients were classified according to number of diseased vessels, the 10-year probabilities of remaining alive in the medical *vs* the surgical group were 85 ***vs*** 85% (NS) with one diseased vessel, 88 *vs* 83% (NS) with two diseased vessels, and 59 *vs* 79% (NS) in the case of three-vessel disease. The mortality of the medical patients with three diseased vessels was higher after the 7-year follow-up, but the difference was not significant (Fig. 5).

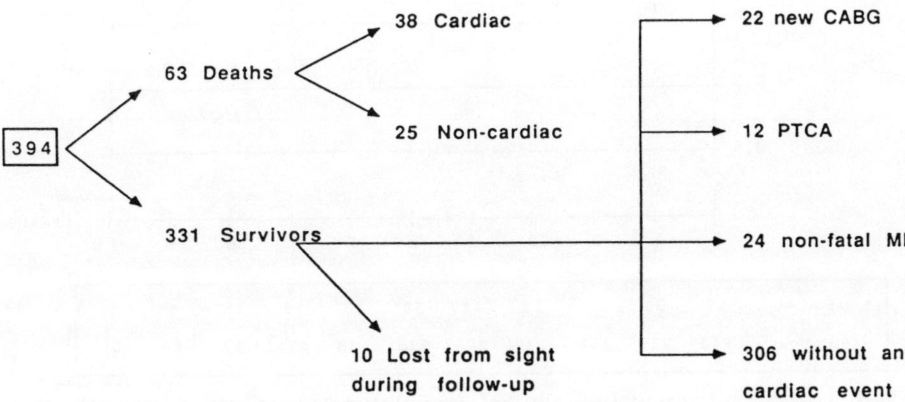

Fig. 3. Follow-up of surgically treated patients (90 ± 27 months).

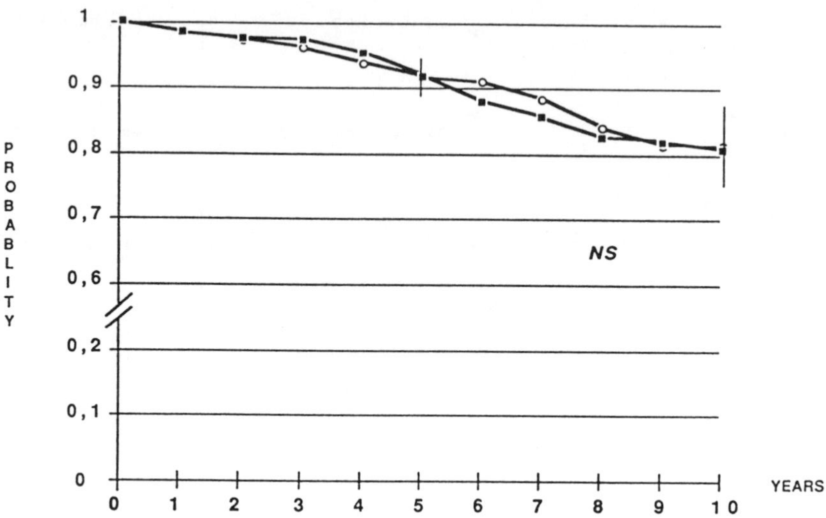

o MEDICAL	397	390	385	380	346	280	205	147	89	40	11
▪ SURGICAL	391	385	382	381	373	359	295	231	157	94	48

Fig. 4. Ten-year survival of medically and surgically treated patients. Numbers of patients at risk are given at the bottom of the figure.

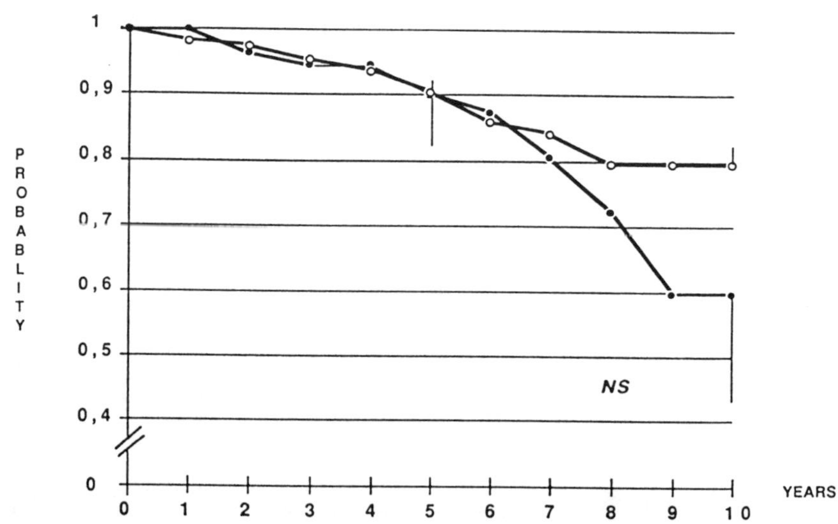

• MEDICAL	55	55	53	52	48	38	27	22	15	6	1
o SURGICAL	243	239	237	232	228	220	169	131	87	46	21

Fig. 5. Ten-year survival of medically and surgically treated patients with three diseased vessels.

Table 4
Summary of 10-year actuarial follow-up in medically and surgically treated patients

	Medical ($n = 397$)	Surgical ($n = 394$)	P
Survival	82%	81%	NS
Cardiac deaths	8%	12%	NS
Myocardial infarction	10%	8%	NS
CABG	26%	9%	—
PTCA	8%	5%	—
No cardiac event	60%	70%	—

Non-fatal cardiac events

The occurence of myocardial infarction was exactly the same in both groups: 5% at 5 years and 10% at 10 years (Table 4). At 10 years, 8% of the medical patients and 5% of the surgical patients had undergone PTCA. In the medically treated group, CABG was the most frequent event: 19% at 5 years and 26% at 10 years in actuarial probabilities. Of the angiographic data, the number of diseased vessels ($P < 0.0005$), a proximal stenosis in the left anterior descending artery ($P < 0.0001$) and the Friesinger score ($P = 0.0006$) were identified as

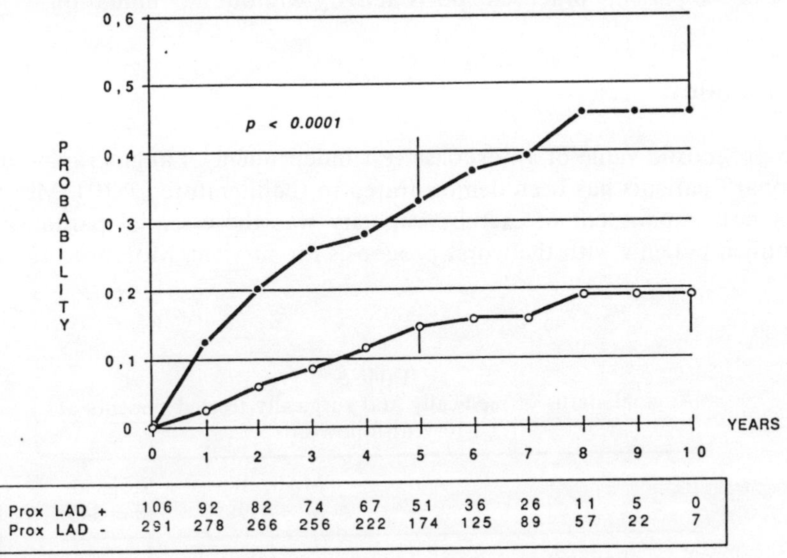

Fig. 6. Ten-year occurrence rates of CABG in medically treated patients subdivided on the presence or absence of proximal stenosis in the left anterior descending artery (Prox LAD).

being independently predictive of CABG by using log-rank tests and Cox's regression model. The presence of proximal stenosis in the left anterior descending artery was particularly predictive of early CABG, the difference being significant from the first 18 months of follow-up (Fig. 6). Triple-vessel disease was the main cause of late CABG. In the surgical group, 9% of patients had had repeat CABG at 10 years. 8% of patients in the medical group and 5% of patients in the surgical group had undergone PTCA. At the end of the follow-up, 60% of the medically treated patients who were eligible for surgery and 70% of the surgically treated patients had had no major cardiac event at 10 years.

Anginal status and quality of life

At the end of the follow-up, 80% of the surgical patients and 58% of the medical patients were free of angina in daily life; 20% of the surgical group and 34% of the medical group were stabilized but showed no improvement in their anginal status. Worsening angina was noted in 8% of the medical patients and 0.2% of the surgical patients who had not been operated on a second time at the end of follow-up (Table 5).

In terms of quality of life (Table 6), 7% of the medically treated patients and 0.3% of the surgically treated patients had their daily activities severely limited; 30% of the medical group and 8.2% of the surgical group were autonomous but without recreational activity. Recreational activity was feasible for 39% of the medical patients and for 68% of the surgical patients. In both groups, about 24% of the patients practised sports activity without any limitation.

Discussion

The prognostic value of an exercise test independent of angiographic data in coronary patients has been demonstrated in the literature [7–10]. More often than not, impairment of exercise capacity was the essential parameter that identified patients with the worst prognosis for survival. Moreover, the results

Table 5
Anginal status of medically and surgically treated patients at 10-year follow-up

	Medical ($n = 339$)	Surgical ($n = 348$)
Free of angina in daily life	58.0%	80.0%
Stabilized but not improved	34.0%	19.8%
Worsened angina	8.0%	0.2%

Table 6
Quality of life in medically and surgically treated patients at 10-year follow-up

Limitation to activity	Medical ($n = 281$)	Surgical ($n = 267$)
Severe: no moving about	7.0%	0.3%
Important: no recreational activity	30.0%	8.2%
Mild: recreational activity	39.0%	68.0%
None: sporting activity	24.0%	23.5%

of multi-centre randomized studies indicate unequivocally that CABG should be performed in some well-defined groups of coronary patients [1–3]. There is no doubt that these data influenced our decision to operate or to defer surgery. It was therefore not surprising to find that the exercise test results and coronary lesions were very different between the medically treated and surgical patients in the study. Baseline variables clearly indicated that the patients from the surgical group had a bad prognosis without CABG. In everyday medical practice there is no question of randomization. The only way to find out if a particular type of treatment is satisfactory is to assess the results with a suitably long follow-up in a sufficiently large population. This was the object of our study. Considerable experience in using long-term physical training in coronary patients long before coronary surgery became commonplace has shown us that coronary patients with sometimes very severe lesions can live a long and comfortable life. In addition, any decision to undertake surgery in the case of patients with early single-vessel disease should be carefully thought through. The progression of lesions and the recurrence of symptoms after 5 or 10 years often means that other arteries will need to be operated on when the graft is in a satisfactory state; angioplasty is not always possible nor successful in the long term.

Survival rates were the same for the two groups, with annual cardiac mortality estimated at 1%. We consider that this study shows that a cautious attitude in the case of moderate forms of coronary disease and an aggressive attitude in the case of very serious forms results in a favourable and identical prognosis. This could probably be improved if some of the patients with lesions on proximal LAD or with triple-vessel disease had been operated on sooner. For these patients, in addition to annual symptom-limited exercise tests, a coronary angiography should be performed again 5 years later, which could eventually lead to a preventive CABG in the case of a creeping progression of lesions. The survival rates reported here are similar to those in the CASS study [2], probably because the characteristics of the CASS patients [11] were much the same as the patients in our study.

The occurrence of late myocardial infarction was the same (about 10%) in both groups at 10 years. This is not surprising: Ambrose [12] reports that myocardial infarction occurs more frequently in areas of previously mild or insignificant coronary lesions, which have been complicated by a ruptured plaque and thrombosis.

Subsequent CABG occurred in about one-fifth of the medically treated patients at 10 years, whereas all the patients were angiographically eligible for surgery. During the same period, 8% of the medical patients underwent PTCA. These results suggest that medical therapy is effective for several years in mildly symptomatic coronary artery disease, even if critical stenosis is observed on proximal artery segments or on the three vessels. Nevertheless, some of our patients with unstable angina due to proximal stenosis of the LAD, which we left to medical treatment because of easy and early stabilization and a favourable exercise test, could have been grafted as a first choice, as suggested by the European Coronary Surgery Study [3]. In addition, patients with three-vessel disease were also more likely to be operated upon later than the others. These results suggest that medical therapy is not always the best treatment for these categories of patients. At the end of the follow-up period, the majority of patients had had no major cardiac event: 60% in the medical group and 70% in the surgical group.

The CASS study showed that indices of quality of life and anginal status in patients assigned to surgery compared to medically treated patients are less apparent in the long term than initially observed [13]. In our study, the surgically treated patients were more frequently free of angina with a better quality of life than the medically treated patients. However, a large number of patients in the medical group were free of angina or had stabilized and 24% of them (compared to 23.5% in the surgical group) were not limited in their range of activities.

The use of internal mammary artery as a graft [14] has been systematically introduced since 1985. Perhaps the natural history of patients will improve in the future.

Conclusion

The two groups of patients studied showed considerable differences in coronary score, exercise test score and clinical presentation of their coronary disease at the time of first assessment. Such differences, as shown in the literature, are clearly predictive of a very significant difference in long-term prognosis. Our study shows that coronary surgery techniques have levelled this difference in a beneficial way, since the non-surgical group evolved favourably. This facts lead us to two conclusions: myocardial revascularization, whether by surgical means or by angioplasty, should only be offered to patients who are really in need of it and not to all those for whom it is technically feasible. Abstaining from revascularization, even after myocardial infarction, is perfectly legitimate in a great number of cases. In addition, this position can always be revised depending on how things evolve subsequently and on the information collected during careful monitoring.

References

1. The Veterans Administration Coronary Artery Bypass Surgery Cooperative Study Group. Eleven-year survival rate in the Veterans Administration randomized trial of coronary bypass surgery for stable angina. *N Engl J Med* 1984; **311:** 1333–1339.
2. Alderman EL, Bourassa MG, Cohen LS, *et al.* Ten-year follow-up of survival and myocardial infarction in the randomized Coronary Artery Surgery Study. *Circulation* 1990; **82:** 1629–1646.
3. Varnauskas E, and the European Coronary Surgery Study Group. Twelve-year follow-up of survival in the randomized European Coronary Surgery Study. *N Engl J Med* 1988; **319:** 332–337.
4. Braunwald E. Effects of coronary-artery bypass grafting on survival: implications of the randomized Coronary Artery Surgery Study. *N Engl J Med* 1983; **309:** 1181–1184.
5. Koch M. Essai de prédiction de la sévérité de l'atteinte coronarienne par l'épreuve d'effort quantifiée. Analyse multivariée. *Thèse: Méd.: Bordeaux* 1988; **2:** 284.
6. Fiesinger GC, Page E, Ross R. Prognostic significance of coronary arteriography. *Trans Assoc Am Physician* 1970; **83:** 78–89.
7. Weiner DA, Ryan TJ, McCabe CH, Chaitman BR, Sheffield LT, Ferguson JC, Fisher LD, Tristani F. Prognostic importance of a clinical profile and exercise test in the medically treated patients with coronary artery disease. *J Am Coll Cardiol* 1984; **3:** 772–779.
8. Bonow RO, Kent KM, Rosing DR, Lan KKG, Lakatos E, Borer JS, Bacharach SL, Green MV, Epstein SE. Exercise-induced ischemia in mildly symptomatic patients with coronary artery disease and preserved left ventricular function. *N Engl J Med* 1984; **311:** 1339–1345.
9. Podrid PJ, Graboys TB, Lown B. Prognosis of medically treated patients with coronary artery disease with profound ST-segment depression during exercise test. *N Engl J Med* 1981; **305:** 1111–1116.
10. Bogaty P, Dagenais GR, Cantin B, Alain P, Rouleau JR. Prognosis in patients with a strongly positive exercise electrocardiogram. *Am J Cardiol* 1989; **64:** 1284–1288.
11. CASS Principal Investigators and Their Associates. Coronary Artery Surgery Study (CASS): A randomized trial of coronary artery bypass surgery. Survival data. *Circulation* 1983; **68:** 939–950.
12. Ambrose JA, Tannenbaum MA, Alexopoulos D, Hjemdahl-Monsen CE, Leavy J, Weiss M, Borrico S, Gorlin R, Fuster V. Angiographic progression of coronary artery disease and the development of myocardial infarction. *J Am Coll Cardiol* 1988; **12:** 56–62.
13. Rogers WJ, Coggin CJ, Gersh BJ *et al.* Ten-year follow-up of quality of life in patients randomized to receive medical therapy or coronary artery bypass surgery. The Coronary Artery Surgery Study (CASS). *Circulation* 1990; **82:** 1647–1658.
14. Loop FD, Lytle BW, Cosgrove DM *et al.* Influence of internal-mammery-artery graft on ten-year survival and other cardiac events. *N Engl J Med* 1986; **314:** 1–6.

7 Stratification of Risk after Myocardial Infarction

Luigi Tavazzi[1*], Alberto Volpi[2], Augusto Cavalli[2]

[1]Fondazione Clinica del Lavoro, Centro Medico di Riabilitazione, Divisione di Cardiologia, Via S. Boezio 26, 27100 Pavia, and *[2]Ospedale G. Fornaroli, Divisione di Cardiologia, Magenta (Milano), Italy*

Introduction

The accurate definition of the long-term outcome after recovery from acute myocardial infarction (AMI) is important for selecting optimal clinical strategies, to widen our current knowledge of pathophysiological components of risk and to plan secondary prevention trials.

In the 1960s and 1970s, prognostic indices calculated by scoring clinical variables were proposed [1,2]. More recently, a new approach primarily pointing to the pathophysiological determinants of prognosis and their interaction has gained wide acceptance. Much effort has also been directed towards the prediction of the individual risk of evolution of the disease, based on the combined effect of several non-cardiac risk factors (such as abnormal lipid profile, hyperfibrinogenaemia, arterial hypertension, psychological profile, etc.) or the characteristics of coronary artery lesions. Unfortunately, the results reported in the literature are rarely unequivocal and the combination effect of recently identified risk factors is unknown. Hence, at this time, risk prediction following myocardial infarction still needs to be based mainly on three major areas of functional risk, namely the extent of myocardial damage or the degree of global pump dysfunction, the extent and severity of residual myocardial ischaemia and the propensity to electrical instability.

*To whom all correspondence should be addressed.

Proceedings of the Vth World Congress on Cardiac Rehabilitation

Demographic variables

It is generally accepted that *age* is an important factor for long-term prognosis in patients surviving the hospital phase of AMI, independently of other known risk factors [3]. It has been suggested that advancing age might act as a surrogate indicator for the presence of a higher incidence of significant multi-vessel coronary obstruction in older patients [4]. However, MDPIT investigators could not find an indication of this in a higher incidence of reinfarction [5]. Hence at this time, mechanisms underlying the effect of age on mortality remain only speculative.

The impact of *sex* on both in-hospital and long-term prognosis following acute myocardial infarction has long been debated. In some epidemiological studies and recent large multi-centre trials the in-hospital crude mortality rates for females exceeded those for males [6,7]. However it is controversial whether this sex-related excess of mortality may be entirely explained by differences in known risk factors for subsequent mortality.

With respect to long-term outcome after hospital discharge, only two studies have so far indicated female sex as an independent risk factor for mortality [8,9], whereas other studies have found an equivalent [10] or even better prognosis [11] in women.

Electrocardiographic variables

It is well known that patients with *anterior myocardial infarction* have a more complicated course during index hospitalization, lower mean values for left ventricular ejection fraction and higher post-hospital mortality rates in comparison with those with inferior or inferior-posterior infarction. The poorer outcome of anterior infarct might result either from a larger amount of myocardial necrosis [12] or a greater propensity to acute regional dilatation and thinning of the infarct zone, which would set the stage for post-acute progressive ventricular remodelling, despite an initial similar loss of myocardium [13]. However, the latter hypothesis is not supported by a recent study in which anterior infarct location was not found to be an independent mortality risk predictor [14].

A number of studies have shown a less favourable post-hospital outcome with respect to survival for patients with non-Q-wave than for those with Q-wave infarction [15]. This excess has been ascribed to a relatively high propensity to recurrent myocardial ischaemia and infarction following hospital discharge. However, according to the findings of recent databases [13,14] and a review of 18 studies [16], long-term survival seems comparable for both types of myocardial infarction. Moreover, survivors of a non-Q-wave infarction are known to exhibit prognostic heterogeneity with high- and low-risk subsets. Elderly patients [17] and patients with ST-segment depression, particularly when persistent on serial ECGs obtained during the index hospitalization [18], have been shown to represent high-risk subsets.

Recurrent myocardial ischaemia

From recent studies it can be estimated that *early post-infarction angina* occurs in one-third of survivors of myocardial infarction and that half of them have concomitant changes on electrocardiogram (Table 1) [19–24]. Contrary to expectations, GISSI-2 findings suggest a reduced frequency of this complication in patients given a thrombolytic drug in the acute phase [25]. In some studies, electrocardiographic evidence of ischaemia (i.e. transient ST-T changes) was related to a greater extent of myocardium at jeopardy, a higher frequency of multi-vessel coronary artery disease [22] and a poorer long-term prognosis [26]. However, it is worth recalling that in the MPIP study [23], only the rare occurrence of high-frequency anginal episodes was a predictor of mortality and in GISSI-2 only very early angina was predictive of subsequent coronary events [27]. Accordingly, the widely held view that the occurrence of angina early in the course of myocardial infarction would establish the need for urgent coronary angiography irrespective of the clinical context and the severity of recurrent ischaemia, should be carefully reviewed and specifically addressed in appropriate studies.

Traditionally, *exercise testing* (ET) has been the most popular method of predicting the risk of subsequent cardiac events after AMI. However, in a recent survey article of 24 studies with a total of more than 5300 patients who underwent either a pre-discharge (sub-maximal) or a post-discharge (maximal) exercise test, the limits of the prognostic information carried by the test have been pointed out (28). Only an inadequate blood pressure response and a low exercise capacity appeared to identify a high-risk group, and in most studies the highest mortality rates were found in patients excluded from exercise testing. Moreover, only in the subset of patients with inferior-posterior AMI were exercise-induced ST-segment shifts of prognostic relevance. These findings, however, can hardly be generalized, as they refer to highly selected samples of patients and no firm conclusions can be drawn with respect to the independent prognostic significance of exercise test variables.

Table 1
Incidence of early post-infarction angina

Authors	Year	No.of patients	Incidence % (*n*)	Incidence with ST-T changes, % (*n*)
Chaturvedi *et al.* [19]	1974	275	12.0	—
Schuster and Bulkley [20]	1981	400	—	17.5 (70)
Fioretti *et al.* [21]	1986	616	21.0 (132)	13.0 (82)
Bosch *et al.* [22]	1987	449	36.5 (164)	18.0 (79)
Benhorin *et al.* [23]	1988	867	33.0 (286)	—
Ross *et al.* [24]	1989	1848	16.6 (307)	—
GISSI-2 [25]	1990	12,381	—	9.6(1.195)

A negative exercise test is believed to represent a reasonably reliable predictor of good outcome [29], though in high-risk patients outcome has been reported to be still poor even if the exercise test is negative [30]. The low predictive value of exercise test markers of ischaemia not including a workload criterion was confirmed in large studies carried out before and after the advent of thrombolysis [23,29,31].

Cardiac *imaging techniques* and ET-independent stress testing procedures have been proposed as more accurate risk stratifiers. The sensitivity, specificity and predictive accuracy of exercise thallium scintigraphy in the detection of multi-vessel coronary artery disease after AMI are increased 8, 18 and 15%, respectively, compared with exercise testing alone [32]. As far as the prognostic value of thallium imaging after AMI is concerned, multiple coronary vascular territory defects, non-infarct zone perfusion defects, transient defects or lung uptake of isotope (indicating pulmonary congestion) have been reported as independent predictors of cardiac events. The few studies to investigate the relative prognostic merits of thallium scintigraphy and conventional exercise testing have shown a higher sensitivity and predictive accuracy, despite a lower specificity, for thallium imaging [32].

Recently, *stress echocardiography*, particularly dipyridamole echocardiographic testing, has gained wide attention as an alternative test to nuclear imaging techniques to stratify risk after AMI. According to recent studies, echocardiographic monitoring during dipyridamole infusion would be more sensitive and specific for ischaemia detection than exercise-related ST-segment changes [31,33] and would allow a quantitative analysis and location of ischaemic myocardium [33].

Table 2 reports the findings of a number of studies addressing the issue of the prognostic significance of *coronary angiographic anatomy* [33–39]. No uniform conclusion can be drawn as regards both the morphology and the severity of coronary stenoses which appear to be elusive predictors of coronary events. In this respect, it is worth recalling that even angiographically minor coronary lesions may subsequently become the site of an occlusive coronary thrombus, and current diagnostic schemes are not reliable in predicting the occurrence and timing of plaque rupture or fissuring and thrombosis.

Left ventricular function

A growing body of evidence indicates that at least two independent indicators of the extent of post-infarction myocardial damage should be taken into account in predicting long-term survival, namely clinical or radiographic evidence of early left ventricular (LV) failure and an objective measure of LV function, obtained near hospital discharge [40].

Despite much investigation, there is still debate regarding the independent prognostic significance of *early left ventricular failure*. This complication might result from the concomitant presence of both an ischaemia-dependent reversible

Table 2

Prognostic significance of coronary angiography after AMI

Authors	No. of patients	Sex	Multivariate analysis	Estimated variables: No. of diseased vessels	Estimated variables: Extent of myocardium at jeopardy	Estimated variables: Severity of coronary stenosis	Impact on survival of tested var.	Follow-up (years)	CAGB (% pts)
Sanz *et al.* [34]	259	Males only	+	+	–	–	+	3	—
DeFeyter *et al.* [35]	179	10% female	–	+	–	–	+	2	13
Roubin *et al.* [36]	229	15% female	–	+	–	–	+	2	10
Taylor *et al.* [37]	106	26% female	+	+	–	–	–	3	18
Schulman *et al.* [38]	143	ns	+	+	+[c]	–	+	5	17
White *et al.* [39]	605	Males only	+	+	+[d]	+	–	6	32
Simoons *et al.* [40]	422	ns	+	+	–	+	+	3–7	35[a] 27[b]

[a] Thrombolysed patients; [b] non-thrombolysed patients; [c] risk segment = variable considered; [d] occlusion and stenosis score = variable considered; ns, not specified.

left ventricular dysfunction and permanent damage from infarcted myocardium [42], or alternatively reflect both acute systolic and diastolic ventricular dysfunction [41,43]. Whatever the responsible mechanism for pulmonary congestion following AMI may be, it should be emphasized that this indicator increases the mortality risk almost eight times, when it is associated with a depressed pre-discharge left ventricular ejection fraction [42].

In several post-myocardial infarction studies, radionuclide or contrast angiography *left ventricular ejection fraction* (LVEF) consistently emerged as a powerful predictor of survival. An inverse curvilinear relationship between resting LVEF and 1-year mortality has repeatedly been shown [42,44,45]. The mechanism that leads to a poor prognosis once LVEF falls is not unique. Both sudden death and pump failure death are common terminal events.

Volume enlargement following AMI has also been shown to be a powerful predictor of reduced survival. In one study [39], angiographic *end-systolic volume* was shown to be the most accurate indicator of the extent of left ventricular damage and the strongest predictor of long-term outcome in male survivors of infarction when LVEF fell below 0.50.

Electrical instability

Frequent and repetitive *ventricular arrhythmias* (VAs) are commonly observed after AMI. In the last 10 years several large clinical and epidemiological studies have allowed a more accurate definition of their prevalence by Holter monitoring. Table 3 sets out a summary of the findings of the most important studies [46–50].

The MILIS [47], MPIP [48] and BHAT [46] studies in the pre-thrombolytic era and GISSI-2 [50] in patients treated with thrombolytic drugs have shown the independent prognostic significance of VAs. However, it must be emphasized that in patients recovering from AMI, the sensitivity and predictive value

Table 3
A summary of findings of the most important studies on ventricular arrhythmias

		Ventricular arrhythmias				
Study	No. of patients	≥ 1/h	>10/h	Complex	NSVT[a]	Recording time (days)[b]
BHAT [46]	1640	84%	13%	20%	—	2–21
MILIS [47]	533	86%	15%	26%	—	10
MPIP [48]	819	86%	21%	28%	11%	—
CAMIAT [49]	649	80%	19%	21%	8%	6–36
GISSI 2 [50]	8676	64%	20%	33%	7%	6–36

[a] NSVT, non-sustained ventricular tachycardia; [b] recording time = Holter timing after AMI.

of VAs are low. Indeed, more than half of all patients who die from sudden death have less than 10 PVCs/h, and only about 10% of all patients with 10 PVCs/h or more will die suddenly within 1–2 years [51]. Thus VAs cannot be used alone as a risk stratifier after AMI and the role of Holter monitoring in uncomplicated patients has been challenged.

Low amplitude *late potentials* in the terminal QRS complex are considered markers for an arrhythmogenic substrate. Their prevalence in healing MI has been reported to vary from 26 to 45% [51]. Lower figures have been reported after successful early reperfusion with thrombolytic agents [52]. In AMI survivors, late potentials have been shown to be independent predictors of both spontaneous and electrically induced ventricular tachycardia and to be also associated with subsequent sudden death events, despite their low positive predictive value [53,54]. The screening for detection of late potentials may be useful for the identification of patients at low risk of spontaneous arrhythmic events, as absence of late potentials has a very high predictive value for uneventful follow-up.

Both experimental [55] and clinical [56] findings suggest that *depressed baroreflex* sensitivity, a marker of depressed vagal reflexes, is associated with a higher risk of developing potentially fatal arrhythmias or sudden death after MI. In a large sample of post-MI patients enrolled in the MPIP, it was also shown that another index of vagal-sympathetic balance, *heart rate variability*, was correlated with mortality [57]. Specifically, either standard deviation of R-R intervals, a global measure of all-source heart rate variability or the prevalence of low-frequency components (mainly sympathetic-dependent) in the power spectral pattern of heart rate variability are strongly associated with death during follow-up after MI [58].

In an attempt to further refine the methods that identify patients at high risk of sudden death, *programmed ventricular stimulation* has been proposed and tested. In a recent meta-analysis of 12 reports dealing with patients with non-sustained ventricular tachycardia, sensitivity, specificity, positive and negative predictive accuracy of the test for sudden death or sustained arrhythmic event were 54, 70, 18 and 93%, respectively [59].

Epilogue

Despite the abundance of reports on post-MI prognostic stratification, several practical issues remain unclear or unresolved. There are many reasons for this. First, quite apart from some methodological limitations, current knowledge is largely based on studies carried out during the "pre-revascularization, pre-thrombolitic era" [28]. Thus it would be essential to know whether available information and proposed prognostic criteria are still applicable in an era in which patients are being treated with thrombolitic drugs as well as aspirin and beta-blockers during the acute phase of MI. Secondly, the patient populations we are dealing with are likely not to be comparable in terms of treatment strategies and more specifically of the incidence rates of revascularization procedures.

Thirdly, as Kotler and Diamond [32] have pointed out, available studies frequently focused on the discriminant accuracy of a test in isolation rather than on its incremental discriminant accuracy (that is, the marginal improvement in predictive accuracy the test can provide). Further, while a single variable may be a weak predictor, clusters of variables may have a much stronger predictive power. For instance, late potentials, complex premature beats and reduced heart rate variability may be markers of different components of the risk of electrical instability (substrate, trigger and "environment", respectively). In isolation, their predictive accuracy is low; together they represent a strong predictor, which increases in power if ventricular function is also taken into account.

Fourthly, it is now clear that there are several subsets of post-MI patients at very different risk of death or infarct recurrence and several simple historical, clinical and instrumental findings can help in a patient's stratification. The recognition of the need for further stratification, selection of the most appropriate tests and validation of their impact on medical decision making and patient outcome are important future goals. For instance, individuals recovering from an infarction treated with thrombolysis make up a growing subset of patients. Thrombolysis increases the patency of infarct-related coronary vessels, making, for this specific aspect, the coronary pattern somewhat different from that found in patients who have not undergone thrombolysis. An immediate effect is a slightly increased risk of early reinfarction, but this seems ruled out simply by the systematic administration of aspirin [7]. There are no other reasons to consider differently those patients treated and those not treated by thrombolitic drugs with respect to prognostic assessment. Thus, we do not consider thrombolytic treatment *per se* as an indication for specific risk stratification or therapeutic strategies and, specifically, for coronary angiography. Admittedly, there remain a number of unresolved pathophysiological issues.

As stressed in the Introduction, the prediction of the evolution of the coronary artery lesions (i.e. their growth, diffusion or instability) is obviously crucial but unfortunately almost impossible. Until we are able to develop reliable paradigms for predicting the progression (or regression) of coronary artery disease, our prognostic skills will remain dangerously approximate, at least in patients who are not severely ill.

More data are also needed to establish the prognostic significance of different degrees of myocardial jeopardy (inducible ischaemia in myocardial regions with preserved wall motion, stunned myocardium, hybernated myocardium) and whether the sensitive tests now available (high-dose dipyridamole, adenosine, re-injection imaging) can provide more accurate prediction of new cardiac events.

The dilatation and distortion of the left ventricle that may occur as a consequence of myocardial infarction is associated with increased adverse cardiovascular events. Infarct expansion is an early phase of a more global process of ventricular remodelling which can progress for months or years before that deterioration in cardiac performance precipitates clinical events. We need more detailed information about this process in order to predict its subsequent evolution soon after AMI and to plan preventive strategies.

Finally, we desperately need data from large randomized trials comparing the relative value of revascularization with the presently available medical therapy in mildly symptomatic or asymptomatic post-MI patients with myocardium at jeopardy. Without such up-to-date therapeutic data, prognostic stratification may ultimately prove to be meaningless for many patients.

References

1. Peel AAF, Semple T, Wang I *et al.* A coronary prognostic index for grading the severity of infarction. *Br Heart J* 1962; **4:** 745–760.
2. Norris RM, Gaughey DE, Deeming LW *et al.* Coronary prognostic index for predicting survival after recovery from acute myocardial infarction. *Lancet* 1970; **ii:** 485–487.
3. Rich MW, Bosner M, Chung MK. Is age an independent predictor of early and late mortality in patients with acute myocardial infarction? *Am J Med* 1992; **92:** 7–13.
4. Tofler GH, Muller JE, Stone PH *et al.* Factors leading to shorter survival after acute myocardial infarction in patients aged 65 to 75 years compared with younger patients. *Am J Cardiol* 1988; **62:** 860–867.
5. Markus FI, Friday K, McCans J *et al.* Age-related prognosis after acute myocardial infarction (the Multicenter Diltiazem Postinfarction Trial). *Am J Cardiol* 1990; **65:** 559–566.
6. Cairns JA, Singer J, Gent M *et al.*. One year mortality outcomes of all coronary and intensive care unit patients with acute myocardial infarction, unstable angina or other chest pain in Hamilton, Ontario, a city of 375,000 people. *Can J Cardiol* 1989; **5:** 239–246.
7. Gruppo Italiano per lo Studio della Streptochinasi nell' Infarto Miocardico Acuto (GISSI). Effectiveness of intravenous thrombolytic treatment in acute myocardial infarction. *Lancet* 1986; **i:** 397–402.
8. Tofler GH, Stone PH, Muller JE *et al.* Effects of gender and race on prognosis after myocardial infarction: Adverse prognosis for women, particularly black women. *J Am Coll Cardiol* 1987; **9:** 473–482.
9. Greenland P, Reicher-Reiss H, Goldbourt U, *et al.* In-hospital and 1-year mortality in 1524 women after myocardial infarction. *Circulation* 1991; **83:** 484–491.
10. Fiebach NH, Viscoli CM, Horwitz R, *et al.* Differences between women and men in survival after myocardial infarction. *JAMA* 1990; **263:** 1092–1096.
11. Wong ND, Cupples LA, Ostfeld AM *et al.* Risk factors for long-term coronary prognosis after initial myocardial infarction: The Framingham study. *Am J Epidemiol* 1989; **130:** 469–480.
12. Geltman EM, Ehsani AA, Campbell MK *et al.* The influence of location and extent of myocardial infarction on long-term ventricular dysrhythmia and mortality. *Circulation* 1979; **60:** 805–814.
13. Stone PH, Raabe DS, Jaffe AS *et al.* Prognostic significance of location and type of myocardial infarction: Independent adverse outcome associated with anterior location. *J Am Coll Cardiol* 1988; **11:** 453–463.

14. Benhorin J, Moss AJ, Oakes D *et al.* The prognostic significance of first myocardial infarction type (Q-wave *vs* non Q-wave) and Q wave location. *J Am Coll Cardiol* 1990; **15:** 1201–1207.
15. Gibson RS. Non-Q wave myocardial infarction: Pathophysiology, prognosis and therapeutic strategy. *Ann Rev Med* 1989; **40:** 395–410.
16. Edlavitch SA, Crow R, Burke GL *et al.* Secular trends in Q-wave and non-Q wave acute myocardial infarction: The Minnesota Heart Survey. *Circulation* 1991; **83:** 492–503 .
17. Nicod P, Gilpin E, Dittrich H *et al.* Short- and long-term clinical outcome after Q-wave and non-Q wave myocardial infarction in a large patient population. *Circulation* 1989; **79:** 528–536.
18. Schechtman K, Capone JR, Kleiger RE *et al.* Risk stratification of patients with non-Q wave myocardial infarction: The critical role of ST segment depression. *Circulation* 1989; **80:** 1148–1158.
19. Chaturvedi NC, Walsh MJ, Evans A *et al.* Selection of patients for early discharge after acute myocardial infarction. *Br Heart J* 1974; **36:** 533–535.
20. Schuster EH, Bulkley BH. Early post-infarction angina: Ischemia at a distance and ischemia in the infarct zone. *N Engl J Med* 1981; **305:** 1101–1105.
21. Fioretti P, Brower RA, Balakumaran K. Early post-infarction angina. Incidence and prognostic relevance. *Eur Heart J* 1986; **7:** 73–77.
22. Bosch X, Theroux P, Waters DD *et al.* Early postinfarction ischemia: Clinical, angiographic, and prognostic significance. *Circulation* 1987; **75:** 988–995.
23. Benhorin J, Andrews LA, Moss AJ. Occurrence, characteristics and prognostic significance of early postacute myocardial infarction angina pectoris. *Am J Cardiol* 1988; **62:** 679–685.
24. Ross J, Gilpin EA, Erling B *et al.* A decision scheme for coronary angiography after acute myocardial infarction. *Circulation* 1989; **79:** 292–303.
25. GISSI 2 Study. A factorial randomised trial of alteplase versus streptokinase and heparin versus no heparin among 12,490 patients with acute myocardial infarction. *Lancet* 1990; **336:** 65–71.
26. Bosch X, Theroux P, Guy B *et al.* Clinical and angiographic features and prognostic significance of early postinfarction angina with and without electrocardiographic signs of transient ischemia. *Am J Med* 1991; **91:** 493–501.
27. The GISSI 2 IRES Group. Prognostic significance of early postinfarction ischemia. *J Am Coll Cardiol (Abstr.)* 1991; **2:** 231A.
28. Froelicher VF, Perdue S, Pewen W *et al.* Application of meta-analysis using an electronic spread sheet to exercise testing in patients after myocardial infarction. *Am J Med* 1987; **83:** 1045–1054.
29. Chaitman BR, Younis LT Shaw LS *et al.* Exercise ECG test results in the TIMI 2 trial. *J Am Coll Cardiol* 1990; **15:** 251A.
30. Krone RJ. The role of risk stratification in the early management of a myocardial infarction. *Ann Intern Med* 1992; **116:** 223–237.
31. Bolognese L, Sarasso G, Aralda D *et al.* High dose dipyridamole echocardiography early after uncomplicated acute myocardial infarction: Correlation with exercise testing and coronary angiography. *J Am Coll Cardiol* 1989; **14:** 357–363.
32. Kotler TS, Diamond GA. Exercise thallium- 201 scintigraphy in the diagnosis and prognosis of coronary artery disease. *Ann Intern Med* 1990; **113:** 684–702.
33. Picano E, Simonetti I, Masini M *et al.* Transient myocardial dysfunction during pharmacologic vasodilatation as an index of reduced coronary reserve: A coronary hemodynamic and echacardiographic study. *J Am Coll Cardiol* 1986; **8:** 84–90.
34. Sanz G, Castaner A, Betriu A *et al.* Determinants of prognosis in survivors of myocardial infarction: A prospective clinical angiographic study. *N Engl J Med* 1982; **307:** 306–310.

35. DeFeyter PJ, VanEenige MJ, Dighton DH *et al.* Prognostic value of exercise testing coronary angiography and left ventriculography 6–8 weeks after myocardial infarction. *Circulation* 1982: **65:** 527–532.
36. Roubin GS, Harriz PJ, Bernstein L *et al.* Coronary anatomy and prognosis after myocardial infarction in patients 60 years of age and younger. *Circulation* 1984; **67:** 743–745.
37. Taylor GJ, Humphries J, Mellits ED *et al.* Predictors of clinical course, coronary anatomy and left ventricular function after recovery from acute myocardial infarction. *Circulation* 1980; **62:** 960–970.
38. Schulman SP, Achuff SC, Griffith LS *et al.* Prognostic cardiac catheterization variables in survivors of acute myocardial infarction: A five year prospective study. *J Am Coll Cardiol* 1988; **11:** 1164–1172.
39. White HD, Norris RM, Brown M *et al.* Left ventricular end-systolic volume as the major determinant of survival after recovery from myocardial infarction. *Circulation* 1987; **76:** 44–51.
40. Simoons ML, Vos J, Tijssen JG *et al.* Long-term benefit of early thrombolytic therapy in patients with acute myocardial infarction: 5 year follow-up of a trial conducted by the Interuniversity Cardiology Institute of the Netherlands. *J Am Coll Cardiol* 1989; **141:** 609–615.
41. Gottlieb S, Moss AJ, McDermott M *et al.* Interrelation of left ventricular ejection fraction, pulmonary congestion and outcome in acute myocardial infarction. *Am J Cardiol* 1992; **69:** 977–984.
42. The Multicenter Postinfarction Research Group. Risk stratification and survival after myocardial infarction. *N Engl J Med* 1983; **309:** 331–336.
43. Nicod P, Gilpin E, Dittrich H *et al.* Influence of prognosis and morbidity of left ventricular ejection fraction with and without signs of left ventricular failure after acute myocardial infarction. *Am J Cardiol* 1988; **61:** 1165–1171.
44. Gadsboll N, Hoilund-Charlsen PF, Marving J *et al.* Right and left ventricular ejection fraction: Relation to one-year prognosis in acute myocardial infarction. *Eur Heart J* 1987; **8:** 1201–1209.
45. Serruys PW, Simoons ML, Suryapranata H *et al.* Preservation of global and regional left ventricular function after early thrombolysis in acute myocardial infarction. *Am J Cardiol* 1986; **7:** 729–742.
46. Kostis JB, Friedman LM, Goldstein LM *et al.* Prognostic significance of ventricular ectopic activity in survivors of acute myocardial infarction. *J Am Coll Cardiol* 1987; **10:** 231–242.
47. MILIS Study Group. Risk factors for sudden death after acute myocardial infarction: Two year follow-up. *Am J Cardiol* 1984; **54:** 31–36.
48. Bigger JT, Fleiss JL, Kleiger R *et al.* The relationship among ventricular arrhythmias, left ventricular dysfunction and mortality in the 2 years myocardial infarction. *Circulation* 1984; **69:** 250–258.
49. Connolly SJ, Cairns JA. Prevalence and predictors of ventricular premature complexes in survivors of acute myocardial infarction. *Am J Cardiol* 1992; **69:** 408–412.
50. Maggioni A, Zuanetti G, Santoro E *et al.* Prevalence and prognostic significance of ventricular arrhythmias in 8676 patients treated with fibrinolytic agents after myocardial infarction in the GISSI 2 trial. *Circulation* (Abstr.) 1991; **84:** II-349.
51. Win-Kuang Shen, Hammill SC. Survivors of acute myocardial infarction: who is at risk for sudden cardiac death? *Mayo Clin Proc* 1991; **66:** 950–962.
52. Gang ES, Lew AS, Hong M *et al.* Decreased incidence of ventricular late potentials after successful thrombolytic therapy for acute myocardial infarction. *N Engl J Med 1*989; **321:** 712–716.
53. Breithardt G, Borggrefe M. Recent advances in the identification of patients at risk of ventricular tachyarrhythmias: role of ventricular late potentials. *Circulation* 1987; **75:** 1091–1096.

54. Middlekauff HR, Stevenson AG, Tillisch J. Prevention of sudden death in survivors of myocardial infarction: A decision analysis approach. *Am Heart J* 1992; **123:** 475–480.
55. Schwartz PJ, Vanole E, Stramba-Badiale M *et al.* Autonomic mechanisms and sudden death: New insights from the analysis of baroreceptor reflexes in conscious dogs with and without a myocardial infarction. *Circulation* 1988; **78:** 969–979.
56. La Rovere MT, Specchia G, Mortara A *et al.* Baroreflex sensitivity, clinical correlates and cardiovascular mortality among patients with a first myocardial infarction: a prospective study. *Circulation* 1988; **78:** 816–824.
57. Kleiger RE, Miller JP, Bigger JT Jr, and the Multicenter Post-Infarction Research Group. Heart rate variability: A predictor of mortality following acute myocardial infarction. *Am J Cardiol* 1987; **59:** 256–262.
58. Bigger JT Jr, Fleiss JC, Steinman RC *et al.* Frequency domain measures of heart period variability and mortality after myocardial infarction. *Circulation* 1992; **85:** 164–171.
59. Kowey PR, Taylor JE, Marinchak RA *et al.* Programmed stimulation does really help in the evaluation of patients with non sustained ventricular tachycardia? A result of a meta-analysis. *Am Heart J* 1992; **123:** 481.

II Viability of Myocardium

8 Study of Myocardial Viability with Thallium-201 and New Tracers Labelled with 99m Technetium

Alain Bertrand, Pierre Y. Marie

Service de Médecine Nucléaire, Hopital de Brabois, Rue du Morvan, 54500 Vandoeuvre-les-Nancy, France

Introduction

Though the first studies of myocardial perfusion using thallium-201 only date back to 1975, 1.5 million myocardial scintigraphies with thallium-201 were carried out in the USA in 1990. This reflects the growing place of nuclear cardiology in the daily management of patients with coronary artery disease. Indeed, scintigraphic or tomoscintigraphic studies of myocardial perfusion and, more recently, of myocardial metabolism have been increasingly developed in recent years. This may be related to methodological and technical progress, to the discovery of new molecules such as those labelled with 99m technetium and, moreover, to the demonstration of the importance of these techniques for the management of cardiac patients.

Today, the principal clinical signs are: (1) the detection of coronary artery disease, (2) prognostic information concerning the extent and severity of stress ischaemia and (3) monitoring of patients after the establishment of a treatment (detection of coronary bypass dysfunction after surgery, detection of restenosis after angioplasty, etc.). Myocardial scintigraphic studies have also proven useful in the management of patients showing left ventricular dysfunction. This is as a consequence of the ability of these techniques to distinguish viable from non-viable myocardium.

Indeed, left ventricular (LV) dysfunction in patients with coronary artery disease does not always correspond to total myocardial destruction such as

Proceedings of the Vth World Congress on Cardiac Rehabilitation

necrosis or fibrosis. In many cases, depressed LV function may be at least partly due to "hibernating myocardium", which resolves after coronary revascularization [1]. Precise identification of those patients in whom coronary revascularization would lower LV dysfunction is particularly warranted, since in patients with coronary artery disease, the severity of LV dysfunction remains a strong predictor of cardiac mortality [2, 3].

The assessment of myocardial viability using radionuclide techniques

A worse prognosis accompanies LV dysfunction in patients with coronary artery disease [2, 3], but coronary revascularization may improve cardiac contractility in a number of cases [4]. However, revascularization procedures such as coronary angioplasty or especially surgical bypass grafting remain a major risk for patients with LV dysfunction. That is why many efforts have been made in recent years to identify subsets of patients in whom LV performance could be enhanced by coronary revascularization.

Two pathophysiological situations may lead to viable but dysfunctional myocardium. *Stunned myocardium*, which is due to an acute ischaemia followed by reperfusion, is frequently observed after successful thrombolytic therapy of a myocardial infarction. Its mechanism remains poorly understood [5], but its main characteristics are that no ischaemia persists and that myocardial contractility returns spontaneously to normal after a delay that does not generally exceed 10 days [1]. By contrast, *hibernating myocardium* is a myocardial dysfunction due to a persisting chronic ischaemia. This corresponds to a mechanism of self-protection of the myocardium, which only performs work according to the amount of energy it receives: "little blood, little work" [6]. In contrast to stunned myocardium, hibernating myocardium represents a pathophysiological situation which is particularly useful to identify, since only by performing a coronary revascularization (angioplasty or bypass grafting) will myocardial contractility be restored.

In nuclear cardiology, several techniques may be used to differentiate between viable and non-viable myocardial segments. Like other methods of assessing LV function (echocardiography, magnetic resonance imaging, X-ray angiography), first-pass or equilibrium angioscintigraphy are of little interest in this setting; and this is despite the vast amount of prognostic information obtained with these techniques in patients with LV dysfunction [7, 8]. However, the assessment of myocardial viability using radionuclide ventriculography may be enhanced in certain conditions, such as during isoproterenol infusion [9] or in the post-exercise period [10]. Nevertheless, nuclear cardiology allow us to analyse the myocardial uptake of metabolic or perfusion myocardial markers, and this allows direct evaluation of myocardial viability, independent of function. A number of these markers require the use of expensive equipment for positron emission tomography. However, some of them, such as thallium-

Table 1
Characteristics of thallium-201, ^{99m}Tc-sestamibi and ^{99m}Tc-teboroxime

	^{201}Tl	^{99m}Tc-sestamibi	^{99m}Tc-teboroxime
Charge	Cation	Cation	Neutral
Clearance time	Intermediate	Prolonged	Rapid
Redistribution	Yes	Minimal	—
Begin imaging	5 min	1 h	1 min
Complete rest-stress	4 h	4 h	1.5 h
SPECT	Good	Good	Difficult
First-pass study	No	Yes	Yes

201 or ^{99m}Tc-sestamibi (Cardiolite*), are routinely available, since they only require the use of a classical gamma-camera.

Of the cardiac scintigraphic tracers, thallium-201 remains the most popular. Its uptake by myocardial cells is greatly dependent on the mechanisms of active transport (Na/K ATPase), which require the presence of an intact sarcolemma [11]. These properties explain the efficiency of thallium-201 in the assessment of myocardial viability. However, some experimental studies have shown that thallium-201 uptake is too dependent on blood flow to be a perfect marker of cell viability [12]. In addition, because of its low photon energy, thallium-201 is not an ideal agent for myocardial scintigraphic or tomoscintigraphic imaging in man. This limitation has led to the synthesis of perfusion markers labelled with technetium (^{99m}Tc).

Like thallium-201, ^{99m}Tc-sestamibi and ^{99m}Tc-teboroxime are blood flow tracers whose myocardial uptake depends predominantly on regional flow distribution. Concerning the detection of myocardial viability, a substantial body of data has been published on ^{99m}Tc-sestamibi (Cardiolite). One of the main properties of ^{99m}Tc-sestamibi is its long myocardial residence time, which allows one to perform image acquisition several hours after the intravenous injection [13]. The mechanism of ^{99m}Tc-sestamibi uptake involves passive distribution across the plasma and mitochondrial membranes, so that at equilibrium this agent is sequestered within the mitochondria by the large negative transmembrane potential [14]. Like thallium-201, the uptake of ^{99m}Tc-sestamibi is dependent on cell viability and on the integrity of the sarcolemma; however, to a lesser extent, it is also dependent on aerobic metabolism [15]. However, ^{99m}Tc-sestamibi does not possess the properties of an ideal marker of viability. This is mainly because its uptake is greatly dependent on blood flow, and this could constitute an important limitation for the identification of viability in the case of severe ischaemia [16].

Routine assessment of myocardial viability using thallium-201

Initially, the presence on thallium-201 (tomo)scintigraphy of a myocardial stress defect which persisted on redistribution imaging performed 3–4 h later, was considered to be indicative of irreversible damage. However, several reports have demonstrated that those irreversible defects were in fact frequently viable, as evidenced by the presence of glucose analogue uptake (as assessed by PET [17]) or by the normalization of thallium-201 uptake after coronary revascularization (bypass grafting or angioplasty [11]). Secondly, it has been established that late imaging at 12–48 h (late redistribution) might demonstrate a significant redistribution in many defects that were identified as irreversibly damaged after only 3–4 h of redistribution [18]. And, more recently, several studies have pointed to the usefulness of performing – after 3–4 h redistribution imaging – a new acquisition 10 min after rest-reinjection of 1 mCi of thallium-201. In such conditions, 30–49% of irreversible defects after 3–4 h redistribution demonstrate normal or at least improved thallium activity after rest-reinjection [11, 19].

Today, the analysis of thallium uptake after 3–4 h redistribution and rest-reinjection scans constitutes the reference method for the assessment of myocardial viability using thallium-201. This is the consequence of the results of several studies, which have shown a good correlation between this technique and the assessment of viability using the reference metabolic markers of PET [17] and, moreover, the satisfactory predictive value of the thallium-201 reinjection method with regard to improvements in wall motion abnormalities after coronary revascularization [11, 19]. However, it must be pointed out that, though rest-reinjection imaging allows us to identify more viable segments than early redistribution scans, the sole analysis of rest-reinjection leads us to underestimate the amount of viability. Indeed, about 10% of thallium stress defects exhibit increased uptake on early or late redistribution scans but not after reinjection [11]. That is why the most accurate method for assessing myocardial viability with thallium consists of a combination of rest-reinjection imaging with early (3–4 h) or late (20–48 h) redistribution imaging.

Routine assessment of myocardial viability using ^{99m}Tc-sestamibi

Less data are available concerning the assessment of myocardial viability with ^{99m}Tc-sestamibi. However, recent studies have shown that ^{99m}Tc-sestamibi is an accurate marker of viability in the case of stunning myocardium. This is illustrated by the good predictive value of the extent of the myocardial defect, assessed early after fibrinolytic therapy of myocardial infarction using ^{99m}Tc-sestamibi, on the spontaneous evolution of LV function [16]. In this case, no ischaemia persists and LV dysfunction resolves partly or totally spontaneously. However, in the case of hibernating myocardium, where a chronic hypoperfusion persists, some data strongly suggest that ^{99m}Tc-sestamibi is less efficient at assessing viability [16]. In this setting, some studies [20, 21] have clearly shown that a number of myocardial segments, without significant uptake of rest-injected ^{99m}Tc-sestamibi, were still identified as being viable with thallium-201 using the rest-reinjection technique. This lower efficiency of ^{99m}Tc-sestamibi in the case of chronic hypoperfusion could be secondary to the strong flow dependence of its myocardial uptake [16]. However, this apparent under-estimation of viability using ^{99m}Tc-sestamibi with regard to thallium-201, implies that all ^{99}mTc-sestamibi irreversible defects showing thallium uptake are actually viable. In fact, this can only be established with studies that compare the respective values of those tracers in the prediction of post-revascularization improvements in LV function. Such studies have not been carried out to date.

References

1. Schaper W. Adaptation to and defense against myocardial ischemia. *Cardiology* 1990; **70:** 367–372.
2. Mock MB, Riingqvist I, Fischer LD. Survival of medically treated patients in the coronary artery surgery study (CASS) registery. *Circulation* 1982; **66:** 562–568.
3. The Multicenter Postinfarction Research Group. Risk stratification and survival after myocardial infarction. *N Eng J Med* 1983; **309:** 331–336.
4. Dilsizian V, Bonow RO, Cannon RO. The effect of coronary artery bypass grafting on left ventricular systolic function at rest: Evidence for preoperative subclinical myocardial ischemia. *Am J Cardiol* 1988; **61:** 1248–1254.
5. Greenfield RA, Swain JL. Disruption of myofibrillar energy use: Dual mechanisms that may contribute to post-ischemic dysfunction in stunned myocardium. *Circ Res* 1987; **60:** 283–289.
6. Reduto LA, Smalling RW, Freund GK, Gould KL. Intracoronary infusion of streptokinase in patients with acute myocardial infarction: Effect of reperfusion on left ventricular performance. *Am J Cardiol* 1981; **48:** 403–409.
7. Hung J, Goris ML, Nash E, Kraemer HC, Debusk RF, Berger WE, Lew H. Comparative value of maximal treadmill testing, exercise thallium myocardial perfusion scintigraphy and exercise radionuclide ventriculography for distinguishing high and low risk patients soon after myocardial infarction. *Am J Cardiol* 1984; **53:** 1221–1227.
8. Morris KG, Palmeri ST, Califf RM. Value of radionuclide angiography for predicting specific cardiac events after acute myocardial infarction. *Am J Cardiol* 1985; **55:** 318.
9. Nesto RW, Cohn LH, Collins JJ, Wynne J, Holman L, Cohn PF. Inotropic contractile reserve, a useful predictor of increased 5 year survival and improved postoperative left ventricular function of patients with coronary artery disease and reduced ejection fraction. *Am J Cardiol* 1982; **50:** 39–44.
10. Rozanski A, Berman D, Gray R. Preoperative prediction of reversible myocardial asynergy by postexercise radionuclide ventriculography. *N Engl J Med* 1982: **307:** 212–216.
11. Bonow RO, Dilsizian V. Thallium 201 for assessment of myocardial viability. *Sem Nucl Med* 1991; **3:** 230–241.

12. Forman R, Kirk ES. Thallium 201 accumulation during reperfusion of ischemic myocardium: dependence on regional blood flow rather than viability. *Am J Cardiol* 1984, **54:** 659–663.
13. Okada RD, Glover DT, Gaffney T, William S. Myocardial kinetics of technetium-99m-hexakis-2-methoxy-2- methylpropyl-isonitrile. *Circulation* 1988; **77:** 491–498.
14. Piwnica-Worms D, Kronauge JF, Chiu ML. Uptake and retention of hexakis (2-methoxyisobutil isonitrile) technetium in cultured chick myocardial cells. *Circulation* 1990; **82:** 1826–1838.
15. Beanlands RSB, Dawood F, Wen-Hu W, McLaughin PR, Butany J, D'Amati G, Liu PP. Are the kinetics of technetium-99m methoxisobutylisonitril affected by cell metabolism and viability? *Circulation* 1990; **82:** 1802–1814.
16. Bonow RO, Dilsizian V. Thallium 201 and technetium 99m SESTAMIBI for assessing viable myocardium. *J Nucl Med* 192; **33:** 815–818.
17. Bonow RO, Dilsizian V, Cuocolo A, Bacharach SL. Identification of viable myocardium in patients with chronic coronary artery disease and left ventricular dysfunction: Comparison of thallium scintigraphy with reinjection and PET imaging with 18F-fluorodeoxyglucose. *Circulation* 1991; **82:** 26–37.
18. Yang LD, Berman DS, Kiat H, Resser KJ, Friedman JD, Rozanski A, Maddahi J. The frequency of late reversibility in SPECT thallium-201 stress redistribution study. *J Am Coll Cardiol* 1990; **15:** 334–340.
19. Dilsizian V, Rocco TP, Freedman NMT, Leon MB, Bonow RO. Enhanced detection of ischemic but viable myocardium by the reinjection of thallium after stress-redistribution imaging. *N Engl J Med* 1990; **323:** 141–146.
20. Cuocolo A, Pace L, Ricciardelli B, Chiariello M, Trimarco B, Salvatore M. Identification of viable myocardium in patients with chronic coronary artery disease: Comparison of thallium-201 scintigraphy with reinjection and technetium-99m methoxyisobutil isonitrile. *J Nucl Med* 1992; **33:** 505–511.
21. Rocco TP, Dilsizian V, Strauss HW, Boucher CA. Technetium-99m isonitril myocardial uptake at rest. II. Relation to clinical markers of potential viability. *J Am Coll Cardiol* 1989; **14:** 1678–1684.

9 Identification of Viable Myocardium After Infarction with Labelled Free Fatty Acids

Pierre-Yves Marie[1,2], Nicolas Danchin*[1], Yves Juillière[1], Gilles Karcher[2], Alain Bertrand[2], François Cherrier[1]

[1] *Department of Cardiology* and
[2] *Department of Nuclear Medicine, CHU Nancy-Brabois, 54500 Vandoeuvre-lès-Nancy, France*

Introduction

The assessment of myocardial viability after acute myocardial infarction remains a challenge. Many efforts have been made in recent years to try and differentiate between hibernating or stunned myocardium and truly necrotic tissue. In clinical practice, such methods as left ventricular angiography or two-dimensional echocardiography after pharmacological tests or after extrasystolic beats are used to detect potentially viable myocardium in an infarcted area [1,2]. Among the radionuclide methods, exercise thallium-201 tomoscintigraphy, particularly when associated with rest-reinjection of thallium-201, can identify a number of patients with residual myocardial viability after acute myocardial infarction. However, because it is largely dependent on coronary blood flow, thallium uptake by myocardial cells cannot constitute an ideal marker of myocardial viability [3]. In contrast, the uptake of free fatty acids, which constitute one of the main substrates of myocardial cell metabolism, is closely dependent on myocardial viability [4]; ischaemic but viable cells show both an increased serum extraction and a slower clearance of certain free fatty acids.

Among free fatty acids, iodine methylhexadecanoic acid (IMHA) can be used in man and permits the use of computed tomography [5]. The purpose of the

*To whom all correspondence should be addressed.

Proceedings of the Vth World Congress on Cardiac Rehabilitation

present study was to compare IMHA rest single photon emission tomography (SPECT) with thallium-201 redistribution followed by rest-reinjection to detect residual myocardial viability after acute myocardial infarction.

Patients and methods

Patients

Sixty patients who had suffered a first episode of acute myocardial infarction and who had undergone subsequent coronary angiography showing a higher than 50% residual stenosis (reduction of intraluminal diameter) on the infarct-related artery, judged suitable for percutaneous transluminal coronary angioplasty (PTCA) or recanalization, were included in the study. They were 52 men and 8 women, with a mean age of 53 $\pm$ 8 years. The infarct was located in the anterior territory in 32 patients (53%); 52 patients had had a Q-wave infarction (87%) and 13% a non-Q-wave infarct evidenced by the association of prolonged chest pain and a rise in cardiac enzymes (CK value higher than twice the upper limit of normal). At the acute stage of myocardial infarction, 31 patients had received thrombolytic therapy (52%). Residual angina was present in 15 patients (25%). On coronary angiography, the infarct-related artery was found patent in 33 patients (55%); 52 (87%) had single-vessel coronary artery disease. The mean left ventricular ejection fraction calculated on the 30° right anterior oblique projection according to the area-length method was 52 $\pm$ 13%.

Radionuclide studies and exercise test protocol

The exercise test and radionuclide protocol was carried out 32 $\pm$ 26 days after the acute episode. The exercise test was performed on a bicycle ergometer, with the patient in the upright position, and with 12-lead ECG monitoring at each minute of exercise and with continuous monitoring of leads V1, V5 and aVF. The protocol began at 40-W and increased by 30-W increments every 3 min. Exercise endpoints were physical exhaustion, development of angina pectoris, sustained ventricular tachyarrhythmia, exertional hypotension or achieving maximal predicted heart rate. The stress ECG was considered positive if there was $>$2 mm ST-segment depression at 0.08 sec after the J point on any of the surface ECG leads.

One minute before the termination of exercise, one mCi of thallium-201 per 25 kg body weight (without exceeding 3 mCi) was injected intravenously. Stress imaging was initiated 10 min later; redistribution studies were made 3–5 hours later and were followed by rest-reinjection imaging 10 min after a second dose of 1 mCi of thallium-201 was reinjected.

Tomographic acquisitions were performed using a rotating gamma camera equipped with a low-energy, high-resolution, parallel hole collimator, interfaced with a computer system (Sopha Medical). A 20% energy window was positioned on the 80 KeV photopeak. In a 180° arc-rotation, from a 30° left posterior oblique to a 60° right anterior oblique projection around the cranio-caudal axis of the patient, 32 projections were obtained for 30 s each and stored in a 64 × 64 matrix. The raw data were smoothed using a 9-point weighted averaging system. Filtered back projection was performed using a Haming-Hann filter. After reconstruction, the data were reorganized to contiguous short axis, vertical long axis and horizontal long axis slices (8 mm thick) encompassing the left ventricle.

Analysis of tomographic scans

Analysis of the reconstructed tomographic slices was performed qualitatively on a 20-segment division of the left ventricle by consensus of two experienced observers who were unaware of the patients' clinical data. A segment was considered to have a stress defect when thallium-201 uptake appeared markedly reduced on the stress scans. Residual myocardial viability of a given segment was considered present if this segment showed a detectable increase of uptake, compared to the stress image, on either thallium-201 redistribution, thallium-201 reinjection or IMHA scans.

Results

Segment analyses

For the 60 patients, 1200 segments were analysed. Among them, 373 exhibited a stress defect on thallium-201 scans. Of these, 103 (28%) were considered viable because of increased uptake at rest.

Residual myocardial viability was identified by thallium-201 redistribution scans in 49 segments (48%) and by thallium redistribution or rest-reinjection in 79 (77%). A significant increase of tracer uptake was observed in 100 segments (99%) using IMHA rest scans. On the whole, as compared to the use of both redistribution and rest-reinjection thallium-201 scans, IMHA permitted the identification of an additional 27% presumably viable segments.

Patient analyses

When considering individual patients, 38 of the 60 patients (63%) had residual myocardial ischaemia, because of the presence of significant tracer uptake at rest on at least one ischaemic stress segment. The residual viability was identified using thallium-201 redistribution in 21 cases (55%), using both thallium-201 redistribution and rest-reinjection in 31 cases (82%) and using IMHA rest scans in 37 cases (97%).

Only 16 patients (27%) had moderate or severe residual ischaemia, defined as the presence of increased tracer uptake on at least three left ventricular segments. In eight of these patients, the extent of residual viability appeared similar on thallium and IMHA scans. In the remaining eight patients, however, thallium scans underestimated the extent of residual viability; in four patients, the extent of residual viability was largely underestimated with 2–4 segments exhibiting increased uptake on IMHA scans not detected by thallium-201 redistribution or rest-reinjection scans.

Discussion

The presence of residual myocardial ischaemia after myocardial infarction is an important prognostic index. Both residual angina or a positive exercise test are strongly related to an adverse prognosis [6,7]. However, neither clinical angina nor ECG positivity during an exercise test can differentiate between myocardial ischaemia caused by coronary stenoses outside the infarct-related area or by persisting myocardial viability in the infarct-related area.

In routine clinical practice, the presence of residual viability in the infarct-related area can be estimated from the extent of left ventricular dyskinesia on left ventricular angiography compared to the location of coronary obstruction on selective coronary arteriography; in addition, in the case of total coronary occlusion, the presence of a well-developed collateral circulation can predict the presence of viable myocardium in the infarct area [8]. However, such estimations are partly subjective; they are, at best, gross indicators of residual viability and they cannot be used to quantify the extent of viable myocardium.

In contrast, exercise thallium-201 computed tomography can predict the location of stress residual ischaemia after myocardial infarction. However, though the presence of rest reversibility in the infarct-related area is considered to represent viable myocardium, non-reversible perfusion defects after exercise may be associated with normalized thallium-201 uptake after successful revascularization [9,10]. Similarly, myocardial viability may be demonstrated by positron emission tomography in myocardial areas showing no reversibility during standard exercise thallium-201 SPECT [11,12]. Therefore, efforts have been made to improve the reliability of thallium-201 exercise SPECT to detect residual myocardial viability, and both late (24 h) redistribution studies and rest-reinjection protocols have been shown to enhance the detection of residual ischaemia in infarct-related areas [13,14]. When comparing rest-reinjection and late redistribution studies, we found that both techniques yielded similar results [15].

The present study confirms that, compared to standard redistribution, rest-reinjection increases the ability of thallium-201 SPECT to detect reversible defects. However, a number of segments showing no reversibility even after rest-reinjection of thallium-201 exhibited definite uptake on IMHA scans. Therefore, IMHA seems to enhance the detection of viable myocardium in the infarct-related artery territory. More importantly still, 25% of patients with a large amount of residual viability were not diagnosed by thallium-201 SPECT with rest-reinjection, while the amount of residual viability was grossly underestimated in another 25% of these patients.

It remains to be demonstrated, however, that myocardial segments which are not reversible on thallium-201 rest-reinjection but which have definite uptake of IMHA are truly viable. In this regard, correlations with the evolution of left ventricular function after myocardial revascularization are needed.

References

1. Pierard LA, De Landsheere CM, Berthe C, Rigo P, Kulbertus HE. Identification of viable myocardium by echocardiography during dobutamine infusion in patients with myocardial infarction after thrombolytic therapy: Comparison with positron emission tomography. *J Am Coll Cardiol* 1990; **15:** 1021–1031.
2. Papio KA, Gorlin R, Bechtel D, Levine JA. Post-extrasystolic potentiation as a predictor of potential myocardial viability: preoperative analyses compared with studies after coronary bypass surgery. *Am J Cardiol* 1977; **39:** 944–953.
3. Chu A, Murdock RM, Cobb FR. Relation between regional distribution of thallium 201 and myocardial blood flow in normal, acutely ischemic, and infarcted myocardium. *Am J Cardiol* 1982; **50:** 1141–1144.
4. Chappuis F, Meier B, Belenger J, Blaunstein P, Lerch R. Early assessment of tissue viability with radioiodinated heptadecanoic acid in reperfused canine myocardium: Comparison with thallium-201. *Am Heart J* 1990; **119:** 833–841.
5. Fagret D, Wolf JE, Borrel E, Rocca C, Machecourt J, Comet M. I-123-BIMHA SPECT detection of viable tissue in myocardial segments with persistent defect at Tl 201 SPECT in patients with a first Q wave myocardial infarction. *Eur J Nucl Med (Abstr.)* 1991; **18:** 645.
6. Théroux P, Waters DD, Halphen C, Debaisieux JC, Mizgala HF. Prognostic value of exercise testing soon after myocardial infarction. *N Engl J Med* 1979; **301:** 341–345 .
7. Moss AJ, Benhorin J. Prognosis and management after a first myocardial infarction. *N Engl J Med* 1990; **322:** 743–753.
8. Fujita M, Ohno A, Wada O, *et al.* Collateral circulation as a marker of the presence of viable myocardium in patients with recent myocardial infarction. *Am Heart J* 1991; **122:** 409–414.
9. Gibson RS, Watson DD, Taylor GJ *et al.* Prospective assessment of regional myocardial perfusion before and after coronary revascularization surgery by quantitative thallium-201 scintigraphy. *J Am Coll Cardiol* 1983; **1:** 804–815.
10. Liu P, Kiess MC, Okada RD, *et al.* The persistent defect on exercise thallium imaging and its fate after myocardial revascularization: Does it represent scar or ischemia ? *Am Heart J* 1985; **110:** 996–1001.
11. Brunken R, Schwaiger M, Grover-McKay M, Phelps ME, Tillisch J, Schelbert HR. Positron emission tomography detects tissue metabolic activity in myocardial segments with persistent thallium perfusion defects. *J Am Coll Cardiol* 1987; **10:** 557–567.
12. Takeishi Y, Tono-oka I, Kubota T *et al.* Functional recovery of hibernating myocardium after coronary bypass surgery: Does it coincide with improvement in perfusion? *Am Heart J* 1991; **122:** 665–670.
13. Kiat H, Berman DS, Maddahi J *et al.* Late reversibility of tomographic myocardial thallium-201 defects: An accurate marker of myocardial reversibility. *J Am Coll Cardiol* 1988; **12:** 1456–1463.

14. Dilsizian V, Rocco TP, Freedman NMT, Leon MB, Bonow RO. Enhanced detection of ischemic but viable myocardium by the reinjection of thallium after stress redistribution imaging. *N Engl J Med* 1990; **323:** 141–146.
15. Marie PY, Danchin N, Karcher G *et al.* Exercise redistribution SPECT Tl-201 after myocardial infarction: Is late redistribution analysis still useful when early rest-reinjection is performed ? *Eur Heart J (Abstr.)* 1991; **12:** 36.

III Exercise Testing

10 Prolongation of Corrected Q Peak T with Exercise Testing Provides Improved Diagnostic Power

M. H. Ellestad, J. A. Queiroz, R. H. Startt-Selvester, A. H. Shandling

Memorial Heart Institute, Long Beach Memorial Medical Center, Long Beach, CA 90801-1428, USA

Introduction

Prolongation of the QT interval has been known to occur with ischaemia for many years [1–3]; however, its use in exercise testing has never been well-accepted because it failed to add significantly to the diagnostic power of the test [4,6]. The overlap of the P- and T-waves with rapid heart rates has created problems in measuring the T duration; therefore, this paper proposes the use of the interval from the onset of the Q-wave to the peak of the T-wave as an index of the QT interval. These measurements and changes in the QPTc from rest to exercise are correlated with coronary angiographic data.

Materials and methods

Exercise tests of 241 patients who have also had angiograms were selected from our files for retrospective analysis. The exercise tests were done on a treadmill with a continuous progressive protocol to a symptom-limited endpoint. The QPT duration was measured in one of the resting standing V_4 to V_6 leads and at peak exercise in the same lead using a 5 × magnifier.

The angiograms were done with the femoral approach using standard methodology. The films were read by a cardiac radiologist, grading the percentage of cross-sectional narrowing by using callipers. Those with narrow-

Proceedings of the Vth World Congress on Cardiac Rehabilitation

Table 1
Patient population

	Healthy	No CAD Normal angiogram	CAD
Males (*n*)	23	10	98
Females (*n*)	22	20	27
Mean age (years)	23 ± 10.7	54 ± 11.6	59 ± 9.6
Previous MI			38
Ca^{2+} blocker			46
Beta-blocker			9
Indications for angiogram and exercise test			
Chest pain		20 (66)	75 (66)
Evaluation of angioplasty			20 (17)
Evaluation of CABG			4 (3)
Evaluation of MI			15 (13)
Other			41 (27)

Note: Figures in parentheses = % of group with angiograms.

ing of at least one artery of ≥70% were designated as abnormal. Those with lesions 30–70% were excluded from the study, and those with lesions ≤30% were designated as normal (Table 1).

Besides the 241 patients who had angiograms, the treadmills of 50 healthy volunteers were also analysed and designated as normals. When the initial 150 patients who had angiography were analysed, the exclusions included those with left ventricular hypertrophy (LVH), left bundle branch block (LBBB), right bundle branch block (RBBB), and those on digitalis. Subsequently, 69 more subjects were analysed who were selected because they were excluded according to the above criteria and are presented separately.

Heart rate corrections and statistics

The QPT intervals were corrected for heart rate by Bazett's formula [6] and the statistical significance by chi-square on Systat software.

Results

An abnormal QPTc was considered to be an increase of 5 ms from resting to peak exercise. The sensitivity of the QPTc for the total cohort was 184/196 = 93%, and specificity was 85/93 = 91%. The sensitivity and specificity for the 200 subjects when the 91 patients with digitalis, LBBB, RBBB and LVH were

Table 2
Results

	No CAD	CAD	SEN	P	SPEC	P	+PV
All patients ($n = 200$)	75	125		P		P	
QVTc normal	67	8			89 ⌉		
QPTc abnormal	8	117	94 ⌉			0.05	94
ST normal	56	29		<0.001	75 ⌋		
ST abnormal	19	96	77 ⌋				83
Women ($n = 69$)	42	27					
QPTc normal	38	6			90 ⌉		
QPTc abnormal	7	21	78 ⌉			0.05	84
ST normal	30	8		NS	71 ⌋		
ST abnormal	12	19	70 ⌋				61
Men ($n = 131$)	33	98					
QPTc normal	29	2			88 ⌉		
QPTc abnormal	4	96	98 ⌉			NS	96
ST normal	26	21		<0.001	79 ⌋		
ST abnormal	7	77	79 ⌋				92
Previous MI ($n = 38$)		38					
QPTc normal		1					
QPTc abnormal		37	97 ⌉				
ST normal		12		0.001			
ST abnormal		26	68 ⌋				

excluded was 94 and 89%, respectively. Sensitivity and specificity for the group originally excluded because of the digitalis, LBBB, RBBB and LVH was 92 and 89% (Tables 2 and 3).

When using an ST depression of 1 mm on the treadmill as a marker for ischaemia in the first 200 patients, sensitivity and specificity were 77 and 75%, respectively.

Scatter plots for the QPTc data in all patients are shown in Fig. 1. These are followed by plots for each sub-group in those patients developing LBBB, RBBB, LVH and for those on digitalis (Fig. 2).

Table 3
Sensitivity and specificity by severity

	1 Vessel	2 Vessels	3 Vessels
QPTc			
Sensitivity	95%	92%	96%
Specificity	92%	92%	92%
PPV	76%	88%	90%
SI			
Sensitivity	65%	74%	84%
Specificity	76%	76%	76%
PPV	42%	67%	72%

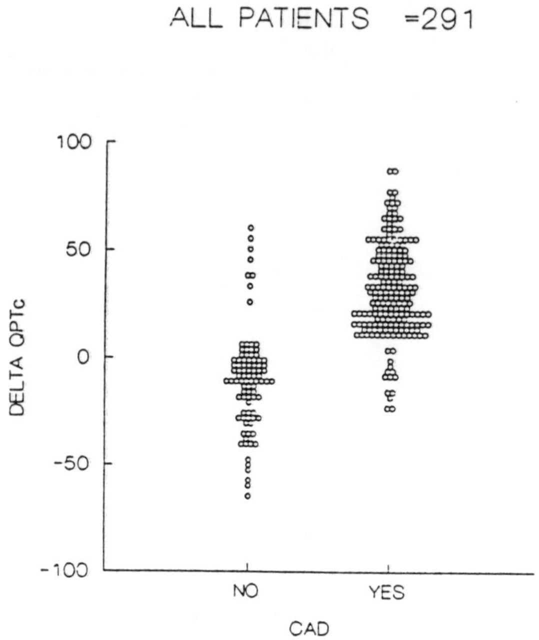

Fig. 1. This scatter plot depicts the change in QPTc from rest to maximum exercise in subjects with CAD as compared to normals. The values in the vertical axis are millisecond differences from rest to exercise for each subject.

Discussion

Prolongation of the QT interval with ischaemia was suggested by Burchell *et al.* [7] as early as 1948 and by Yu *et al.* in 1950 [1]. Mechanical systole, which closely correlates with the QT interval, was shown to be prolonged in ischaemia by Pauget *et al.* in 1971 [8]. The overlapping T- and P-waves did not deter attempts to use the information in exercise testing as evidenced by a number of authors who correlated the QT and the QX-QT with angiograms in the 1980s [9, 10].

We first proposed the use of the QPT interval as an index of the QT in 1983 and selected an increase of 40 ms with exercise as a marker for ischaemia [11]. Only recently have we revisited this work and found that an increase of only 5 ms increases the sensitivity and preserves the specificity.

In 1985, O'Donnell and colleagues [12] examined the terminal slope of the T-wave and reported that it increased with ischaemia. This shift would tend to increase the Q peak T more than the QT, and thus tends to support our thesis. Because ST analysis is of reduced value in patients with LBBB, RBBB, LVH and those on digitalis, analysis of the QPTc in these groups was the next logical step. Because of the inherent problems in ST analysis in these patients,

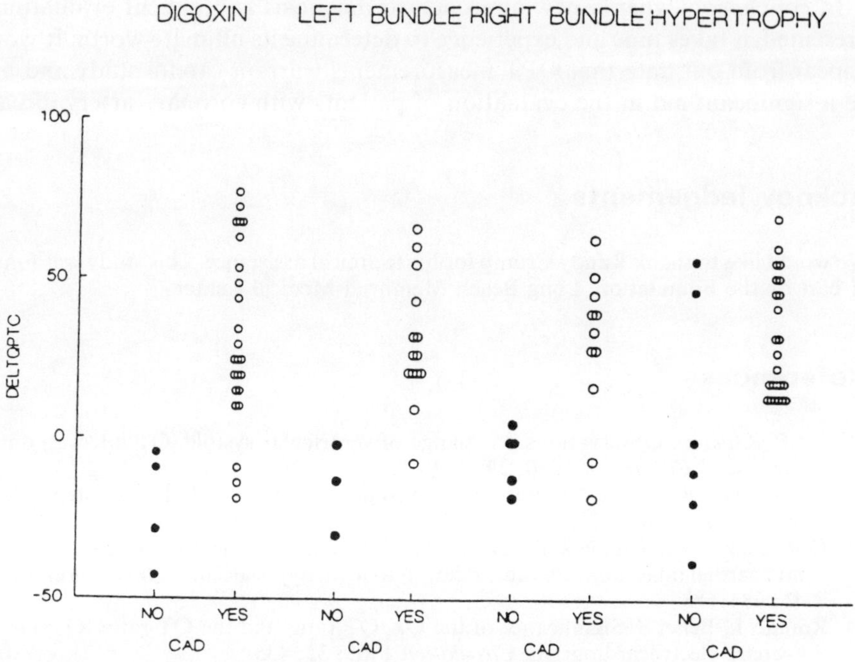

Fig. 2. Scatter plot using the same format as in Fig. 1 for patients in digitalis and with LBBB, RBBB and LVH. Note high specificity except for LVH.

few get referred for exercise testing, so we have relatively small numbers in the sub-groups, especially in those with normal coronary angiograms. Be that as it may, our preliminary data suggest that QPT measurements may also be useful in these patients. It appears that the QPT will almost certainly outperform ST measurements.

The weaknesses of this study are due to its retrospective nature and the inherent bias found in any study where coronary angiograms are used as the gold standard. Our use of a coronary lesion of $\geq 70\%$ to describe our ischaemic patients and $\leq 30\%$ for normals is somewhat at variance with most published studies. We believe that the patients with coronary stenosis from 30–70% may or may not have an ischaemic response to exercise. By excluding them, we think our results may be more reliable than if we arbitrarily selected 50 or 70% stenosis as a dividing line between normal and abnormal angiograms.

Further work to validate the utility of QPT measurements needs to be done and is now underway. A prospective study should give us a better measure of its clinical usefulness. We also need to better understand the mechanism of exactly how the ischaemic process alters the QT and QPT. We also need to know how the changes in the various leads correlate with ischaemia in various parts of the heart and with various locations in the coronary tree.

In conclusion, when a new approach to diagnosis and patient evaluation is presented, it takes time and experience to determine its ultimate worth. It would appear from our data that QPT measurements warrant careful study and may be a significant aid in the evaluation of patients with coronary artery disease.

Acknowledgements

We would like to thank Randy Crump for his technical assistance. This study was funded in part by the Foundation, Long Beach Memorial Medical Center.

References

1. Yu PNG, *et al.* Observations on change of ventricular systole (QT interval) during exercise. *J Clin Invest* 1950; **29:** 279.
2. Master AM, Rosenfeld J. Criteria for the clinical application of the two-step exercise test. *JAMA* 1961; **178:** 283.
3. Doroghazi RM, Childers R. Time-related changes in the Q-T interval in acute myocardial infarction: Possible relation to local hypocalcemia. *Am J Cardiol* 1978; **41:** 684–688.
4. Roman L, Bellet S. Significance of the QX/QT ratio and the QT ratio (QTr) in the exercise electrocardiogram. *Circulation* 1965; **32:** 435.
5. Robb GP, Marks HH. Postexercise electrocardiograms in arteriosclerotic heart disease: Its value in diagnosis and prognosis. *JAMA* 1967; **200:** 918.
6. Bazett HC. An analysis of the time relations of electrocardiograms. *Heart* 1920; **7:** 353–370.
7. Burchell HB, Pruitt RD, Barnes AR. The stress and the electrocardiogram in the induced hypoxemia test for coronary insufficiency. *Am Heart J* 1948; **36:** 373–389.
8. Pauget JM, Harris WS, Mayron BR, Naughton JP. Abnormal responses of the systolic time intervals to exercise in patients with angina pectoris. *Circulation* 1971; **43:** 289–298.
9. Greenberg PS, Friscia DA, Ellestad MH. Predictive accuracy of Q-X/Q-T ratio, Q-Tc interval, S-T depression and R-wave amplitude during stress testing. *Am J Cardiol* 1979; **44:** 18–23.
10. Lepeschkin E, Surawicz B. Characteristics of true-positive and false-positive results of electrocardiographic exercise tests. *N Engl J Med* 1958; **258:** 511.
11. Vasilomanolakis EC, Baron DB, Famularo MA, Redd RM, Paliwal YK, Ellestad MD. Identification of exercise induced ischemia by measurement of Q to peak T interval (Abstr.). AHA 56th Scientific Session, Anaheim, CA, November 1983.
12. O'Donnell J, Lovelace E, Knoebel SB, McHenry PL. Behavior of the terminal T-wave during exercise in normal subjects, patients with symptomatic coronary artery disease and apparently healthy subjects with abnormal ST segment depression. *J Am Coll Cardiol* 1985; **5:** 78–84.

11 Interpretation and Use of Exercise Testing in Children

F.W. James

Division of Cardiology, Children's Hospital Medical Center, Cincinatti, Ohio 45229-2899, USA

Introduction

The interpretation of an exercise study provides clinical information for rational and productive use of the procedure in the diagnostic evaluation and management of children and young adults. Typical exercise responses or patterns suggesting a specific diagnosis must be considered a bonus, because some physiological or pathophysiological descriptions are common to several diagnoses.

Several investigators [1,2] have used exercise testing to assess the capacity and adaptive ability of young subjects to external work and growth. Estimates of physical working capacity, oxygen transport, pulmonary ventilation, cardiac performance and function, myocardial perfusion, and rhythm and conduction of the heart can reveal the impact of specific disease upon the cardiovascular system, and perhaps suggest clues to mechanisms of disease.

Surgical treatment can restore cardiovascular anatomy and haemodynamics in many cardiac defects to normal or near normal levels. Despite these successful efforts, significant abnormalities which can be of potential risk to patients with or without significant residual lesions may be detected during exercise testing.

This chapter discusses briefly the rationale for the clinical use of exercise testing in a paediatric population. Also, the benefits and potential use of the exercise procedure in young patients with cardiovascular disease are reviewed.

Proceedings of the Vth World Congress on Cardiac Rehabilitation

Reasons for clinical exercise testing

The exercise procedure supplements sound clinical judgement. The reasons for testing in children and young adults with or without cardiovascular diseases are: (1) to estimate, provoke or describe responses to work under standardized conditions; (2) to explore physiologic mechanisms to explain signs and symptoms; (3) to assess the effects of specific medical and surgical treatments, and (4) To estimate prognosis and functional capacity for reasonable involvement in vocational, recreational and athletic activities.

The exercise procedure contributes to the evaluation of children with the following cardiac conditions: (1) left or systemic ventricular outflow obstruction; (2) chronic left or right ventricular volume overload (i.e. atrioventricular or semilunar valve incompetence or left-to-right shunts); and (3) cardiac rhythm and conduction disturbances. The evaluation of other conditions such as hyperlipidaemia, hypertension, chest pain, palpitations, fainting spells or exercise intolerance benefit from standardized clinical exercise testing.

General

An exercise laboratory [2] for clinical testing should be able to record blood pressure, heart rate, multiple electrocardiographic leads, and estimate working capacity, pulmonary ventilation and gas exchange. Other measurements such as cardiac output, systolic time indices, percent shortening fraction and ejection fraction enhanced the assessment of cardiac performance and function.

Equipment

A cycle or treadmill ergometer, an apparatus for measuring peripheral blood pressure indirectly, a multiple channel electrocardiograph for recording two or more electrocardiographic leads, and an oscilloscope for continuous visualization of the electrocardiogram are basic equipment for performing exercise testing in clinical settings. Other procedures requiring echocardiography, nuclear imaging or mass spectrometry are added based upon availability.

Protocols [8]

Several cycle protocols including normal data are available for routine clinical use in children. In our laboratory, we use a fixed continuous, progressive exercise protocol which is suitable for subjects of different size and age, and problems of varying severity. Treadmill protocols are also available, but the normal data are limited for children. However, with diligence, successful testing can be accomplished using the treadmill ergometer.

Exercise cardiovascular responses in normals

Estimates of *physical working capacity* have been made using PWC_{170} (highest rate of work required to produce a heart rate of 170 beats/min and a breathing rate ≤ 30/min), maximal power output (highest rate of work reached), or total work (accumulated work to exhaustion during exercise). Using James' protocol [3], boys and girls with body surface areas have similar estimates of working capacity. In subjects with a body surface area $\geq 1.2\ m^2$, working capacity is significantly higher in males than height-matched females.

Systolic blood pressure rises promptly with leg exercise with diastolic and mean pressures increasing to a modest degree [3]. The rise in systolic pressure when systemic vascular resistance is falling reflects the increase in the rate of ejection of blood from the left ventricle. Peak exercise systolic pressure is positively related to body size (height) and age in children $< 1.0\ m^2$, and body size only in boys and girls $\geq 1.2\ m^2$.

Exercise electrocardiogram

In normal children with normal blood lipids, 9% may have ST-depression = 1 mm, and 2.7% = 1–2 mm, with the highest frequency among the girls [3]. The R-R interval shortens approximately 56% from rest to peak exercise primarily due to reduced T-P interval and Q-T interval. The ST-segment decreases in duration and is occasionally encroached upon by the initial portion of the T-wave. The QRS interval varies minimally in duration during exertion.

Responses in specific clinical problems

Valvar or discrete subvalvar aortic stenosis

Exercise testing is most helpful in assessing the severity of aortic stenosis, especially in those patients with resting left ventricular-aortic gradients ≥ 30 mmHg (Fig. 1) [4–6]. Working capacity is inversely related to severity of obstruction and is greatly affected in those patients with a resting aortic gradient ≥ 70 mmHg. Peak exercise systolic pressure is lower than normals and is mostly depressed in patients with an aortic gradient > 30 mmHg. The occurrence of exercise-induced ST-depression during submaximal or maximal exercise must be factored in the clinical interpretation of the test. For example, significant ST-depression occurring at maximal exercise with a high heart rate may imply less severity of obstruction as compared to the same amount of ST-depression at submaximal exercise with a low heart rate [6, 7].

After surgery, abnormal pre-operative exercise responses (i.e. ST-depression, low systolic pressure and working capacity) resolve towards normal, and the rate and amount depends upon the presence of residual defects and the post-operative time period.

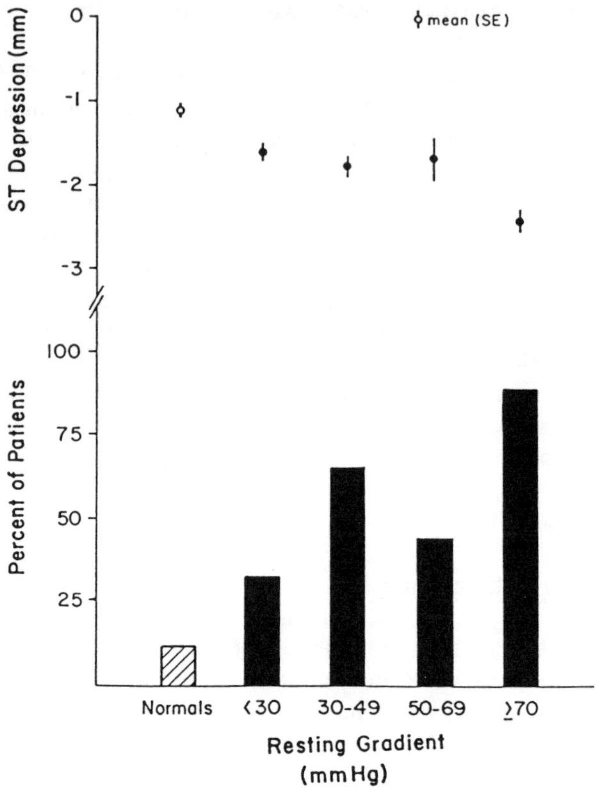

Fig. 1. Mean exercise-induced ST-depression in normal controls and patients with aortic stenosis. Courtesy of James *et al.* [6].

Comments: Exercise-induced ST-depression ≥2 mm, depression or fall in exercise systolic pressure and reduced working capacity are signs of severe left ventricular outflow tract obstruction, with subendocardial ischaemia and serious left ventricular impairment. Satisfactory relief of obstruction without serious residual abnormality can improve the abnormal exercise responses.

Coarctation of aorta

After coarctectomy, some patients may have abnormal systolic blood pressures (Fig. 2) and significant ST-depression during submaximal exercise. These exercise responses can occur in both males and females who may not have significant residual gradients (< 30 mmHg) across the site of anastomosis. The reasons for the abnormal systolic pressure and ST-segment are not clear, but systemic hypertension, residual obstruction, associated defects and premature atherosclerosis are reasonable areas to pursue. *Comments:* In some cases, exercise-induced systolic hypertension may respond to dietary measures and/or

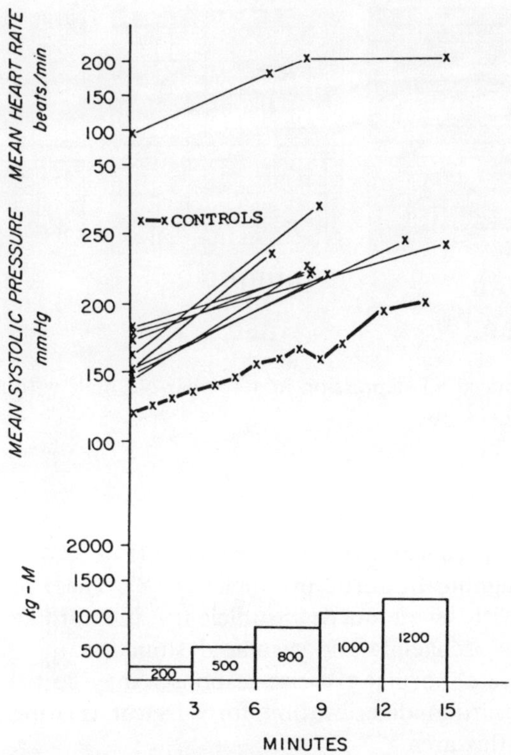

Fig. 2. Exercise mean heart rates and systolic pressures in normal controls and patients with coarctation of the aorta. After James [10].

drug therapy. The clinical approach for resolving or preventing exercise-induced ST-depression in patients with coarctation of aorta is unknown at this time.

Tetralogy of Fallot

Working capacity and heart rate in patients after corrective surgery for tetralogy of Fallot are lower than normal. Exercise testing has identified serious ventricular arrhythmia in patients after corrective surgery for tetralogy of Fallot. Further, sudden death has occurred in patients who have documented serious ventricular arrhythmia. The frequency of ventricular arrhythmia increases with residual defects [2, 8, 9].

Comments: Serious ventricular arrhythmia in patients with or without residual defects after reconstructive surgery of the right ventricular outflow tract must be considered for anti-arrhythmic therapy [7, 8].

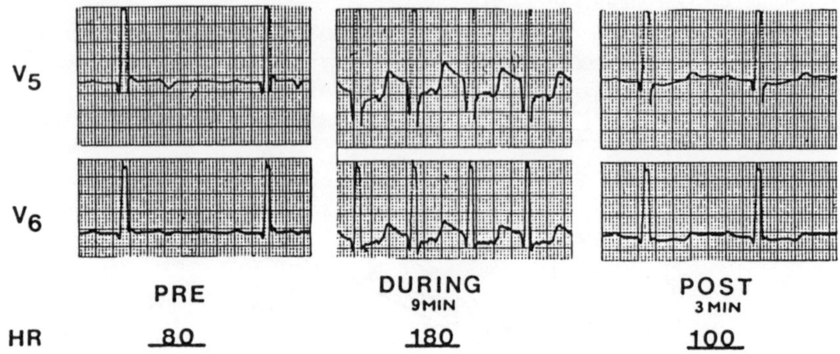

Fig. 3. Exercise-induced ST-depression in a 15-year-old male with aortic insufficiency. Courtesy of James [11].

Aortic valve insufficiency

Exercise systolic hypertension and ST-depression (Fig. 3) are reported responses in patients with significant aortic insufficiency [8]. These findings are usually seen in patients with severe aortic insufficiency and cardiac enlargement and suggest myocardial ischaemia and cardiac dysfunction.

Comment: These abnormal exercise responses may be risk factors for early detection of myocardial deterioration for surgical treatment. Further work will be helpful in this area.

Pulmonic stenosis

Average total work is decreased in patients with a significant resting gradient across the right ventricular outflow tract. In a series of 10 patients with pulmonic stenosis [8], at 41–68% $\dot{V}O_2$max, right ventricular pressures increased 74–92% over resting, and 6 patients had systolic pressures of 75 and 160 mm Hg. ST-depression was recorded in some patients in leads V2, V3, II, III, AVF and elevated in leads AVR and AVF.

Comments: Although increased right ventricular pressure occurs in affected patients during exercise, the clinical significance for surgical treatment of the acute elevation of right ventricular pressure even with ST-depression is not clear.

Ventricular arrhythmia with 'normal heart'

Ectopic ventricular arrhythmia does not carry a high index of suspicion for coronary artery disease in the young patient. Normal patients with ventricular arrhythmias generally have normal working capacities, maximal heart rates and blood pressures during exercise. Exercise may induce ventricular arrhythmia or suppress or aggravate pre-existing arrhythmia (Fig. 4).

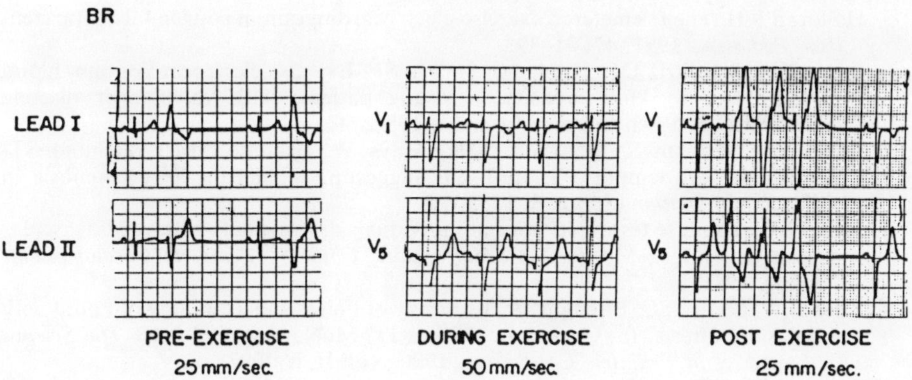

Fig. 4. Exercise-induced ventricular tachycardia in a 13-year-old patient with a 'normal' heart and pre-existing arrhythmia at rest. Courtesy of James [10].

Comments: In asymptomatic patients, anti-arrhythmia therapy is withheld and patients are followed. The author has seen completed resolution of exercise-induced ventricular arrhythmia over time and has permitted subjects to participate in competitive sports.

Summary

This chapter briefly discusses the technology and its rise in the clinical setting. Emphases are placed upon pathophysiological changes which are important for test interpretation. The clinical application of exercise testing for diagnosing the presence, severity and prognosis of diseases affecting the cardiovascular system in the young are reviewed. Exercise testing provides useful data that are not apparent at rest, but must be considered in the clinical evaluation of individuals within the paediatric age range.

References

1. World Health Organization (WHO), Work Group 3, Expert Committee on Rehabilitation of the Patient with Cardiovascular Disease, Geneva, Switzerland (in press).
2. American Heart Association. Standards for exercise testing in the pediatric age group: American Heart Association Council on Cardiovascular Disease in the Young. *Circulation* 1982; **66:** 1387A–1397A.
3. James FW, Kaplan S, Glueck CJ, Tsay J-Y, Knight MJS, Sarwar CJ. Responses of normal children and young adults to controlled bicycle exercise. *Circulation* 1980; **61:** 902–912.
4. James FW. Response to exercise of patients with aortic stenosis. *Prog Pediatric Cardiol* (in press).

5. Halloran KH. The telemetered exercise-electrocardiogram in congenital aortic stenosis. *Pediatrics* 1971; **47:** 31–39.
6. James FW, Schwartz DC, Kaplan S, Spilkin SP. Exercise-electrocardiogram, blood pressure and working capacity in young patients with valvular or discrete subvalvar aortic stenosis. *Am J Cardiol* 1982; **50:** 769–75.
7. James FW, Kaplan S, Mackzum MK, Mays W. Exercise, heart rate and ST-depression – A temporal relationship suggesting significant aortic stenosis in children. *Circulation* (Suppl. 3) 1985; **72.**
8. James FW. Exercise testing in normal individuals and patients with cardiovascular disease. In: Engle, MA (ed.), *Cardiovascular Clinics – Pediatric Cardiovascular Disease.* 1981, p. 227.
9. Neches WH, Park SC, Ettedgui JA. Tetralogy of Fallot and Tetralogy of Fallot with pulmonary atresia. In: Garson A, Bricker JT, McNamara DG (eds), *The Science and Practice of Pediatric Cardiology.* 1990, Vol. II, p. 1097.
10. James FW. Effects of physical stress on adolescents with normal or abnormal cardiovascular function. *Postgrad Med* 1974; **56:** 53–59.
11. James FW. Exercise testing in children and young adults: An overview. In: Wenger NK (ed.), *Cardiovascular Clinics, Exercise and the Heart.* FA Davis, Philadelphia, PA, 1978.

12 Exercise Capacity after Valve Replacement

Kristian Kothe*, Reinhard Aurisch, Andreas Förster

Kardiologische Abteilung, Klinik für Innere Medizin der Medizinische Fakultät (Charité) und Klinik für Nuklearmedizin, Humboldt-Universität zu Berlin, Luisenstrasse 11-13, 0-1040 Berlin, Germany

Introduction

Cardiac valve surgery has made considerable advances in the last decade. This is due especially to the extension of the indication to very aged patients, with severely limited left ventricular function and combination surgery (valve replacement and bypass). An acceptable rate of complications and early mortality has been attained [1, 5, 9, 12–14, 19]. Current international studies [6, 7, 16, 21] are investigating how exercise capacity and the associated quality of life develops post-operatively, especially for the increasing percentage of patients with heart failure despite cardiac valve replacement.

Over the last few years, there has been an increase in our understanding of the pathophysiology of exercise capacity and of the methods for the assessment of exercise capacity with heart failure. Significant advances have also been made in the quantification of exercise capacity with heart failure and after physical conditioning [3, 4, 13, 16–18]. The traditional opinion regarding mobilization following valve replacement has, for example, been abandoned. This has been replaced by a progressive programme of active early mobilization in the first post-operative days, followed by physical conditioning in the subsequent post-operative weeks. This conditioning consists of group calisthenics, cycling and walking.

* To whom all correspondence should be addressed.

Proceedings of the Vth World Congress on Cardiac Rehabilitation

There is, however, growing interest in the individual management of heart failure patients post-operatively, so as to be able to attain at least a minimum peripheral adaptation in the area of skeletal musculature, even if at a considerably later time and at a relatively low level of stress. For that reason, we compared pre-operative exercise capacity with the rate of peri-operative complications, and the early post-operative and subsequent exercise capacity, following physical conditioning, correlated with left ventricular function and lactate dynamics, independent of the locality of the valve disease.

Methods and patients

Pre-operative findings

1. Severity of the valve disease and left ventricular functional impairment;
2. colour Doppler echocardiography;
3. radionuclide ventriculography at rest and during stress in connection with the measurement of lactate dynamics during and after the stress test.

The characteristics of the patients were as follows:

1. *Localization of the valve disease*: mitral valve disease (MVD, $n = 26$, 63% female, 37% male); aortic valve disease (AVD, $n = 20$, 41% female, 59% male); double valve disease (DVD, $n = 16$, 100% male).
2. *Age*: mean 57.6 years (range 42–76 years).
3. *Severity of left ventricular function*: slight risk >45%; moderate risk >30% but <45%; high risk <30%.
4. *Increase in pre-operative risk*: ejection fraction >45%; combined operation >30% but <45% (valve replacement and bypass); reoperation.
5. *Sex and age differences*: the patients were sub-classified into groups aged 42–60 years and 60–76 years, for both men and women as well as men and women combined. These groupings were also classified with respect to localization of valve disease.

Peri-operative monitoring

Monitoring was implemented peri-operatively to identify those patients with low-output syndrome (LOS):

1. Myoglobin (EIA testing time 15 min); myosin-LC (EIA); creatine-kinase (CK) and its cardiospecific isoenzyme (CK-MB) (test kits, Boehringer, Mannheim, Germany); lactic acid level (ALAT) (test kits, Arzneimittel Werk, Dresden, Germany). Blood samples taken every 30 min in the first 4 h post-operation.
2. Assessment of left ventricular ejection fraction (LVEF) in the intensive care unit with In^{113}, and then continuously for patients with LOS.

3. Monitoring of blood pressure and ECG in the first 24 h post-operation, and then continuously for patients with LOS.
4. Classification of patients with LOS according to:
   clinic
   pressure monitoring
   CI $\leq$2.21 m^2/min
   EF dynamics $<$25%
   myoglobin $>$300 μg/l
   CK $\geq$25 μM (at $<$2% CK-MB)
   ALAT $\geq$1.5 μM

Post-operative active early mobilization and physical conditioning

Active early mobilization was conducted in patients with LOS using an 8-stage programme over a maximum of 4 weeks, ending with a symptom-limiting stress test (in a sitting position, up to an average of 50 W for 5 min). The lactate concentration dynamics were determined before stress, at sub-maximal levels of stress, and 3 and 6 minutes after being stressed. A resting radionuclide ventriculography was conducted before release from hospital.

A delayed-stage programme over 7 weeks was implemented for those patients with LOS, whereby patients older than 60 years could not be stressed for 5 min at a work intensity of 50 W at the time of their release from hospital. We continued to observe these patients in the post-operative period with respect to physical conditioning in either a rehabilitation clinic or as out-patients in selected hospitals near their homes. The physical conditioning was conducted as group calisthenics, exercising on a bicycle ergometer and walking. Following physical conditioning, the radionuclide ventriculograph was checked, both at rest and under stress. Simultaneously, exercise capacity and lactate dynamics were measured.

The pre- and post-exercise results were compared for age and sex and by group according to localization of valve disease.

Results

1. *Ejection fraction before valve replacement.* The mean ejection fraction with AVR was within or below the normal range before valve replacement. In contrast, in patients with DVR, it was at 55%, and with MVR significantly below at 50% (Fig. 1).

2. *Pre-operative workload and valve position.* The pre-operative values for the males with AVR were twice those of the females during the stress test. In contrast, the male patients with MVR and a reduced LVEF still exhibited 444 W/min; the females exhibited 301 W/min. The female patients with DVR had a limited workload pre-operatively (Fig. 2).

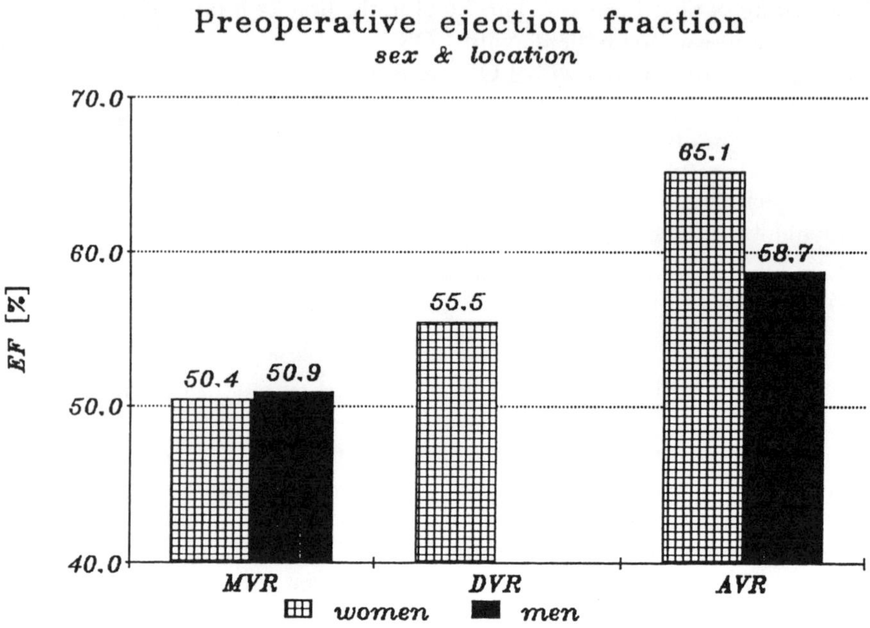

Fig. 1. Pre-operative left ventricular ejection fraction (LVEF).

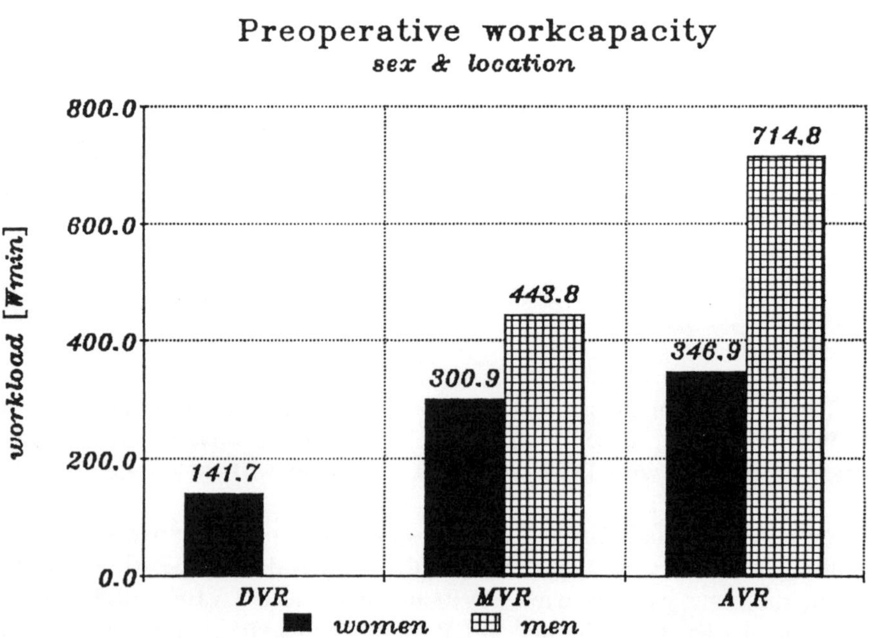

Fig. 2. Pre-operative valve disease in relation to workload.

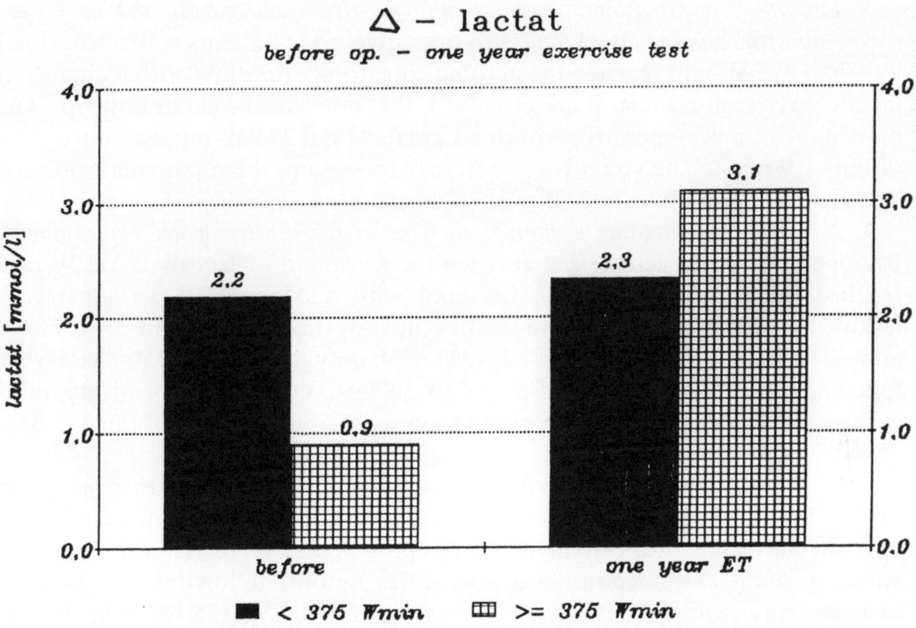

Fig. 3. Lactate concentration dynamics at a workload <375 or ≥375 W/min before the operation and at 1-year follow-up.

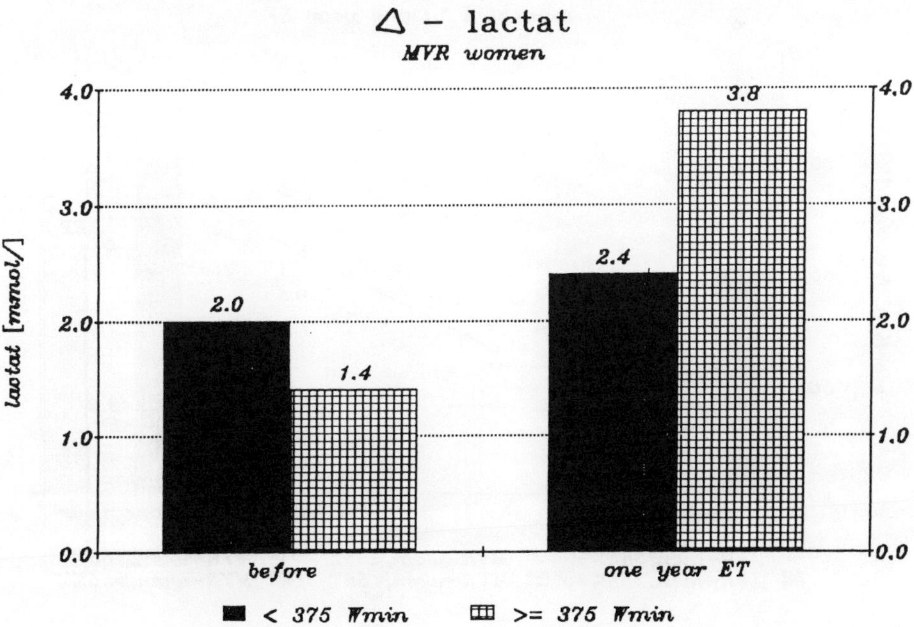

Fig. 4. Lactate concentration dynamics.

3. *Lactate concentration dynamics before valve replacement and at 1-year follow-up with respect to workload.* Pre-operatively, the patients with a workload less than 375 W/min reached the aerobic–anaerobic threshold with a change in lactate (ΔLa) of 2.2 mM. This remained the same at 1-year follow-up. The patients with a pre-operative workload greater than 375 W/min exhibited ΔLa of only 0.9 mM in the stress test. At 1-year follow-up, these patients exhibited a further increase of 3.1 mM (Fig. 3).

4. *Lactate concentration dynamics in females with mitral valve replacement.* Pre-operatively, the female patients with a workload of less than 375 W/min reached the aerobic–anaerobic threshold with a ΔLa of 2.0 mM. At 1-year follow-up, ΔLa increased to 2.4 mM. In contrast, the patients with a workload greater than 375 W/min exhibited a ΔLa of only 1.9 mM (Fig. 4). At 1-year follow-up, ΔLa increased significantly to 3.8 mM. This was more pronounced among the females than in the population as a whole, which attained a ΔLa of only 3.1 mM.

5. *Course of the ejection fraction at 1-year follow-up.* In those men who had undergone aortic valve replacement, the pre-operative LVEF was, at 60%, normal, and then dropped in the early post-operative phase. Pre-operative values were then attained in the course of the 3-month follow-up. A significant increase was exhibited at 1-year follow-up ($P > 0.05$) (Fig. 5). The female patients who had undergone mitral valve replacement and clearly exhibited a

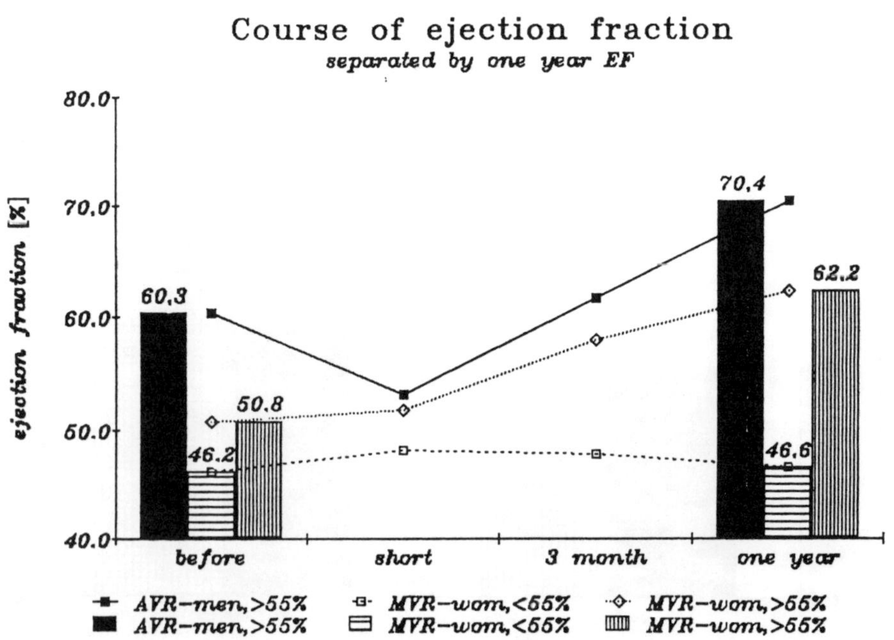

Fig. 5. Course of the ejection fraction up to 1-year post-operation according to sex and localization of valve disease.

reduction in LVEF (<55%), showed a slight reduction in the early post-operative phase. They exhibited a significant increase during the course of the 3-month follow-up, which continued to increase to 62% ($P < 0.001$) at 1-year follow-up. Those female patients with the same valve disease but a mean LVEF of 46% pre-operatively, exhibited constant values throughout the observation period.

6. *Comparison of the ejection fraction at 1-year follow-up with respect to localization of valve disease and workload.* Pre-operatively, a workload of less than 375 W/min was significantly more common among those patients with aortic valve disease and reduced left ventricular function. There was also an increase in LVEF at 1-year follow-up in the group with a clearly impaired workload capability (Fig. 6). This was found to be due to a discontinuity in physical conditioning. There was no significant change in LVEF at the 1-year follow-up of those patients with a workload capability of less than 375 W/min and mitral valve disease. However, the post-operative LVEF following mitral valve replacement among the group with a workload of less than 375 W/min, as well as the group with a workload greater than 375 W/min, was significantly lower than aortic valve replacement.

7. *Lactate concentration dynamics in females with mitral valve replacement and ejection fraction <50%.* Those females who had undergone mitral valve replacement and who had a LVEF of less than 50%, exhibited the smallest

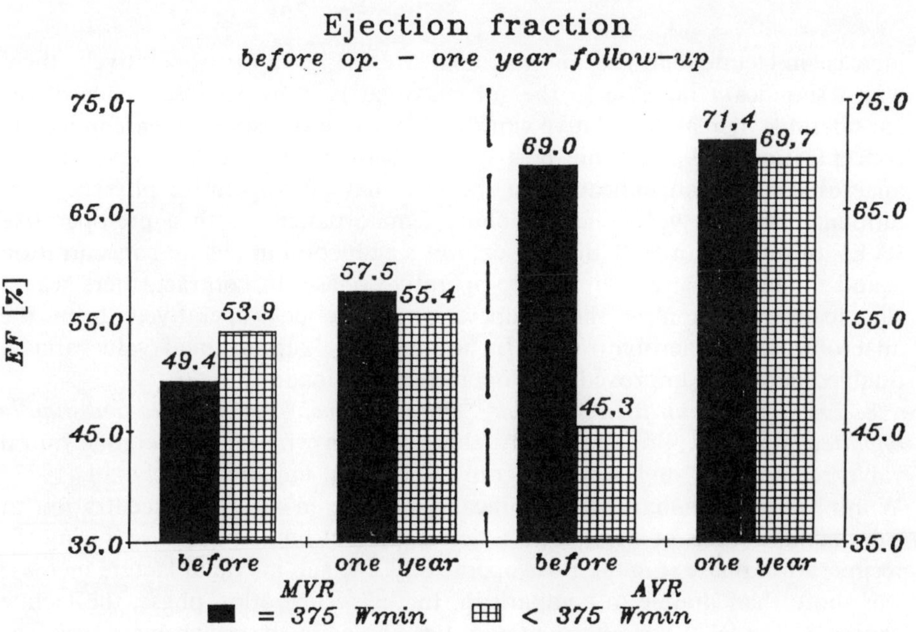

Fig. 6. Comparison of the pre-operative ejection fraction with the 1-year follow-up with respect to workload.

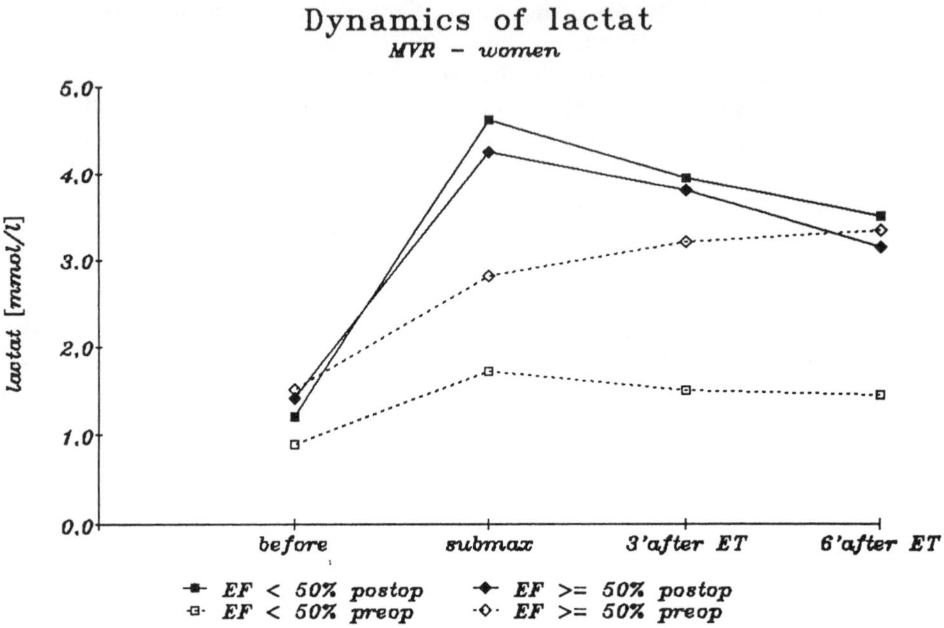

Fig. 7. Lactate concentration dynamics in females with mitral valve replacement in the post-operative period and an ejection fraction <50%.

increase in lactate following sub-maximal stress (Fig. 7). Post-operatively, there was a significant increase to the sub-maximal level as a consequence of the considerable increase in relative workload. There was also a decrease in lactate concentration at 3 and 6 min post-stress. All the values were, however, in the anaerobic range, an indication of the fact that post-operative physical conditioning was not yet sufficient. Those female patients with a pre-operative LVEF of more than 50% did not exhibit a reduction in lactate concentration 3 and 6 min post-stress in the pre-operative phase. In contrast, there was a significant reduction in the recuperation phase post-operatively from the anaerobic to the aerobic range. In addition, the sub-maximal value almost doubled, a sign of improved post-operative workload.

8. *Lactate concentration in females with mitral valve replacement and slightly impaired workload.* Pre-operatively, those women who had undergone mitral valve replacement and who had only a slightly impaired workload (≥375 W/min) showed a markedly significant increase in lactate concentration at sub-maximal levels of stress, with a detectable but limited decrease during the recuperation phase (Fig. 8). Post-operatively, the sub-maximal lactate increase was more than double in comparison. In the recuperation phase, the lactate concentration fell 1 mM after 6 min, but remained in the anaerobic range. The workload increased post-operatively, but physical conditioning was not yet adequate.

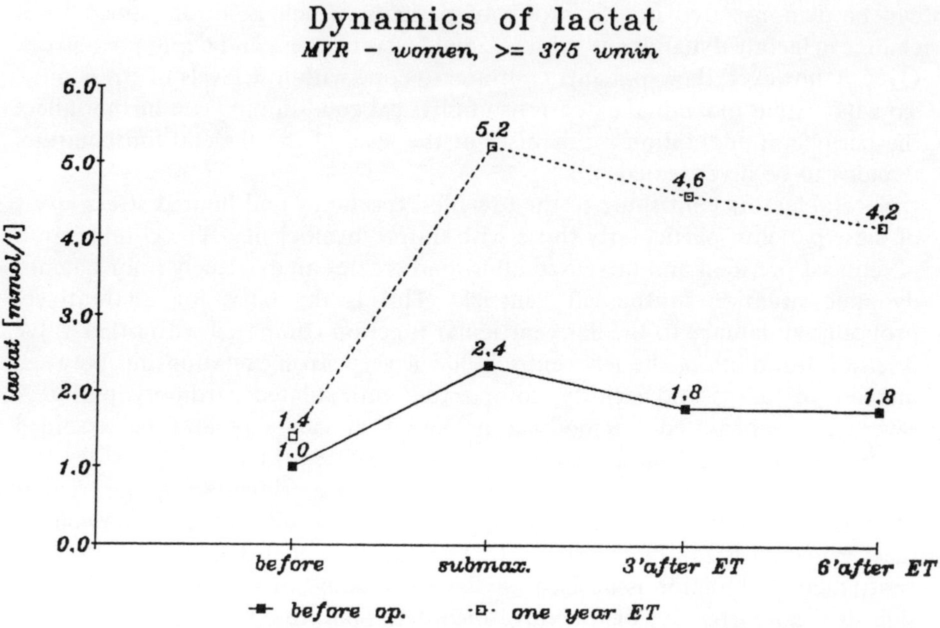

Fig. 8. Lactate concentration dynamics in females with mitral valve replacement in the post-operative period with a workload >375 W/min.

Discussion

According to the results of this study, a prompt, active early mobilization appears to be possible for the majority of adult patients following cardiac valve replacement. With proper implementation and supervision, there are no serious complications in patients who do not exhibit a severe reduction in left ventricular function [2, 6, 15]. Prompt physical conditioning of this group of patients reduces the overall post-operative rehabilitation period and, simultaneously, improves the range of physical performance while offering considerable safety. This holds true to a great extent for patients older than 60 years. There must be considerable modification of any active early mobilization and subsequent physical conditioning in cases of severely reduced left ventricular function, especially following mitral valve replacement or double valve replacement [5, 6, 14].

Patients with mitral valve disease must be monitored closely in the peri- and post-operative periods. Early mortality in this group can reach 10%, twice as high as that observed with other valve diseases. Low-output syndrome is also associated with a 10 times greater risk, as our own results clearly demonstrate. Even pre-operatively, these patients demonstrate a comparatively low LVEF and low physical stress capacity, with a small and insufficient reduction in lactate concentration 6 min post-stress. An increase in physical stress capacity can be demonstrated in this group of patients, which is accompanied by a change in lactate dynamics at sub-maximal levels of stress and 6 min post-stress. Overall, however, these patients continue to cope with low levels of stress only. To what extent individual extensions of physical conditioning can further affect the peripheral adaptation mechanism at the level of the skeletal musculature, remains to be investigated.

Several factors contribute to the low life-expectancy and limited stress levels of these patients, particularly those with mitral insufficiency. The combination of reduced pre-load and increased after-load creates an extremely poor haemodynamic situation in the left ventricle. This is the basis for qualitatively pronounced damage to the left ventricular function compared with other valve diseases. In addition, the left ventricle has a very strong relationship between increase in radius and rigidity, comparable with dilated cardiomyopathy. A severe decompensated haemodynamic situation can therefore be assumed relatively early in the course of the disease [1, 10, 19, 21].

It was also possible to demonstrate in animal experiments that ventricular dysfunction following valve replacement is, to a certain degree, reversible. If these experiences can be translated to human subjects, it would mean that left ventricular dysfunction is at least partially reversible with an individual right-side surgical correction of the valve disorder. The pre-operative constellation of findings, including stress capacity and lactate dynamics, therefore take on an increasingly important role in the timing of operations.

The reduction in cardiac contraction alone does not determine heart failure in the post-operative period, especially the peripheral adaptation of the skeletal musculature. Peripheral vasoconstriction, caused by the activated renin–angiotensin and sympathetic nerve system, reduces the peripheral circulation, especially of the skeletal musculature, and the consequences at the level of the structural and functional proteins of the muscles determine the reduced prognosis and poor stress capacity. Physical conditioning, even after valve replacement, positively influences the latter, as demonstrated by the results of lactate dynamics [3, 4, 8, 17–20].

References

1. Carabello B. Hemodynamic indications for mitral valve surgery in mitral regurgitation. *Controv Cardiol* 1991; **3:** 12–13.
2. Chapell J-P, Allaf Bl-H, Larbuisson R, Limet R, Lamy R, Heusghen C. Improved detection of perioperative infarction after cardiac surgery using CK-MB mass measurements. In: Unger F (ed.), *Coronary Artery Surgery in the Nineties.* Springer-Verlag: Berlin, 1987, pp. 217–223.
3. Coats AJS. Physical conditioning in heart failure patients. *Lancet* 1990; **335:** 63–64.
4. Cohn JN, Raifer SI. Evaluation of functional capacity in heart failure: A consensus conference. *Heart Failure* 1990; **6:** 168–173.
5. David TE. A rational approach to the surgical treatment of mitral valve disease. In: Karp RB, Lake HL, Wechsler AS (eds.), *Advances in Cardiac Surgery.* CV Mosby: Baltimore, MD, 1990; pp. 63–84.

6. Gleichmann U, Körfer R, Mannebach H, Mommsen S, Meffert Ch, Mertens HM. Frühmobilisation und Rehabilitation nach Herzoperation aus der Sicht der Erwachsenenkardiologie. *Z Kardiol* (Suppl. 4) 1990; **790:** 153–161.
7. Goenen M. Severe perioperative cardiogenic shock in open heart surgery: Benefits of combined therapy. In: Unger F (ed.), *Coronary Artery Surgery in the Nineties*. Springer-Verlag: Berlin, 1987, pp. 217–223.
8. Hoffmeister HM, Ley J, Seipel L. Effects of repeated ischemia on the left ventricular myocardium of dilated hypertrophied hearts. In: Jacob R, Seipel L, Zucker IH (eds.), *Cardiac Dilitation*. Gustav Fischer: Stuttgart, 1990, pp. 123–131.
9. Horstkotte D, Delaye F. The limits of central hemodynamic improvement by heart valve replacement. In: Horstkotte D, Loogen F (eds.), *Update in Heart Valve Replacement*. D. Steinkopff Verlag: Darmstadt, 1986, pp. 43–46.
10. Horstkotte D, Schulte HD, Bircks W. Factors influencing prognosis and indication for surgical intervention in acute native-valve endocarditis. In: Horstkote D, Bodnat E (eds.), *Infective Endocarditis*. ICR: London, 1991, pp. 171–197.
11. Kaul TK, Llewellyn M, Khasimi RA, Rasdale D. Myocardial protection in combined coronary bypass and valve procedure. In: Unger F (ed.), *Coronary Artery Surgery in the Nineties*. Springer-Verlag: Berlin, 1987, pp. 164–167.
12. Kothe K, Aurisch R, Butzeck J, Bohm J, Porstmann B, Schönfeld G. Perioperatives Risiko und Rehabilitation bei akuter infektiöser Endokarditis. *Z Klin Med* 1989; **44:** 2013–2016.
13. Kothe K, Porstmann B, Aurisch R, Butzeck J. Herzoperation im höherem Lebensalter. *Z Alternforschung* 1990; **45:** 337–342.
14. Kothe K, Butzeck J, Bohm J, Porstmann B. Perioperative Komplikationen bei Risikopatienten mit Herzklappenersatzoperation. *Z gesamte inn Med* 1990; **45:** 312–314.
15. Kothe K, Butzeck J, Porstmann B, Bohm J. Modifizierte bed-side Diagnostik bei Risikopatienten zur aortokoronaren Venenbypass-Operation. *Anaesthesiol Reanimat* 1991; **16:** 32–36.
16. Messmer BJ. Die körperliche Belastbarkeit herzoperatierter Patienten aus Herzchirugischer Sicht. *Deutsch Z Sportmed* 1989; **40:** 354–362.
17. Metra TE, Raddino R, Cas LD, Visioli O. Assessment of peak oxygen consumption, lactate and ventilatory threshold correlation with resting and exercise hemodynamic data in chronic congestive heart failure. *Am J Cardiol* 1990; **65:** 1127–1133.
18. Morgen JP. Molecular and cellular pathophysiology of heart failure. *Curr Opin Cardiol* 1990; **5:** 271–277.
19. Spotnitz HM, Antunes ML. Effect of aortic and mitral regurgitation on left ventricular structure and function. In: Karp RB, Lake HL, Wechsler AS (eds.) *Advances in Cardiac Surgery*. CV Mosby: Baltimore, MD, 1990, pp. 85–116.
20. Sullicvan MJ, Knight JD, Higginbotham MB, Green H. Relationship of arterial lactate to skeltal muscle metabolism during bicycle exercise in heart failure. *J Am Coll Cardiol* (Abstr.) 1990; **16:** 176.
21. Tirone ED. A rational approach to the surgical treatment of mitral valve disease. In: Karp RB, Lake HL, Wechsler AS (eds.) *Advances in Cardiac Surgery*. CV Mosby: Baltimore, MD, 1990; pp. 117–134.
22. Tsung-Po, Matloff JM. Coronary surgery in the elderly. In: Gray RJ, Matloff JM (eds.), *Medical Management of the Cardiac Surgical Patient*. Williams and Wilkins: Baltimore, MD, 1990, pp. 27–37.

13 Stress Echocardiography in the Diagnosis of Coronary Artery Disease

Thomas Marwick*

Service de Cardiologie, Cliniques Universitaires St Luc, Université Catholique de Louvain, Avenue Hippocrate 10, 1200 Brussels, Belgium

Introduction

Two-dimensional echocardiography (2DE) has become a routine technique for the evaluation of valvular and myocardial diseases. However, as ischaemia usually occurs under stress, resting 2DE in ischaemic heart disease has traditionally been restricted to evaluating the extent and complications of myocardial infarction. The combination of stress (either exercise or pharmacological) with 2DE permits the detection of abnormal wall motion due to ischaemia. The following sections deal with practical aspects of performing the test, the accuracy of exercise and non-exercise methodologies (in comparison with coronary arteriography), and comparisons with the conventional exercise ECG and nuclear imaging approaches.

Methodology

Equipment

Despite recent advances in echocardiography, image quality and video-recording impose practical limitations on the performance and interpretation of stress echocardiograms using routine treatment. Many of these difficulties have been improved by digital technology, which is probably the single most important

* Present address: Academic Department of Cardiology, St. Mary's Hospital Medical School, South Wharf Road, London W2 1NY, UK.

Proceedings of the Vth World Congress on Cardiac Rehabilitation

methodological development behind the growth of stress 2DE. On-line digitization enables rapid acquisition of stress images, enhances the quality of the stored image, and permits easier comparison of pre- and post-stress studies.

Interpretation

Both quantitative and qualitative approaches have been utilized, but the feasibility of the former is limited by considerations relating to image quality and translational cardiac movement. Use of the qualitative approach allows temporal and spatial integration of the image by an experienced observer to compensate for these aspects. The studies reported here all involve qualitative wall motion analysis, whereby the normal response to stress is considered to be hyperkinesis, infarction is identified by akinesis at rest, and ischaemia by either deterioration or failure to improve function after stress.

Stress techniques

As with other imaging modalities, the heart may by stressed by exercise and non-exercise methods. Exercise 2DE may be performed at peak exercise (using a bicycle ergometer) or after exercise (using either a bicycle or treadmill). As ischaemia due to single-vessel disease may resolve rapidly after stress, the post-treadmill technique has a slightly lower sensitivity for ischaemia. Both of the exercise methodologies require imaging at or after peak exercise, with consequent problems imposed by body movement and respiratory excursion. Thus, the exercise approaches are more technically demanding than those using non-exercise stressors (which include pacing, cold pressor and pharmacological tests). The latter are obviously indicated in patients who are unable to perform maximal exercise, but while they avoid the technical problems of exercise 2DE, they are non-physiological, so that their use in patients able to exercise maximally may be questioned.

Echocardiography with exercise stress

The sensitivity, specificity and predictive accuracy of exercise 2DE have been examined at several centres, using coronary arteriography (>50% stenoses) as the "gold standard". We studied a group of 150 consecutive patients undergoing exercise echocardiography, in whom the coronary anatomy was known, and 29 individuals at low risk for coronary artery disease. Abnormal exercise echocardiograms were present in 96 of 114 (84%) patients who had significant coronary stenoses. False-negative results correlated with the performance of sub-maximal exercise, moderate (50–70% diameter) stenoses and single-vessel disease. After the exclusion of 7 patients performing submaximal exercise, the sensitivity of stress echocardiography was 90%; it was 87% in 54 non-infarct patients performing maximal exercise. The sensitivity was 83% in those with single-vessel disease and 95% in patients with multi-vessel coronary disease; but in the latter group, multi-vessel disease was identified as such in only 47%. In post-infarction patients, the diagnosis of multi-vessel disease (identified as "ischaemia as a distance") was more accurate, with a sensitivity of 85%. In the 36 patients without significant coronary disease, stress echocardiography had a specificity of 86%, and of the 29 individuals at low risk of coronary disease, 97% had normal tests. Age, sex, body weight and image quality did not significantly influence the accuracy of stress echocardiography. However, the presence of left ventricular hypertrophy, which constitutes a particular limitation to the accuracy of myocardial perfusion imaging (with respect to both false-positive and false-negative scans), was not examined in that study. The influence of LV mass on the results of stress 2DE was therefore examined separately, in 158 patients selected for adequate image quality for LV mass calculations, and with known coronary anatomy. The specificity and accuracy of exercise echo was found to be significantly higher in patients with LVH (98 and 93%, respectively), than those with normal LV mass (83 and 80%, respectively).

In summary, the sensitivity and specificity of exercise echocardiography reported here are very similar to those previously reported using the same technique at other centres. This correlation responds to concern that previous data on exercise 2DE has been biased by "expertise" and patient selection.

Echocardiography using pharmacological stress

A substantial proportion of individuals are unable to exercise maximally; attempts to employ exercise methodologies in this group are characterized by poor sensitivity. Although pacing and cold pressor stresses have been employed, pharmacological approaches have received most acceptance – the principal choice being between inotropic agents (dobutamine) and coronary vasodilators (adenosine, dipyridamole).

The accuracy of dobutamine stress echocardiography (DE) in the diagnosis of CAD was studied in 85 unselected patients presenting for angiography. This study also compared the accuracy of DE for the diagnosis of ischaemia with that of ^{99m}Tc-MIBI, using the same stress in the same patients (see below). The stress protocol used 5–40 mcg/kg/min i.v. in five stages, with 2DE recorded at each stage, and on-line echo digitization at rest, low and high doses. The endpoints were: attainment of peak dose, severe ischaemia, or side-effects predicating submaximal testing (systolic blood pressure <220 mmHg, BP fall >20 mmHg, intolerable symptoms). The protocol was completed in 63 patients (74%); 7 were limited by ischaemia and 15 had submaximal stress because of the development of hypo- or hypertension; there were no major complications. Significant CAD ($>50\%$ stenosis) was present in 59 patients; the sensitivity of DE was 48/59 (81%), the specificity 22/26 (85%) and the accuracy 70/85 (82%). After exclusion of patients with negative results, who were unable to complete the protocol or on beta-blockers, the sensitivity of DE was 94%. These results are consistent with those of two published series of similar size.

A similar study protocol was used to assess adenosine echocardiography (AE) in 71 consecutive patients without previous infarction. The stress protocol used 0.14 and 0.18 mcg/kg/min in 3-min stages, chosen to equate it with previously reported dipyridamole echocardiography protocols. Endpoints were: BP fall >20 mmHg, severe ischaemia, intolerable symptoms or attainment of peak dose. The peak dose was attained in 53 patients (75%); 3 were limited by ischaemia and 15 by other side-effects, although there were no major complications. Significant CAD (>50% stenosis) was present in 47 patients; the sensitivity of AE was 23/47 (49%), the specificity 20/24 (83%) and the accuracy 43/71 (61%). Thus, the sensitivity of AE in this study was unacceptably poor, despite good results with simultaneous MIBI- SPECT perfusion imaging. These findings parallel those of a previous clinical study, as well as experimental data suggesting that, as a vasodilator, the optimal role of adenosine is as a stress for perfusion imaging rather than with stress 2DE, where the development of ischaemia is necessary.

Stress echocardiography *vs* stress electrocardiography

The most widely used technique for the functional evaluation of coronary artery disease is the exercise ECG. Comparison of the results of stress 2DE with those of stress ECG alone may determine whether the new technique is used to augment the older approach (in patients with LBBB, LVH, etc.) or even replace it.

In the study of post-treadmill stress described above, stress 2DE had significantly higher sensitivity than stress ECG (87 *vs* 63%, $P = 0.01$), after the exclusion of non-diagnostic results. In the 36 patients without significant coronary disease, stress echocardiography has a specificity of 86%, compared with 74% for stress 2DE, after exclusion of non-diagnostic tests (NS). Using similar methodology, studies from other investigators have shown equivalent results. However, the results of these comparisons are obviously dependent upon the methodology employed for exercise test interpretation; exercise 2DE appears to be more sensitive, judged on ST-segment criteria, but the same may not be true in a comparison involving a multivariate analysis of the exercise data, based upon not only the ST-segment response, but also the exercise capacity and haemodynamic responses to stress.

The role of stress ECG testing is less well established with non-exercise stresses. The accuracy of 2DE in patients undergoing adenosine and dobutamine echocardiography was significantly higher than that of the ECG findings during these tests.

Stress echocardiography *vs* other stress imaging techniques

The sensitivity and specificity of exercise 2DE have been found to be equivalent to those of thallium-201 and Tc-MIBI perfusion imaging in several studies. We have concentrated on the comparison of exercise 2DE with thallium-201 SPECT and Rb-82 PET using dipyridamole-stress, as the vasodilator response to dipyridamole is more potent than that of exercise, and therefore always provides the optimal circumstances for their performance, at least in theory. These data, in patients with known coronary anatomy, have shown a high concordance between exercise 2DE and these other techniques, with the former having fewer erroneous results than thallium-201 SPECT (reflecting avoidance of the late thallium redistribution phenomenon).

The results of 2DE and MIBI-SPECT have been compared with dobutamine stress in 85 patients with known coronary anatomy (see above). In that study, ^{99m}Tc-MIBI (20 mCi) was injected at the time of peak stress, with SPECT images 2 h later, and rest MIBI-SPECT was undertaken on another day. The regional diagnoses with DE and MIBI showed a 75% concordance. There was no difference in sensitivity between DE and MIBI (both 81%), and after exclusion of patients with negative results, who were unable to complete the protocol or on beta-blockers, the sensitivity of DE was 94% and that of MIBI 98%. However, the specificity of DE was higher (85 *vs* 65%), though this failed to reach significance. The extent of ischaemia by DE correlated better with that by MIBI ($R = 0.63$) than either DE ($R = 0.43$) or MIBI ($R = 0.40$) correlated with the extent of CAD using an angiographic score.

In the above study of adenosine 2DE, ^{99m}Tc-MIBI was also injected at peak dose, with the same MIBI imaging protocol. In contrast to the results for dobutamine stress, the respective sensitivities of 2DE and MIBI were 49 and 87% ($P < 0.01$), with specificities of 83 and 65% (NS). These findings are consistent with the effect of vasodilators being primarily to induce heterogeneity in the extent of hyperaemia (favouring perfusion imaging), with ischaemia being a less frequent accompaniment.

Conclusion

Stress 2DE has become a clinically useful adjunct to the diagnosis of coronary heart disease. The development of this methodology has been facilitated by technical advances, which are now routinely available, Previous measurements of the accuracy of the test have been reproduced in a sequential group undergoing angiography. Similarly, dobutamine stress has been confirmed as a suitable non-exercise alternative, in those patients unable to exercise. Stress 2DE appears to be superior to ST-segment interpretation alone, irrespective of stress. Finally, the results of the technique appear to be comparable to those of myocardial perfusion imaging, except with the use of a vasodilator stress.

14 Quantifying the Extent of Coronary Disease Using a New Exercise Test Scoring System

Michel Koch[1], Jean-Francois Dartigues[2], Herve Douard[1], Jean-Paul Broustet*[1]

[1] Department of Clinical Cardiology A and Department of Exercise Testing, Hôpital Cardiologique du Haut-Lévêque, Avenue de Magellan, 33604 Pessac and [2] Laboratoire de Statistiques Médicales, Unité Inserm 330, Université de Bordeaux II, Rue Léo Saignat, 33000 Bordeaux, France

Methods and materials

Initial study

Subjects

The subjects were selected from those patients who had attended the Department of Clinical Cardiology between 1984 and 1989 and undergone an exercise test for suspected coronary disease, followed by coronary arteriography within 1 month. The 201 patients were selected at random from a population of 450 consecutive subjects fulfilling the criteria for inclusion. Forty patients (16.6%) were eliminated at the outset because their files were incomplete. The mean age of the remaining patients was 57.4 ± 9.0 years. Males made up 83.2% of the sample and females 16.8%.

The patients with antero-septal, lateral and anterior infarctions were excluded due to exercise-induced ST-segment elevation. The risk of false-positives and false-negatives in the exercise test results were limited by excluding those tests skewed by beta-blockers or digitalis; diseased valves (including mitral valve prolapse); dilated myocardiopathy without a history of chest pain (ejection

* To whom all correspondence should be addressed.

Proceedings of the Vth World Congress on Cardiac Rehabilitation

fraction <0.40); well-established hypertension with left ventricular hypertrophy on resting electrocardiogram (ECG); instances of Wolff–Parkinson–White Syndrome; extensive hypertrophic myocardiopathy (unquestionable electrical left ventricular hypertrophy and/or parietal thickness ≥ 13 mm on the echocardiogram). However, the study did include female patients, true posterior and diaphragmatic infarctions, and patients with normal or not significantly diseased coronary arteries.

Data collection

Data relating to age, sex, parameters of the exercise test and cardiographic data were collected retrospectively from the patients' medical files.

1. Exercise test

The exercise test was performed seated on a bicycle ergometer with an electromagnetic brake, in stages of 30 W per 3 min for the males and 20 W per 3 min for the females. The exercise test was limited by the symptoms, by theoretical heart rate, by a drop in the systolic blood pressure (SBP) ≥ 20 mmHg, or by an irregular ventricular rhythm. The extent of ST-segment depression, the occurrence of an isolated ectopic beat or even a bigeminal ventricular premature beat were not considered sufficient for stopping the test.

The patients were encouraged to perform the test at maximum. Heart rate and blood pressure were measured and recorded every 60 s. The ECG was recorded and digitalized using a Marquette CASE apparatus. The data from the following leads were used in the analysis: bipolar leads CM5 (sensitive to the detection of depression [4] and analysis of the antero-lateral wall) and ML5 (more precise analysis of the diaphragmatic and posterobasal segments, from the sternal manubrium to the fifth lumbar vertebra), and one unipolar V lead (exploring the septum and located on the lower part of the sternum). ST-segment depression was measured automatically by the machine at 0.06 s from point J. The CASE 2 system also gives a curve of evaluation of the depression slope throughout the exercise test. The slope was taken into account by subtracting 25% from the ST-depression when not sloping. The two scores used were as follows: the criteria for stopping (on a scale of 1–8) and the time taken for the depression to recover (on a scale of 1–4).

2. Coronary arteriography

The coronary arteriograms were interpreted visually. The criteria adopted were: (1) the number of vessels significantly damaged (50% stenosis) and (2) the Friesinger index [2, 5], which provides a score from 0 to 15. Each of the main arterial trunks was scored independently from 0 to 5:

0 = no arteriographical abnormalities
1 = mild irregularities
2 = local stenosis of 50–90% of the area of the luminal cross-section (i.e. 30–70% of the diameter)
3 = multiple stenoses on the same vessel of 50–90% of the area of the section
4 = one or several stenoses greater than 90% of the area
5 = proximal thrombosis

The left trunk was scored twice, in the coding of the left anterior descending artery and of the circumflex.

Statistical analysis

For the *univariate analysis*, Pearson's *r*-test and Spearman's test were used for the quantitative variables and Student's *t*-test, variance analysis, the Mann-Whitney U-test and the Kruskall-Wallis test were used for the qualitative variables. The *P*-value took into account Bonferroni's correction. *The multivariate analysis used a multilinear regression incorporating the subset regression procedure* [6]. *The dependent variables were the number of vessels and Friesinger's index.* The parameters chosen for analysis were age, sex, the criteria for cessation (score), duration of exercise (min), maximum heart rate (HR_{max}), maximum blood pressure (BP_{max}), score for CM5 and ML5 ST-depression, ST-segment recovery, variation in heart rate (ΔHR) and variation in systolic blood pressure (ΔBP). The introduction of a formula derived from that of Hollenberg improved the result. The model obtained was a classic formula of the type: $Y = ax + by + \ldots + c$. The goodness of fit of the model was tested by the method of residuals. The model was then proved in terms of prediction of the existence of significant coronary disease or multi-vessel disease. This was done by carrying out an analysis of the sensitivity and specificity of various thresholds of the scoring system.

External validation study

Subjects

The 129 subjects were selected from a consecutive series of patients in the first 4 months of 1991 in the same hospital department as the initial study. The criteria for exclusion were exactly the same. However, the exercise test equipment had changed (Marquette CASE 15), as had the coronary arteriograph equipment (Siemens, Philips: numerization). The analysis of the patients' files and exercise test results was carried out by an independent observer not involved in the initial study. The arteriograms, carried out in the month following the exercise tests, were interpreted by the cardiologists and a consensus reached. Analysis was carried out on the initial exercise test score using the CM5 and ML5 leads, and then on the same score using the V5 and D2 leads.

Results

Initial study

The number of significantly affected vessels was on average 1.9 (0 vessels, 16%; 1 vessel, 22%; 2 vessels, 27%; 3 vessels, 23%; left trunk, 12%) (Table 1). Altogether, 22% of the patients took part in an exercise test after regression of unstable angina. Twenty-three per cent had a previous history of inferior infarction and 64% were smokers. In 14% of cases, the tests were skewed by therapy other than beta-blockers and digitalis or related drugs. The tests were terminated on average at 80% theoretical HR_{max}, The patients' performance on the exercise test was noticeably poor (see Table 2).

Univariate analysis

Classification of the variables was carried out using the threshold ($P = 0.0017$) obtained by the Bonferroni rule and the results are shown in Table 3. The criteria for terminating the test was an interesting predictive factor ($r = 0.53$). Termination due to chest pain was common among the coronary patients (60%

Table 1.
Baseline characteristics[a]

Clinical variables	
Age	57.4 ± 9
Sex: male	83%
Symptoms	
Asymptomatic	3%
Non-specific chest pain	15%
Typical stable angina	26%
Severe stable angina	11%
Unstable angina	22%
Previous myocardial infarction	
without residual angina	8%
with residual angina	15%
Smoking	64%
no. of years	23 ± 2.3
Hypertension	30%
Angiographic characteristics	
Number of vessels diseased	1.9 ± 1.3
0	16%
1	22%
2	27%
3	23%
Left main coronary artery	12%

[a] Data expressed as a mean ± SD or as a percentage.

Table 2
Exercise characteristics of the population[a]

Exercise test	
Criteria for cessation of test	
Leg fatigue	16%
Dyspnoea	12%
Ventricular arrhythmia	5%
Syncope or major ST-depression ($\geqslant$4mm)	4%
Typical chest pain	55%
Effort hypotension (decrease of SBP $\geq$ 20 mmHg)	8%
Performance (kpm)	3875.4 $\pm$ 701.4
Duration of test (min)	9.3 $\pm$ 3.5
HR_{max}	128.2 $\pm$ 22.1
ΔHR	51.3 $\pm$ 19.7
SBP_{max}	182.4 $\pm$ 27.5
ΔSBP	38.2 $\pm$ 21.7
Maximum ST-depression	
CM5 lead	2.5 $\pm$ 1.4
ML5 lead	0.7 $\pm$ 0.8
ST-recovery (min)	
<1 min	28%
>1 min and <3 min	17%
>3 min	54%

[a] Data expressed as a mean $\pm$ SD or as a percentage.

of all cases), whereas it was rare among those patients with no vessels significantly affected (12%). Reductions in systolic blood pressure while exercising also led to early termination. Multi-vessel disease had a specificity of 97.3% with a predictive positive value of 87.5% for 11% sensitivity. The assessment of ST-segment depression using the CM5 and ML5 leads takes into account the slope and amplitude of the R-wave as well as the amplitude of the depression. The improvement in the prediction of coronary lesions using this method was significant, since the coefficient of correlation increased from 0.54 for simple ST-depression to 0.58 for the assessment. The time taken to recover from ST-segment depression was one of the best variables for predicting the extent of lesion by univariate analysis ($r = 0.59$). The intuitive formula H derived from Hollenberg's model [2] also gave results that were the more interesting because they were independent of recovery ($r = 0.60$). This formula is different from the original [2] in that the slope of ST-segment depression and depression of point J are taken into consideration using a simple visual estimate, whereas Hollenberg used the integral of the graph.

Multivariate analysis

Multivariate analysis of the exercise scores was carried out *vs* the extent of coronary lesions. The seven variables with the best predictive value were: (1)

Table 3

Prediction of extent of coronary artery disease: Classification of variables[a]

No predictive value ($P > 0.05$)	Poor predictive value ($0.0017 < P < 0.05$)	Fairly good predictive value ($P < 0.0017$, $r < 0.50$)		Excellent predictive value ($P < 0.0017$, $r > 0.50$)	
Sex	Smoking (years)	Age	($r = 0.3$)	Criteria for cessation	($r = 0.53$)
Exercise arrhythmia	Hypertension (history)	Duration	($r = -0.42$)	ST-CM5	($r = 0.54$)
DBP_{max}	SBP_{max}	Performance	($r = -0.4$)	Qot. CM5 + M15	($r = 0.59$)
ΔDBP		HR_{max}	($r = -0.45$)	ST-recovery	($r = 0.59$)
		ΔHR	($r = -0.45$)	H formula*↓ $\frac{(CM5 + ML5) \cdot 10/(R)}{\text{Duration } HR_{max}/THR_{max}}$	($r = 0.6$)
		ΔSBP	($r = -0.38$)		
		ST-M15	($r = 0.26$)		
		ST-VE	($r = 0.35$)		

[a] Criteria for cessation of test = scoring system from 1 to 8 (see Appendix).
ΔDBP, change in diastolic blood pressure; ΔHR, change in heart rate during exercise; ΔSBP, change in systolic blood pressure; H formula, derived from Hollenberg formula; DBP_{max}, maximum diastolic blood pressure; HR_{max}, maximum heart rate; SBP_{max}, maximum systolic blood pressure; THR, theoretical heart rate (220 − age); Qot.CM5 + M15 = ST-depression in CM5 (−20% if ascending slope) + ST-depression in ML5 (−20% if ascending slope); R ampl, R-amplitude (in mm); ST-CM5, ST-depression in CM5 lead; ST-M15, ST-depression in ML5 lead; ST-recovery, scoring system from 1 to 4 (see Appendix); ST-VE, ST depression in VE lead.

Table 4
Distribution of exercise test score by number of vessels[a]

Vessels diseased	Exercise score ($\bar{x} \pm$ SD)
0	3.8 ± 2.2
1	9.5 ± 3.6
2	12.0 ± 3.3
3	14.0 ± 3.0
Left main trunk	15.0 ± 2.7

[a] Overlapping between classes is inevitable given the rigidity of classification by number of vessels.

sex, (2) criteria for stopping, (3) variations in heart rate, (4) variations in SBP, (5) ST-depression, (6) time to recover from depression and (7) the formula derived from Hollenberg (see Appendix).

The model is able to predict the number of vessels involved with a coefficient of correlation of 0.73. The means and standard deviations for the five groups of patients are shown in Table 4. The model can also predict the Friesinger index ($r = 0.78$) (Fig. 1). An analysis of the residuals showed that the distribution of the points around the line of regression was homogeneous and rather dense.

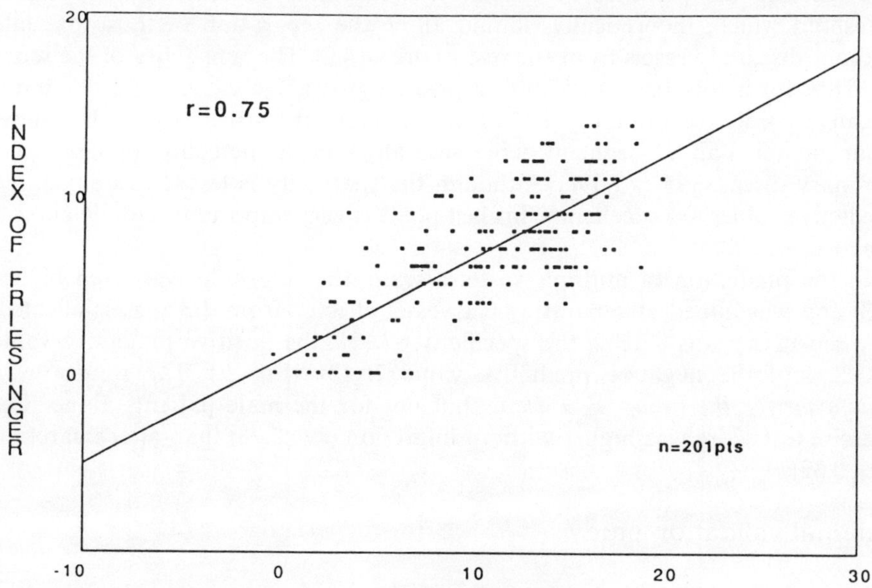

Fig. 1. Correlation between exercise test and coronary arteriography. The Friesinger index is more accurate than the number of diseased vessels.

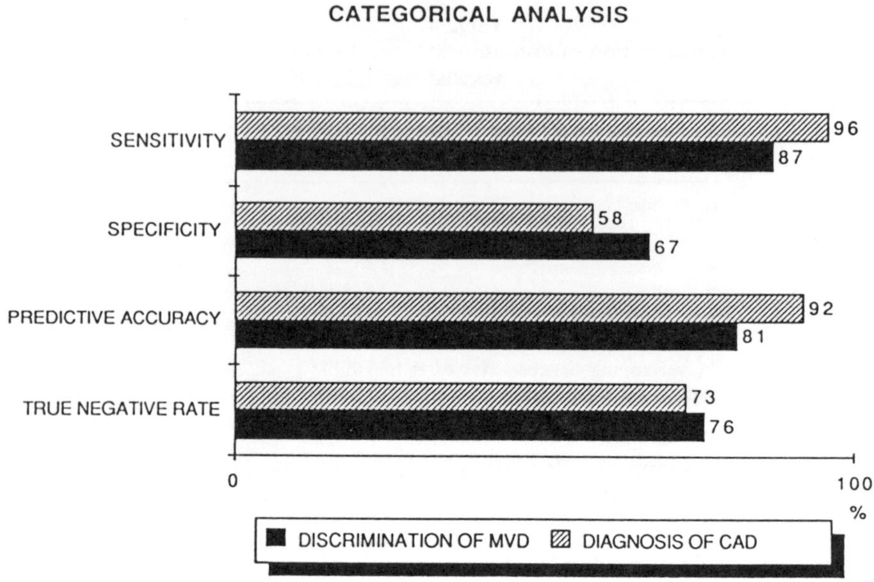

Fig. 2. Categorical analysis. Predictive accuracy, which is one of the more important parameters, is fairly good.

Predicting the presence of coronary disease was obtained by defining a threshold which, theoretically, should allow the separation of those patients without diseased vessels from the rest (score = 4.2). The sensitivity of the score is 95.8% for a specificity of 57.6%, a positive predictive value of 92.0% and a negative predictive value of 73.1% (Fig. 2). Thus, the sensitivity of the model is far greater than ST-segment depression alone in the detection of significant coronary disease (95 *vs* 80%). Although the specificity is less (58 *vs* 80%), the predictive values are excellent. This last point is very important in daily clinical practice.

In the prediction of multiple-vessel disease, the threshold was fixed higher (9.3) and was aimed at separating 0/1 vessel affected from 2/3 vessels affected. The sensitivity was 87.2%, the specificity 67.1%, the positive predictive value 81.3% and the negative predictive value 76.1% (Fig. 2). *The results were significant for the group as a whole*, but not for the male patients alone. The exercise test score was higher without infarction ($r = 0.78$) than after infarction ($r = 0.62$).

External validation study

Of the original 129 patients chosen for analysis, a number were rejected at the outset: 11 revascularized patients for whom it was not possible to calculate a Friesinger index; 26 patients whose exercise test was skewed by anti-anginal medications; 5 patients whose exercise test protocol was not standard (abrupt test) and therefore could not be analysed; and 1 patient who had undergone permanent electrosystolic training. Of these 86 remaining patients, a further 16 were excluded for the following reasons: 6 had a left bundle branch block (9.3%); 8 because of left ventricular hypertrophy (7%); and 2 for recent myocardial infarction (<3 week) (2.3%). Therefore, only 70 patients were finally included. Their mean age was 59 ± 10 years, the mean number of affected vessels was 1.5 ± 0.87, the mean Friesinger index was 6.1 ± 3.5 and the mean exercise test score was 7.7 ± 3.7. The sample included 12 women (17.1%) and 58 men (82.9%). The percentage of the patients who had had a previous myocardial infarction was 37.1%. The initial test gave the correlations shown in Table 5.

The exercise test scores using the V5 and D2 leads gave similar results at all levels. Thus, for the correlation with the Friesinger index: whole sample ($r = 0.80$, $P < 0.0001$); patients having already had an infarction ($r = 0.70$, $P < 0.001$); patients with no infarction ($r = 0.90$, $P < 0.0001$). In an analysis by category, the scores produced similar results. Therefore, in the detection of significant coronary lesions, sensitivity was 92% in this study *vs* 95% in the initial study, specificity was 78 *vs* 58%, the positive predictive value was 96 *vs* 93% and the negative predictive value was 58 *vs* 69%.

Discussion

Numerous studies have shown that multivariate analysis is a prerequisite for the successful interpretation of the results of exercise tests. Certain exercise test scoring systems are intuitive [1–3, 7–14] and give excellent results. Thus Hollenberg's score, in the form of a derived formula, was used in our scoring system. Other models are the fruit of multivariate statistical analysis [15–22]. The variables most often used in these models include: the notion of angina, ST-segment depression and performance during effort. Our results are in

Table 5
Results of the initial exercise test

	Friesinger index		No. of vessels	
	r	*P*	*r*	*P*
Total sample ($n = 70$)	0.812	<0.0001	0.70	<0.00001
Patients having had an infarction ($n = 26$)	0.62	<0.001	0.43	<0.029
Patients not having had an infarction ($n = 44$)	0.88	<0.0001	0.80	<0.0001

agreement with these studies. In a study of coronary artery surgery [19], Fischer *et al.* showed how powerful these procedures can be. And, finally, yet others have used Bayes' method of analysis of probabilities with success [22]. In fact, the quantification of lesions is not always approached in a precise way and is often limited to the prediction of multi-vessel disease [10, 18, 19]. Furthermore, the formulae giving the best results are often difficult to use in practice (they may be very complex or require a specific computer system) or are difficult to apply to populations which are too restricted because they are too highly selective.

The sample obtained was homogeneous and, as regards extent of coronary disease, intermediate between those of Hollenberg *et al.* [2] (more patients with triple-vessel disease), Lachterman *et al.* [23] (fewer patients with triple-vessel disease or left main trunk disease) and Fischer *et al.* [19] (more patients with no vessels affected). The rate of myocardial infarction was the same as that in Lachterman *et al.* [23]. Using univariate analysis, the best predictive variables were ST-segment depression, the *H* formula derived from Hollenberg ($r = 0.60$ *vs* 0.71 in the initial study) and the time to recover of the ST-segment. This confirms the work of Fuller and Movahed [24] and Savage *et al.* [25]. As Hollenberg *et al.* [2, 3] and Cohn *et al.* [18] stress, the ratio of the ST-segment depression to the amplitude of the R-wave and to the ST-slope is an important variable that is rarely taken into account. With multivariate analysis, the two criteria (number of affected vessels and Friesinger index) were the same as in Hollenberg *et al.* [1]. The correlation coefficient of 0.76 was similar to the 0.71 obtained by Hollenberg and co-workers.

What does this index represent? It is a quantitative measure for estimating the severity of coronary disease. It should not be fractionated; however, it does enable a well-known qualitative criterion to be obtained and this can be used as a pointer for the clinician. How it corresponds to the number of affected vessels is shown in Table 4. For the detection of significant coronary disease, the model fares well when compared with other studies (Fig. 3). Although the specificity was not as great in our study, the sensitivity was greater. This was because of the cut-off value that we chose. The relevant parameters in clinical practice are the positive and negative predictive values – these were high.

The score can easily be adapted to exercise tests carried out on a bicycle ergometer. It therefore enables quantification and follow-up of patients in exercise labs using this method. A study is being carried out at present using the Bruce protocol. The exercise score we have devised can be used at the patient's bedside using an ordinary pocket calculator and requires only the exercise test report. The external validation study confirmed the results in an independent series and with equipment currently on the market. Overall, the results were similar (slightly higher in the initial study in the absence of infarction and slightly lower in the case of previous myocardial infarction, but this sample was small). However, use of the V5 and D2 leads gave almost identical results to the CM5 and ML5 leads. However, the system does have a number of *limitations.*

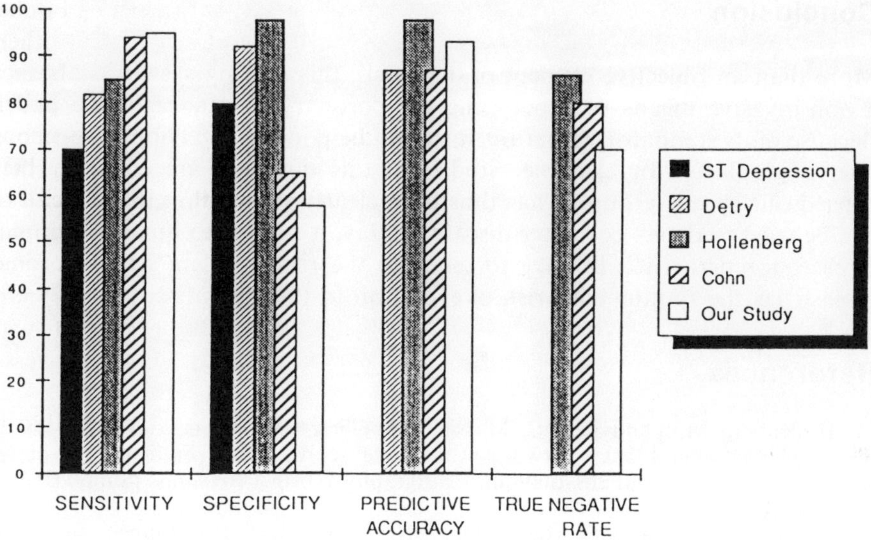

Fig. 3. Comparative analysis. Results for sensitivity and predictive accuracy were better than for the other parameters.

First, this retrospective study must be completed by an external validation study using an independent sample. Secondly, although the criteria for inclusion were not particularly strict (women were included, as were patients with no affected vessels and patients with inferior infarctions), this scoring system cannot be used for the time being for infarctions other than inferior or posterior ones or for tests skewed by beta-blockers, digitalis and related drugs or for severe myocardial hypertrophy. The low number of bypass patients in the sample (only 4 out of 201) means that the system should be used with great care in this type of patient if no selection study has been carried out. The predictive value of the formula is slightly better when the subject has no history of infarction; however, it is still accurate if this is not the case. The exercise test indicates ischaemia rather than lesions, which explains the less than perfect correlation. The exercise test, therefore, should be used in conjunction with a coronary arteriogram to predict survival and heart failure. Finally, when compared to isotopic examinations and stress echocardiography, which give a diagnostic performance which is at least as good, the quantified exercise test offers a number of advantages: it gives additional information on the circulatory response, the risk of arrhythmia during exercise, and functional capacity. Above all, it is less expensive as regards both equipment and time. And this factor cannot be overlooked at a time when investigative costs are a major burden to health service budgets.

Conclusion

More than an objective element of diagnosis, this scoring system is above all a non-invasive means of supervising the coronary resistance of the patient. Because of its standardized nature, it should help in the detection of re-stenosis after angioplasty, for example. Studies in this direction are currently being carried out by our group. It has thus been clearly shown that the exercise test can be used to detect coronary disease. Today, it is used to quantify coronary disease; tomorrow it will have to relate to the real problem set by coronary disease, i.e. the spontaneous risk of evolution to the patient.

References

1. Hollenberg M, Vandyke DC, Massie BM, Gertz EW, Wisneski JA. Myocardial ischemia quantified by two new exercise scores based on computer-derived ECG response and 201-thallium scintigraphy. Abstr. *Circulation* (Suppl. II) 1981; **64:** 185.
2. Hollenberg M, Mateo G, Massie BM, Wisneski JA, Gertz EW. Influence of R-wave amplitude on exercise-induced ST depression: Need for a "gain factor" correction when interpreting stress electrocardiograms. *Am J Cardiol* 1985; **56:** 13–17.
3. Hollenberg M, Zoltick JM, Mateo G *et al.* Comparison of a quantitative treadmill exercise score with standard electrocardiographic criteria in screening asymptomatic young men for coronary artery disease. *N Engl J Med* 1985; **10:** 600–606.
4. Blackburn H. The exercise electrocardiogram: Technological, procedural, and conceptual developments. In: Blackburn, H (ed.), *Measurements in Exercise Electrocardiography*. Thomas: Springfield, IL, 1969, p. 220.
5. Friesinger GC, Page E, Ross R. Prognostic significance of coronary arteriography. *Trans Assoc Am Physician* 1970; **83:** 78–89.
6. Wilson RW. Regressions by leaps and bounds. *Technometrics* 1974; **16**.
7. Dagenais GR, Rouleau JR, Christen A, Fabia J. Survival of patients with a strongly positive exercise electrocardiogram. *Circulation* 1982; **65:** 452–458.
8. Cole JP, Ellestad MH. Significance of chest pain during treadmill exercise: Correlation with coronary events. *Am J Cardiol* 1978; **41:** 227–232.
9. Ellestad MH. Can stress testing identify the severity of coronary disease? In: Corday E, Swan HJC (eds), *Clinical Strategies in Ischemic Heart Diseases*. Williams and Wilkins: Baltimore, MD, 1979, p. 208.
10. Berman JL, Wynne J, Cohn PF. A multivariate approach for interpreting treadmill exercise tests in coronary artery disease. *Circulation* 1978; **58:** 505–512.
11. Elamin MS, Mary DA, Smith DR, Linder R. Prediction of severity of coronary artery disease using slope of submaximal ST segment heart rate relationship. *Cardiovasc Res* 1980; **14:** 681–691.
12. Okin PM, Kligfield P, Ameisen O, Goldberg HL, Borer JS. Improved accuracy of the exercise electrocardiogram: Identification of three-vessel coronary disease in stable angina pectoris by analysis of peak rate-related changes in ST segments. *Am J Cardiol* 1985; **55:** 271–276.
13. Okin PN, Kligfield P, Ameisen O, Goldberg HL, Borer JS. Identification of anatomically extensive coronary artery disease by the exercise ECG ST segment/heart rate slope. *Am Heart J* 1988; **115:** 1002.
14. Okin PN, Anderson K, Levy D, Kligfield P. Heart rate adjustment of exercise ST segment depression for improved risk prediction in the Framingham offspring study. *Circulation* (Suppl. II) 1989; **80:** 1652.

15. Mark DB, Mark AH, Harrell FE, Lee KL, MacCaliff RM, Pryor DB. Exercise treadmill score for predicting prognosis in coronary artery disease. *Ann Intern Med* 1987; **106:** 793–800.
16. Mark DB, Shaw L, Frank E *et al.* A new prognostic treadmill score stratifies risk in out-patients. *Circulation* (Suppl. II) 1989; **80:** 1651.
17. MacCaliff RM, Mark DB, Harrell FE *et al.* Importance of clinical measures of ischemia in the prognosis of patients with documented coronary artery disease. *J Am Coll Cardiol* 1988; **11:** 20–26.
18. Cohn K, Kamm B, Feteih N, Brand R, Goldschlager N. Use of treadmill score to quantify ischemic response and predict extent of coronary disease. *Circulation* 1979; **59:** 286–296.
19. Fischer LD, Kennedy JW, Chaitman BR *et al.* Diagnostic quantification of CASS (Coronary Artery Surgery Study). Clinical and exercise test results in determining presence and extent of coronary artery disease: A multivariate approach. *Circulation* 1981; **63:** 987–1000.
20. Goldman L, Cook EF, Mitchell N *et al.* Incremental value of the exercise test for diagnosing the presence or absence of coronary artery disease. *Circulation* 1982; **66:** 945–952.
21. Kansal S, Roitman D, Bradley EL, Sheffield LT. Enhanced evaluation of treadmill tests by means of scoring based on multivariate analysis and its clinical application: A study of 608 patients. *Am J Cardiol* 1983; **52:** 1155–1160.
22. Detry JM, Robert A, Lunaert RJ *et al.* Diagnostic value of computerized exercise testing in men without previous myocardial infarction: A multivariate, compartmental and probabilistic approach. *Eur Heart J* 1985; **6:** 227–238.
23. Lachterman B, Lehmann K, Detrano R, Neutel J, Froelicher VF. Comparison of ST segment/heart rate index to standard ST criteria for analysis of exercise electrocardiogram. *Circulation* 1990; **82:** 44–50.
24. Fuller T, Movahed A. Current review of exercise testing; Application and interpretation. *Clin Cardiol* 1987; **10:** 189–200.
25. Savage MP, Squires LS, Hopkins IT, Raichlen JS, Park CH, Chung EK. Usefulness of ST segment depression as a sign of coronary artery disease when confined to the post exercise recovery period. *Am J Cardiol* 1987; **60:** 1405–1406.

Appendix

$$\textbf{Exercise score} = 5 - (2.7\ \ \text{sex}) + (0.6\ \text{CS}) - (0.03\ \ \Delta\text{HR}) - (0.03\ \ \Delta\text{SBP}) + (0.5\ \text{CM5}) + (1.3\ \text{Rec}) + 4.6\ \frac{(\text{CM5} + \text{ML5})\cdot 10/(\text{R})}{\text{Duration}\ \text{HR}_{max}/\text{THR}_{max}}$$

Sex: −0, where sex is 0 for men and 1 for women.

CS: criteria for cessation to be assessed by the operator:

1. leg fatigue
   or pain in articulations
   or inability to maintain 60 rpm
   or theoretic HR reached
2. Dyspnoea
3. Supraventricular arrythmia
4. Ventricular arrhythmia

5. Quasi syncope
   or major ST depression
   or absence of increased blood pressure
6. Chest pain
7. Hypotension ($\geq$20 mmHg for SBP)

ΔHR = HR_{max} recorded during test minus resting HR
ΔSBP = SBP_{max} recorded during test minus resting SBP (mmHg)
CM5 = absolute value for ST-depression or ST-elevation in CM5 lead less 25% if the slope is ascending. [**N.B.:** Absolute value: a depression or an elevation of less than 1 mm has an absolute value of 0. Thus only significant modifications of the ST-segment are taken into consideration. The slope is judged globally with the naked eye against the integral of the slope graph.]
ML5 = same as for ML5 derivation
Rec = recovery from significant ST depression

1. Recovery from a depression in <1 min
2. Recovery from a depression in >1 min and <3 min
3. Appearance of a depression in the 3rd min which did not exist in the 1st
4. Recovery >3 min

R = R-amplitude, at rest, in CM5 (mm)
Duration = duration of test (min)
HR_{max} = maximum heart rate recorded during test
THR_{max} = 220 minus age

The score can in theory reach values of about 40. In practice, the maximum indices we obtained were about 25 for extremely severe lesions. This formula can easily be calculated *a posteriori*, at the patient's bedside using a programmable pocket calculator. The formula gives an estimate of the coronary index.

IV Exercise Training

15 Cardiac Complications of Exercise

John D. Cantwell

Cardiac Rehabilitation and the Internal Medicine Residency Program, Georgia Baptist Medical Center, 300 Boulevard, N.E., Atlanta, GA 30312, USA

Introduction

The many benefits from aerobic exercise have been extolled in recent position papers by the American Heart Association [1] and the American College of Sports Medicine [2]. As with any form of therapy, complications can and do arise. We recently reviewed our 20-year experience with such cardiac complications, focusing on those which occur during exercise testing, physical training and cardiac rehabilitation. We also reviewed severe cardiac complication of a specific sport, basketball, during two consecutive seasons in our state.

Cardiac complications during exercise testing

From 1972 to 1992, we have performed 10,556 treadmill exercise tests on 6519 people. Significant cardiac complications, defined as an event requiring prompt medical attention, are noted in Table 1.

Supraventricular tachyarrhythmias were observed in two subjects. One, a 39-year-old man, had a past history of these. He developed A-V nodal re-entrant tachycardia during the test and converted to sinus rhythm after a 5-mg intravenous dose of verapamil. A 51-year-old man developed atrial fibrillation during the test and this persisted for 24 h converting with oral digoxin, atenolol and quinidine gluconate.

Proceedings of the Vth World Congress on Cardiac Rehabilitation

Table 1
Cardiac complications during exercise testing: 10,556 tests, 1972–92

Complication	*n*
Supraventricular tachyarrhythmias	3
Ventricular tachycardia	2
Transmural ischaemia	3
Acute myocardial infarction	2
Deaths	0

Two patients had sustained ventricular tachycardia, terminated by thumpversion. One was an apparently normal 28-year-old man, whose echocardiogram subsequently revealed mitral valve prolapse. The other was a 62-year-old patient with prior coronary bypass surgery and mitral valve prolapse. He eventually had surgical repair of his mitral valve.

Two additional patients had combined ventricular arrhythmias with ST-segment elevation. One, a 28-year-old man, had transient ST-segment elevation

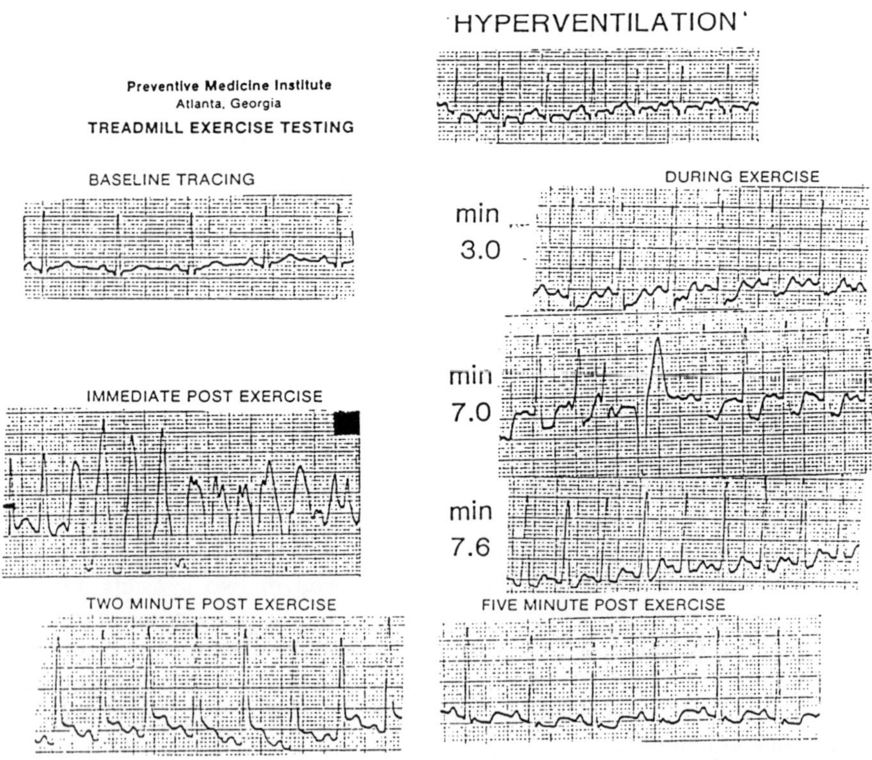

Fig. 1. Transient ST-segment elevation and non-sustained ventricular tachycardia in a 28-year-old man.

associated with non-sustained ventricular tachycardia (Fig. 1). He noted a prior transit burning sensation in the anterior chest, along with dyspnoea, while pushing a stalled car. Several similar episodes had occurred during sexual intercourse and while awaiting a stressful interview. He was taken directly to the cardiac catheterization laboratory following the treadmill test and the study showed a 95% lesion of the proximal left anterior descending (LAD) coronary artery. Coronary angioplasty was successfully performed and follow-up treadmill tests have been normal over the ensuing 6 years of follow-up.

A 47-year-old man with mild hypertension had an exercise test because of midscapular back pain which developed after walking half a mile and subsided within a 1 min of rest. The discomfort had also occurred while watching a football game and was associated with gas and belching, and aggravated by lying on his back. During a thallium stress scan, he developed the mid-back discomfort 5.8 min into the Bruce protocol, followed by ST-segment elevation and non-sustained ventricular tachycardia. The thallium scan showed a large reversible perfusion defect involving the anterior wall, apex and septum. Prompt cardiac catheterization indicated a 95% proximal LAD coronary lesion and coronary angioplasty was successfully carried out.

Two patients had acute myocardial infarctions (MIs) during treadmill testing. One, aged 69, had a 1 year history of right anterolateral chest discomfort which could last a day or so. In recent weeks, he had noticed a "soreness" across the mid-chest, radiating to the neck, and this could last for several hours and would be improved after stretching his arms. During the Bruce treadmill test, he experienced mild anterior chest tightness after 2 min, not associated with ECG changes. The test was stopped at 4.7 min when his pain increased. His blood pressure fell to 74/54 mmHg, associated with pallor and diaphoresis. The ECG showed transient ST-segment elevation in level V5 at 2 min after exercise and depression by 10 min after (Fig.2). A 12-lead ECG taken 10 min post-exercise showed marked ischaemia (Fig. 3). Emergency cardiac catheterization revealed total occlusion of the proximal LAD coronary artery and of the mid-obtuse marginal branch of the left circumflex artery. Intra-coronary streptokinase was administered and coronary angioplasty of the LAD artery performed. The following day the patient had an exacerbation of his pain and repeat catheterization showed re-occlusion of the LAD artery. Coronary bypass surgery was subsequently performed, with good results.

The other patient who had an acute MI during treadmill testing was a 54-year-old man who underwent a routine exercise test prior to entering into a fitness centre. He exercised for 10 min on the Bruce protocol, stopping because of mild fatigue. His exercise ECG was normal until 5 min post-exercise, when ST-segment elevation was noted in lead V1 (Fig. 4). A 12-lead ECG (Fig. 5) showed acute anterior wall injury. Emergency cardiac catheterization revealed total occlusion of the LAD artery. Attempts to open the vessel with thrombolysis and angioplasty were unsuccessful, so bypass surgery was performed. The patient made a good recovery and has participated in our cardiac rehabilitation programme without subsequent problems.

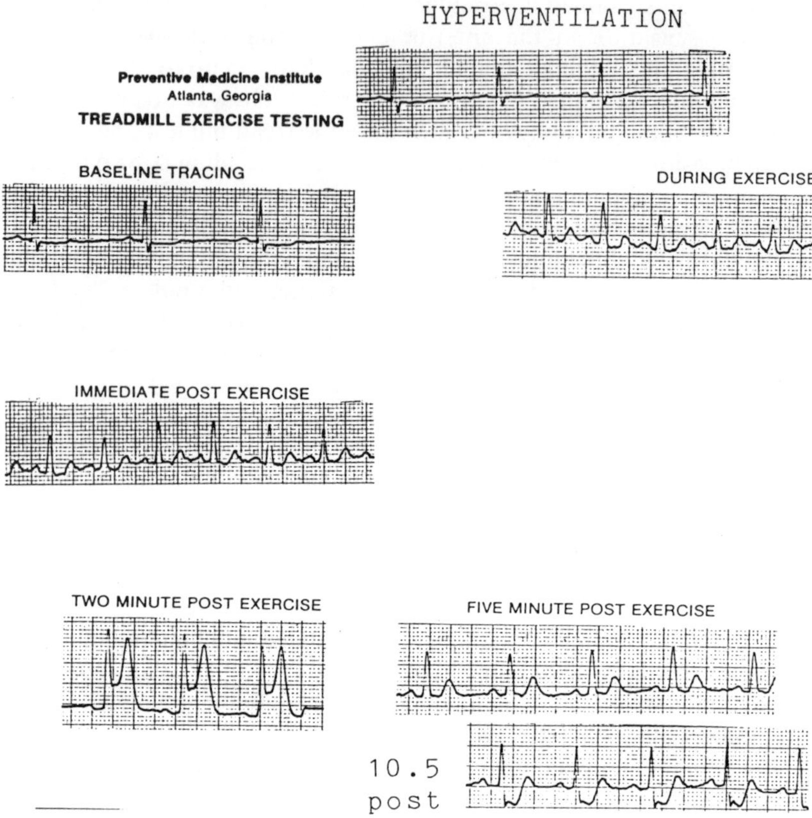

Fig. 2. Acute myocardial injury post-exercise test in a 69-year-old man.

Cardiac complications during physical training

Exercise programmes were prescribed for 5050 subjects seen at our Preventive Medicine Center during the 20-year period between 1972 and 1992. All individuals had a thorough medical history and cardiovascular examination to exclude known contraindications to physical training, such as aortic stenosis, hypertrophic cardiomyopathy and poorly controlled arrhythmia or hypertension.

Only one known major cardiac event occurred in subjects without a prior history of coronary artery disease. That person, age 46, had been a jogger for 20 years, typically running 12 miles per week without any symptoms. His mild hypertension, present for 15 years, was controlled with 2.5 mg of enalapril and 20 mg of propranolol twice daily.

He was found unresponsive, in jogging clothes, in another city. A treadmill test 4 months previously had shown junctional ST-segment depression, so a

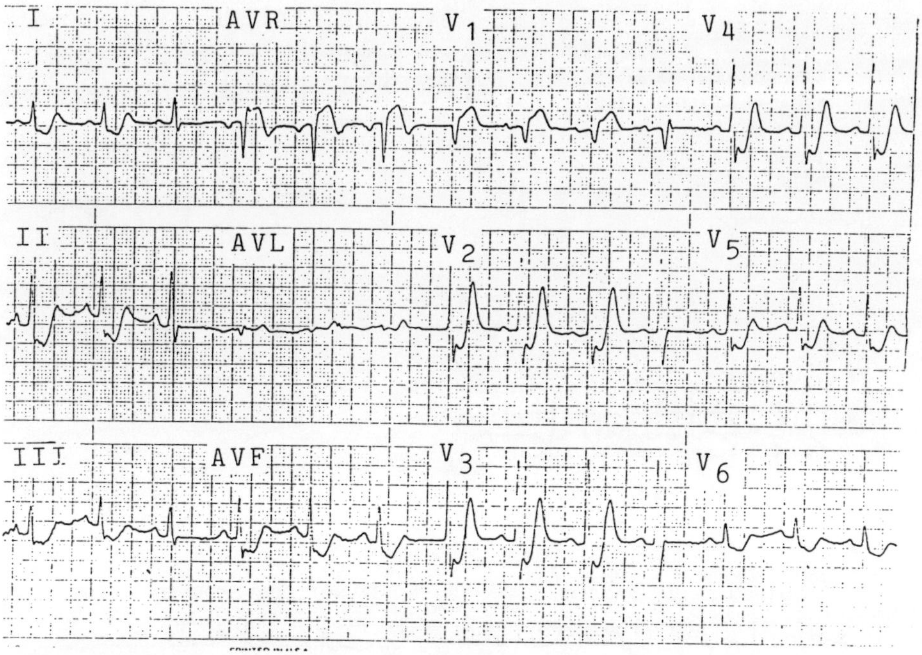

Fig. 3. 12-Lead 10 min post-exercise in a 69-year-old man.

thallium stress scan was obtained and was normal. The autopsy showed total atheromatous occlusion of the circumflex coronary artery. The heart weighed 400 gm and there was no evidence of muscle scarring.

Two other patients with known coronary artery disease had severe cardiac events while jogging. One, age 51 years, had a fatal cardiac arrest during this activity 16 months after an anterior wall myocardial infarction. He had been participating sporadically in a cardiac rehabilitation programme without symptoms, increasing his treadmill test time from 6.4 to 13.0 min (Bruce protocol) and lowering his serum cholesterol level from 250 to 203 mg/dl. The cause of death was attributed to a ventricular arrhythmia, without acute infarction, in the setting of underlying coronary artery disease.

Another patient with known coronary disease had a cardiac arrest while jogging on a beach. He was aged 56 and had had two prior heart attacks at ages 46 and 48. Cardiac catheterization was done a year prior to his arrest, and following a brief syncope episode in a gym, and showed total occlusion of the right coronary artery, a 90% occlusion of a large posterolateral branch of the circumflex coronary artery, and 50% narrowing of the left anterior descending artery, just beyond the first septal perforation. A ventriculogram revealed inferior akinesis and anteroapical hypokinesis. The ejection fraction was low at 25%.

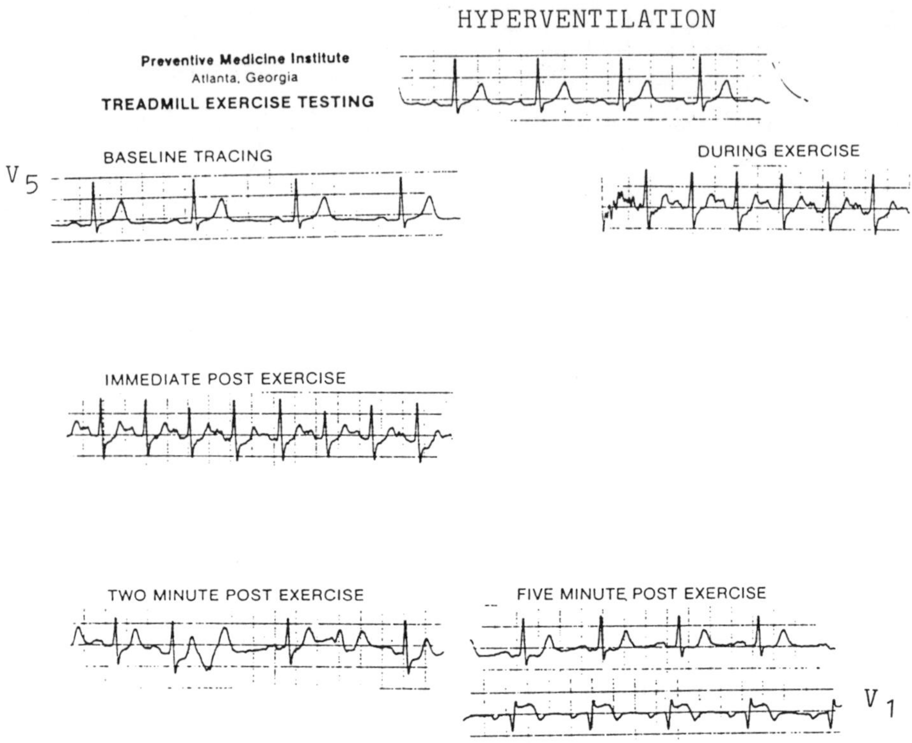

Fig. 4. ST-segment elevation in a 54-year-old man.

The patient continued to jog on his own, despite advice to the contrary. He was resuscitated from his cardiac arrest, with some difficulty, and suffered permanent damage to the central nervous system, requiring nursing home care. He died of a cardiac event in the nursing home 5 years after the arrest.

Cardiac events during cardiac rehabilitation

From 1970 to 1977, we had five cardiac arrests (Fig. 6) in 79,875 patient-hours of exercise, for an incidence of one per 15,975 patient-hours. All five events were primary ventricular fibrillation, without acute myocardial infarction, in patients with documented coronary heart disease. Prompt defibrillation was done and there were no deaths.

From 1980 to 1990, there were three events in 93,679 patient-hours of exercise. One was a case previously alluded to, with transient syncope and no documented arrhythmia. The second case was a 64-year-old man with a prior myocardial infarction and coronary bypass procedure (with plication of a ventricular aneurysm). He had participated in cardiac rehabilitation for 12

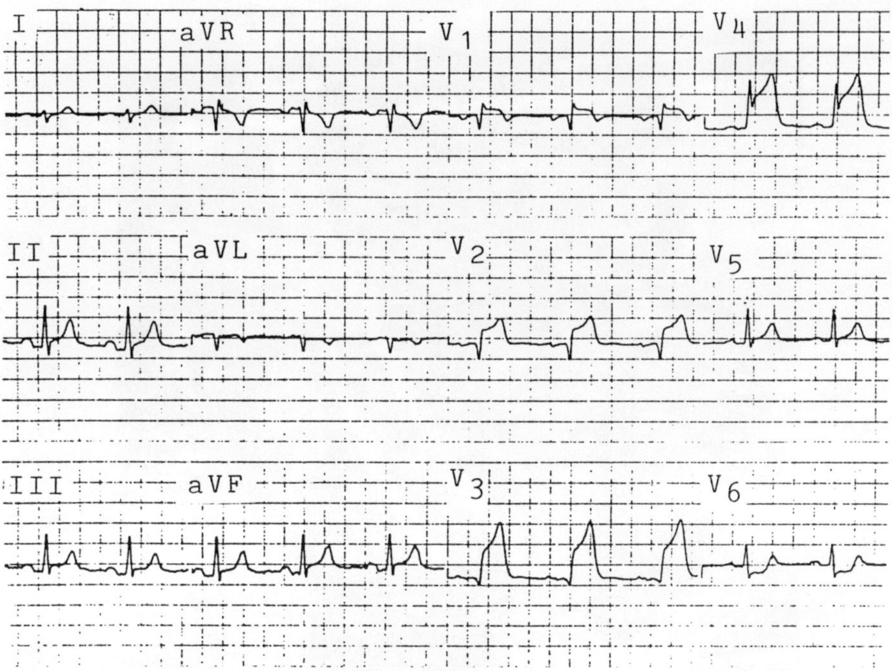

Fig. 5. 12-Lead ECG in a 54-year-old man.

years. During his usual 3-mile brisk walk, he suddenly collapsed. Cardiopulmonary resuscitation was begun and an ECG rhythm strip revealed ventricular fibrillation. He was successfully defibrillated and admitted to the hospital, where serial ECGs and enzyme levels did not show acute myocardial injury or infarction. Subsequent electrophysiology studies were performed and he was eventually treated with amiodarone. Unfortunately, he developed pulmonary complications from the drug and died as a result.

The third event occurred in a 49-year-old executive who had undergone an exercise test prior to entry into a corporate fitness programme. He had smoked for 22 pack-years and was taking clofibrate for an initial cholesterol level of 325 mg/dl. The treadmill ECG showed borderline ST-segment depression without symptoms. Because of the latter, his exercise was confined to a cardiac rehabilitation programme. Over an 8-month period, he had worked up to walking 1 mile, jogging a quarter of a mile and using the stationary bicycle for 15 min, three times per week. At the completion of a routine exercise session, the patient had come out of the shower area complaining of dizziness, sweating and chest discomfort. An electrocardiographic rhythm strip showed normal sinus rhythm. The patient's dull substernal discomfort seemed similar to his "oesophageal" pain, secondary to the oesophageal spasm diagnosed ten years earlier; however, while changing his clothes, he developed an exacerbation of

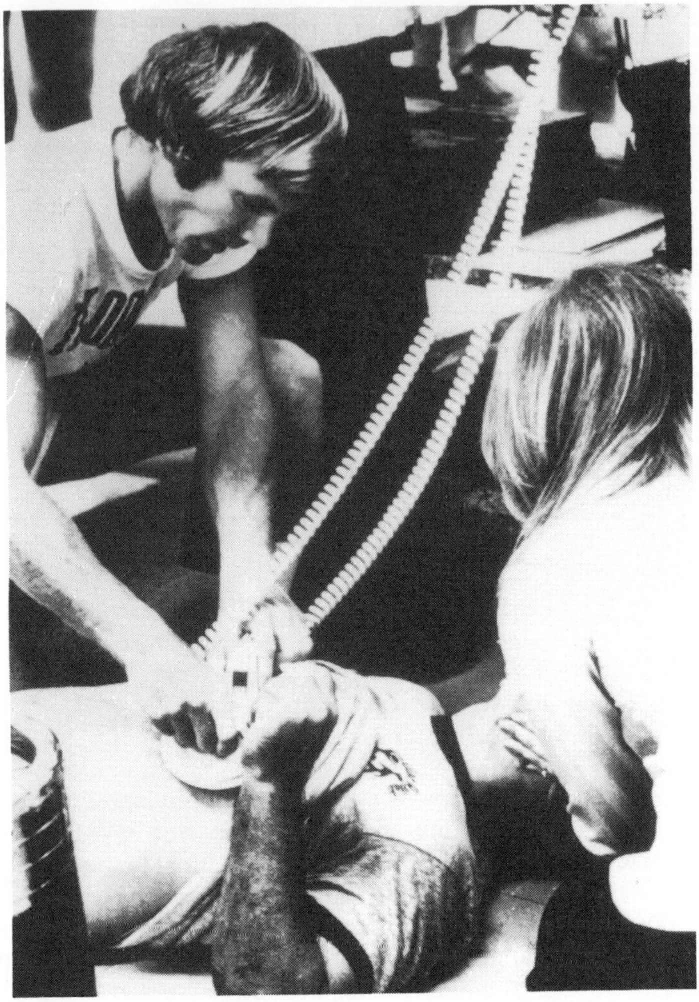

Fig. 6. Cardiac arrest during cardiac rehabilitation activity.

the chest pain. His blood pressure was difficult to obtain. Emergency treatment was initiated. The patient was transported to the hospital by ambulance, receiving cardiopulmonary resuscitation en route. He was pronounced dead at the hospital. An autopsy was not obtained.

Cardiac deaths during basketball games

Exercise-related sudden cardiac death is rare among young athletes. We investigated four such events which occurred in male basketball players in

Georgia, during the 1986–88 seasons. One occurred among approximately 13,500 high school athletes and two among approximately 1300 college athletes; one was a college student playing a pick-up game. Pre-participation screening failed to diagnose cardiac disease in three of the four athletes.

Case 1 was a 16-year-old black athlete who was 68 inches tall and weighed 169 lb. He became very tired and lethargic after a 90-min workout with his team. He complained of chest discomfort and then vomited and suddenly collapsed. The coach initiated resuscitative measures after a brief delay, to no avail. The autopsy showed anomalous origin of the left coronary artery (from the right rather than the left sinus of Valsalva). A flap-like ostium was also observed. The cause of death was attributed to an ischaemic-related arrhythmia caused by the patient's anomalous coronary artery.

Case 2 was a 19-year-old black man, 75 inches tall and weighing 200 lb, who suddenly became confused and collapsed at basketball practice. Cardiac resuscitation was unsuccessful. The autopsy showed hypertrophic cardiomyopathy with a cardiac weight of 520 g and a septal to left ventricular posterior wall ratio of 1:3.

Case 3 was an 18-year-old black athlete who collapsed and had seizures during a pick-up basketball game. Resuscitation measures were begun, after a brief delay, without benefit. Autopsy revealed a 600 g heart with a septal to left ventricular posterior wall ratio of 1:3. Muscular subaortic stenosis was observed, along with mitral valve prolapse. Microscopic examination showed disarray of the septal myocardial fibres.

The final case was a 20-year-old white man who suddenly collapsed while playing basketball with friends. He had a prior history of hyperlipidaemia and had undergone cardiac catheterization at age 15 because of a syncopal episode. He was told of moderate aortic stenosis and mild aortic regurgitation and was advised to discontinue participation in sports.

The autopsy showed advanced calcification of the aortic valve and involvement of the left coronary ostium. Sixty percent occlusions were noted in the LAD coronary artery and in the circumflex artery. The cause of death was attributed to an ischaemia-related arrhythmia brought on by his severe aortic stenosis and moderately advanced coronary disease.

Discussion

Our experience with cardiac complications during exercise testing is similar to data published elsewhere. In 1971, Rochmis and Blackburn [3] reported one death per 10,000 tests and a combined mortality–morbidity rate of only 4 per 10,000 tests. In 1980, Stuart and Ellestad [4] published the results of a national survey of exercise test facilities (518,448 tests in 11,375 centres). The mortality rate was 0.5 deaths per 10,000 tests and the combined mortality–morbidity rate was 8.86 per 10,000 tests. Cooper reported only five events in over 20,000 maximal treadmill tests; three were myocardial infarctions which occurred within 24 h of the test and two were instances of ventricular fibrillation related to the test, one reverting spontaneously and the other responding to defibrillation.

Our finding of only one cardiac event during exercise in apparently normal individuals emphasizes the safety of this activity when proper screening measures are conducted. It is possible that other events have occurred, but it is unlikely as such unexpected events are of such magnitude that the physician involved in clearing such a person for exercise is likely to be informed of the adverse outcome.

Gibbon *et al.* [5] reported a $5\frac{1}{2}$ year follow-up of 2935 apparently healthy adults engaged in physical training programmes. They noted only two non-fatal cardiac events in 374,798 person-hours of exercise (which included 1,308,610 miles run).

Participation in cardiac rehabilitation programmes appears to be getting safer. Haskell [6] surveyed 30 programmes between 1960 and 1977, noting an incidence of one cardiac arrest per 32,593 patient-hours, one fatality per 166,402 patient-hours and one myocardial infarction per 232,805 patient-hours. A subsequent survey by Van Camp and Peterson [7] reported data from 167 randomly selected programmes between 1980 and 1984. The rate of cardiac arrest was only 25% of that noted by Haskell and the rate of fatalities only 15%. Our results, comparing the 1970s with the 1980s, also reflects the lower risk of cardiac events, probably due to more aggressive management of patients with ischaemic heart disease (with medications, angioplasty and bypass surgery).

Exercise-related sudden cardiac deaths are fortunately rare in young athletes. Hypertrophic cardiomyopathy has been the leading cause in a prior report, and was the cause of death in half of our cases of young basketball players. The best screening is a careful history and physical examination, routinely checking to see if systolic murmurs increase with Valsalva's manoeuvre and/or with standing [8]. We also do ECGs on all Georgia Tech athletes, looking for inappropriate ventricular hypertrophy, repolarization abnormalities and abnormal Q-waves. When such are detected, we will follow up with echocardiograms. Others have looked at the cost-effectiveness of extensive screening in both white and black basketball players and have found it to be low [9].

Several thoughts come to mind, based on our experience, concerning the safety of exercise. Regarding exercise testing, most of the problems we encountered were in patients with proximal left anterior coronary lesions and atypical symptoms. We tend to be cautious in testing middle-aged people with such atypical symptoms, stopping the test early upon the first evidence of 1 mm ST-segment depression, a 10 mmHg fall in systolic blood pressure from baseline, or progressive chest pain. We are careful to watch for late recovery silent ischaemic events, and don't unhook patients from the ECG machine until the ST-segments are back to baseline. In view of the safety of exercise testing, we are considering the use of well-trained ancillary medical personnel (nurses, exercise technologists) to administer more tests, at lower cost, with availability of a physician in the near vicinity to respond to rare emergencies.

As for physical training, some tend to discourage screening exercise tests, except in those at highest risk. We would caution against this, for we know how safe exercise is when screening tests are done, but lack solid data as to the risk when they are omitted. Our approach is to do treadmill tests with all men aged 40 years and over, and women aged 50 and over, about to embark on an exercise programme more strenuous than walking. We test younger people who have multiple coronary risk factors, such as dyslipidaemia and cigarette smoking. We are also exploring ways, as previously mentioned, to reduce the cost of exercise testing.

In cardiac rehabilitation, we have been impressed with the importance and effectiveness of prompt defibrillation. All but one of our adverse events was ventricular fibrillation, without infarction, and responded to electrical shock. The one fatality was atypical – an acute MI with shock. On-site thrombolytic therapy, probably unnecessary given the proximity of the hospital, was the only therapy we didn't administer. We advise patients with known cardiac disease to avoid jogging in medically unsupervised programmes as this activity is harder to regulate (compared to walking) and environmental factors such as heat and humidity come into play. We also de-emphasize competition in our rehabilitation programme events.

In screening young athletes prior to their respective seasons, we emphasize a thorough history and physical. Too often, these are poorly done, in noisy athletic buildings, and one can miss the often subtle features of hypertrophic cardiomyopathy. When young athletes complain of angina-like pain, in the absence of familial hyperlipidaemia, we do further studies to exclude congenital coronary anomalies [10].

References

1. American College of Sports Medicine. Position Stand on Exercise and Coronary Artery Disease. 1992 (in press).
2. AHA Statement on Exercise. Benefits and recommendations for physical activity programs for all Americans. *Circulation* 1992; **86:** 340–344.
3. Rochmis P, Blackburn H. Exercise tests: A survey of procedures, safety, and litigation experience in approximately 170,000 tests. *JAMA* 1971; **217:** 1061–1066.
4. Stuart RJ, Jr, Ellstad MA. National survey of exercise stress testing facilities. *Chest* 1980; **77:** 94–97.
5. Gibbon LW, Cooper KH, Meyer BM *et al.* The acute cardiac risk of strenuous exercise. *JAMA* 1980; **244:** 1799–1801.
6. Haskell WL. Cardiovascular complications during exercise training of cardiac patients. *Circulation* 1978; **57:** 920–924.
7. Van Camp SP, Peterson RA. Cardiovascular complications of outpatient cardiac rehabilitation programs. *JAMA* 1986; **256:** 1160–1163.
8. Cantwell JD, Wilson KE, Thomas RJ. Hypertrophic cardiomyopathy. *Your Patient and Fitness* 1989; **3:** 12–22.
9. Epstein SE, Maron BJ. Sudden death and the competitive athlete: Perspectives on preparticipation screening studies. *J Am Coll Cardiol* 1986; **7:** 220–230.
10. Taylor AJ, Rogan KM, Virmani R. Sudden cardiac death associated with isolated congenital coronary artery anomalies. *J Am Coll Cardiol* 1992; **20:** 640–647.

16 Ratings of Perceived Exertion (RPE) in Cardiac Rehabilitation: Application and Validation

Robert J. Robertson*, Fredric L. Goss, Kenneth F. Metz

Human Energy Research Laboratory, Health and Physical Education, School of Education, University of Pittsburgh, Pittsburgh, PA 15261, USA

Introduction

This review examines scientific and clinical evidence that supports the use of exertional perceptions in cardiac exercise rehabilitation. Particular emphasis is placed on the validity of perceptual application during graded exercise testing and individualized exercise prescription. The clinical application of perceived exertion in conjunction with physiological responses such as oxygen uptake ($\dot{V}O_2$), heart rate and power output (*PO*) is also discussed.

Perceived exertion: Definition

The perception of physical exertion is defined as the subjective intensity of effort, stress, discomfort and/or fatigue that is experienced during exercise [1]. This definition presents a clear, concise and unequivocal description of those factors that influence the perceptual process during dynamic exercise. The definition also provides a cognitive reference for numerical and semantic assessments of exertional intensity, facilitating the generalizability of perceptual responses across clinical, research and sport settings. Patients, experimental

* Address all correspondence to Robert J. Robertson, 113 Trees Hall, University of Pittsburgh, Pittsburgh, PA 15261, USA.

Proceedings of the Vth World Congress on Cardiac Rehabilitation

subjects and sport participants should be thoroughly acquainted with the foregoing standard definition of perceived exertion before subjective measurements are used in exercise testing and prescription.

Scaling procedures

Exertional perceptions are typically assessed with a category rating scale [2]. The most frequently used category format is Borg's [3] RPE scale (Table 1). The RPE scale contains numbers ranging from 6 to 20 with essentially every other numerical category anchored by a verbal descriptor. During exercise, the patient responds with a numerical rating that corresponds to the perceived intensity of exertion experienced at the moment. The response is termed the rating of perceived exertion, (RPE). Two other commonly used scales having category properties are presented in Table 2. The C-R 10 scale [4] is formatted in categories but also has a zero point giving it restricted ratio properties. The nine-category PITT [5] scale positions verbal descriptors near the extremes of the perceptual response range. This scale was developed at the University of Pittsburgh in the late 1960s.

Perceptually based exercise tests

Graded exercise testing involves the gradual, progressive and systematic administration of an exercise stimulus to assess exertional tolerance in clinical,

Table 1
Fifteen category scale to rate perceptions of exertion (RPE)

6	No exertion at all
7	Extremely light
8	
9	Very light
10	
11	Light
12	
13	Somewhat hard
14	
15	Hard (heavy)
16	
17	Very hard
18	
19	Extremely hard
20	Maximal exertion

Reproduced from Borg[3] with permission.

Table 2
Psychophysical scale to rate perceptions of exertion (RPE)

(a) *Category-ratio scale of perceived exertion*		
0	Nothing at all	
0.5	Very, very weak	(just noticeable)
1	Very weak	
2	Weak	(light)
3	Moderate	
4	Somewhat strong	
5	Strong	(heavy)
6		
7	Very strong	
8		
9		
10	Very, very strong	(almost maximum)
*	Maximal	
(b) *Pittsburgh perceived exertion scale*		
1		
2	Not at all stressful	
3		
4		
5		
6		
7		
8	Very, very stressful	
9		

Part a) reproduced from Borg [4]; part b) reproduced from Robertson *et al.* [6].

research and sport settings. Ratings of perceived exertion are frequently used as an adjunct to standard physiological and clinical responses during a graded exercise test. In this review, clinical application of RPE will be examined using two methodologically similar testing protocols, i.e. a sub-maximal cycle ergometer test and a performance-based running test.

Cycle ergometre protocol

The Sjostrand cycle ergometre protocol systematically increases power output until the test termination criterion is attained [6]. Pedal rate is set at 50 rev/min and power output is incremented by 150–300 kgm/min (25–50 W) every 3 min. In the perceptual modification of this protocol, RPE is measured at the end of each 3-minute exercise stage [7]. The test is terminated when a predetermined RPE is attained, usually a 17 on the Borg scale. RPEs are then plotted as a function of *PO*, providing a reference line that depicts the relation between independent and dependent variables (Fig. 1). A horizontal line is drawn from

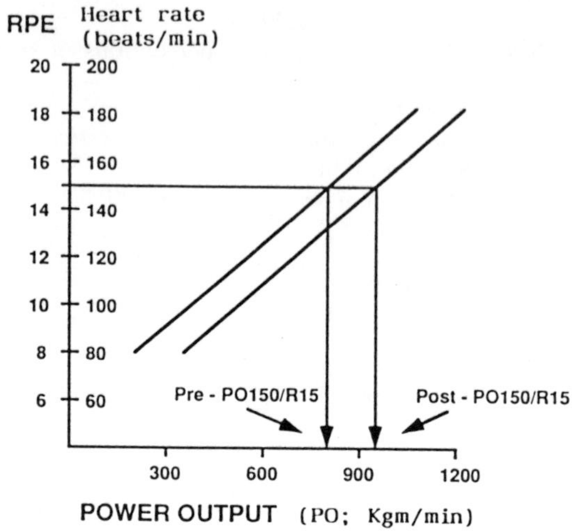

Fig. 1. Perceptually based cycle ergometer test to assess aerobic fitness. Pre-, pre-training; post-, post-training; *PO*/150/R15/ = power output at a heart rate of 150 beats/min and a RPE of 15.

the criterion RPE (i.e. 15) on the y-axis to the reference line. A vertical line is then drawn downward from the point of intersection on the reference line to the x-axis, where *PO* at an RPE of 15 is determined (i.e. PO_{R15}). The same procedure can be applied for any predetermined criterion RPE, i.e. 13, 15, 17.

The perceptually modified Sjostrand protocol can be administered prior to and following an aerobic training programme. Comparisons are made between the PO_R attained prior to and following training. A pre- to post-training increase in PO_R indicates an improvement in functional aerobic power.

Run test protocol

The perceptually based run test is a low-risk, sub-maximal evaluation that can be easily administered as part of a daily training programme to assess therapeutic progress and/or classify aerobic fitness [8]. The run test requires that three separate trials be performed at constant, self-selected velocities. During the first trial, the individual is instructed to run very slowly. In the second trial, the instructions require the individual to run somewhat faster but at a preferred pace. During the third trial, the individual is instructed to run somewhat faster than the previous trial. Normally, the distance for each test trial ranges from 600 to 1200 m. The test distance should be selected such that each trial is 3–5 min in duration, allowing sufficient time to achieve a physiological steady-state.

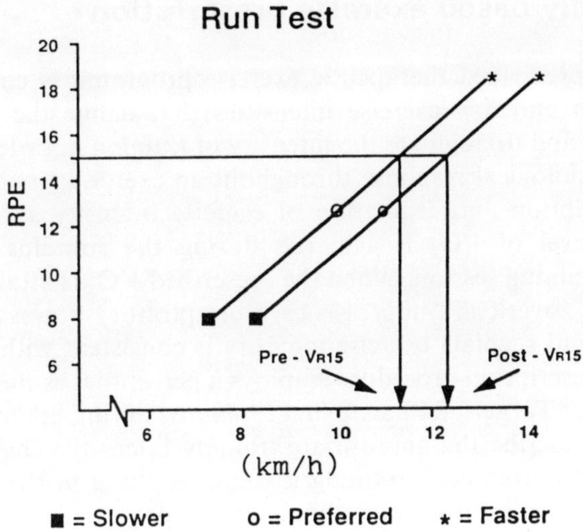

Fig. 2. Perceptually based run test to assess aerobic fitness. Pre-, pre-training; post-, post- training; V_{R15} = velocity of running at a RPE of 15.

The recovery period between test trials is 5 min. A measured running track or gymnasium floor provides the best setting to ensure that the requisite distance has been completed. Shorter lap distances allow more frequent measurement of RPE, reducing test variability.

RPE is determined at the end of each lap. The RPEs for the last two laps are averaged and used to compute test responses. Total time to complete the test distance is recorded and running velocity is calculated. RPEs from the three test trials are then plotted as a function of running velocity (Fig. 2). This procedure can be facilitated by using linear regression. The plotting procedure assumes that RPE is a linear function of the subjectively selected test speeds. A criterion RPE is then identified, usually 13, 15 or 17 on the Borg scale. A horizontal line is drawn from the criterion RPE on the y-axis to the reference line which depicts the relation between independent and dependent variables. A vertical line is then drawn downward from the point of intersection on the reference line to the x-axis, identifying the running velocity (i.e. V_R) that is equivalent to the criterion RPE. The faster the V_R, the higher is the individual's level of aerobic fitness.

The perceptually based run test can be administered immediately before and after a therapeutic training programme designed to improve functional aerobic power. The running velocity attained at the criterion RPE is compared between the pre- and post-training tests. A post-training increase in V_R indicates an improvement in functional aerobic power.

Perceptually based exercise prescription

Individually prescribed therapeutic exercise programmes employ RPE to (a) establish high and low exercise intensities that define the cardiorespiratory training zone and (b) regulate the intensity of training in order to maintain the "target" physiological response throughout an exercise session.

The prescription and regulation of exercise intensity assumes that a pre-determined level of $\dot{V}O_2$ is achieved during the stimulus portion of each therapeutic training session. When the prescribed $\dot{V}O_2$ is attained, the resulting physiological "overload" improves cardiorespiratory fitness. The use of RPE to prescribe and regulate exercise intensity is consistent with this assumption. The actual prescription procedure employs a perceptual estimation–production paradigm [9]. "Target" RPEs are first *estimated* during graded exercise testing in order to prescribe the appropriate training intensity. The target RPEs are then *produced* during each training session, resulting in the requisite physiological stimulus to improve functional aerobic power.

Prescription of exercise intensity

Training intensity is prescribed using RPE and $\dot{V}O_2$ responses to a graded exercise test (i.e. treadmill, cycle ergometer, arm ergometer). RPEs are estimated at the end of each test stage and are subsequently plotted against corresponding $\dot{V}O_2$, i.e. l/min, ml/kg/min or METs. (MET or metabolic equivalent: 1 MET = a $\dot{V}O_2$ of 3.5 ml/kg/min, i.e. the approximate resting $\dot{V}O_2$.) This provides a reference line depicting the relation between independent and dependent variables (Fig. 3). Maximal oxygen uptake ($\dot{V}O_2$ max) is identified as the highest $\dot{V}O_2$ achieved during the graded exercise test. The training zone to improve cardiorespiratory fitness typically ranges from 70 to 85% $\dot{V}O_2$ max [10]. The first step in the prescription process is to calculate the absolute $\dot{V}O_2$ (or METS) that corresponds to the low (i.e. 70% $\dot{V}O_2$ max) and high (i.e. 85% $\dot{V}O_2$ max) ends of the training zone. As shown in Fig. 3, lines are drawn vertically from these absolute $\dot{V}O_2$ levels on the x-axis to the reference line. Horizontal lines are then drawn from the points of intersection on the reference line to the y-axis. The intersection points on the y-axis identify the low and high "target" training RPEs.

Regulation of exercise intensity

Perceptual regulation of exercise intensity during therapeutic training uses a sensory production procedure. Target RPEs that have been estimated during testing are produced during each exercise session, providing an optimal physiological training stimulus. During training, the patient/participant is instructed to titrate exercise intensity (i.e. walk speed, run speed, pedal/crank *PO*) to produce exertional perceptions that fall between the low and high target RPEs. The target perceptual intensity is maintained throughout each therapeutic

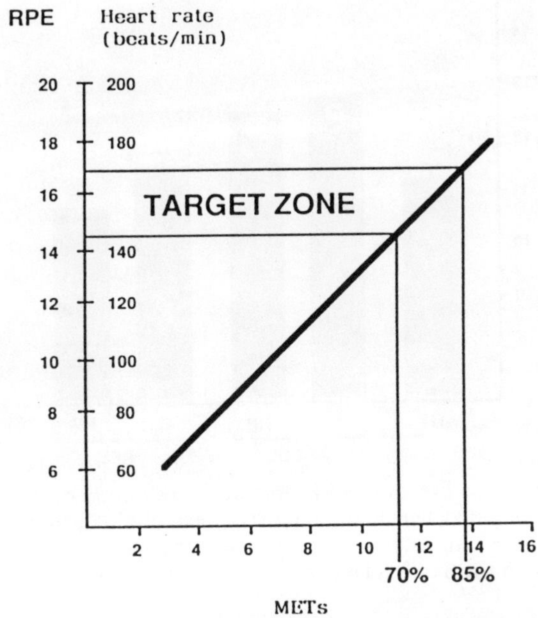

Fig. 3. Prescription of exercise intensity using "target" ratings of perceived exertion (RPE). METs = metabolic equivalents (1 MET = a $\dot{V}O_2$ of 3.5 ml/kg/min).

training session. As functional aerobic power (i.e. $\dot{V}O_2$ max) increases over the course of the training programme, the patient/participant exercises at progressively higher intensities in order to maintain the prescribed target RPEs. The physiological "overload" is correspondingly greater, producing an optimal stimulus to improve functional aerobic power as training adaptation occurs.

Cross-modal exercise prescription

Cross-modal generalization of a therapeutic exercise prescription is especially useful in cardiac rehabilitation and health/fitness programmes that employ *circuit-training* techniques to improve cardiorespiratory fitness. Circuit-training requires that the patient/participant exercise 3–6 min at each exercise station in a series of stations. A different exercise mode is performed at each station, i.e. treadmill, cycle ergometer, automated step, rowing machine, cross-country ski simulator. The exercise intensity that is undertaken at each station in the circuit is typically prescribed using treadmill test responses. It is assumed that the treadmill-based prescription generalizes to all other modes in the exercise circuit.

Cross-modal generalizability of an exercise prescription is valid when heart rate is used as the target physiological response to regulate training intensity [11]. Recent evidence by Robertson *et al.* indicates that cross-modal regulation of exercise intensity using a target RPE is also a physiologically valid procedure

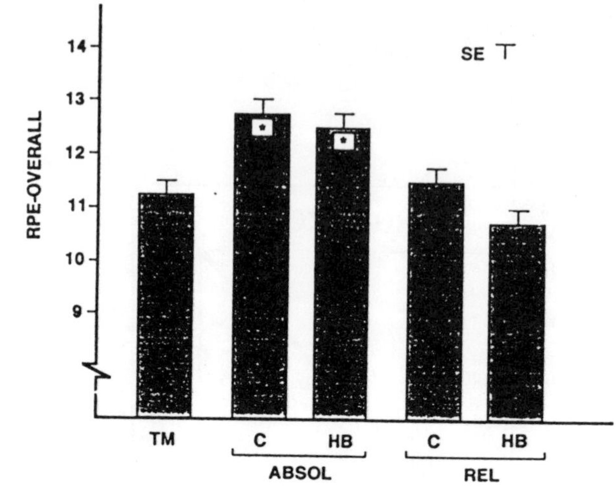

Fig. 4. Ratings of perceived exertion (RPE) for the overall body during treadmill (TM), cycle (C) and hand-weighted bench stepping (HB) exercise at absolute (ABSOL) and relative (REL) intensities. An asterisk indicates that the mean for that mode/intensity is higher ($P < 0.05$) than the treadmill mean. Reproduced from Robertson *et al.* [12] with permission.

[12]. In this experiment, the exercise prescription was derived from perceptual estimates during a graded treadmill test. Exercise training was undertaken using two different modes: (a) a stationary cycle ergometer and (b) rhythmical bench stepping while synchronously pumping light hand-held weights. The intensity of exercise during the testing mode (i.e. treadmill) and the two training modes (i.e. cycle and step/hand weights) was set at 70% of the mode-specific $\dot{V}O_2$ max. It was hypothesized that RPE at 70% $\dot{V}O_2$ max would not differ between the testing and training modes. This was the case. As shown in Fig. 4, RPE was the same during testing on a treadmill and training using a cycle ergometer and bench step with hand-held weights. The findings provide physiological validation of perceptually based cross-modal prescription of exercise intensity.

Conclusion

The experimental and empirical observations presented in this review indicate that ratings of perceived exertion are valid and easily applied measures to assess functional aerobic power and prescribe exercise intensity for clinically normal individuals and cardiac patients.

References

1. Robertson RJ, Falkel JE, Drash AL *et al.* Effect of blood pH on peripheral and central signals of perceived exertion. *Med Sci Sports Exercise* 1986; **18:** 114–122.

2. Goss FL, Robertson RJ, Auble TE *et al.* Are treadmill based exercise prescriptions generalizable to combined arm and leg exercise? *J Cardiopulmonary Rehab* 1987; **7:** 551–555.
3. Borg G. Psychophysical studies of effort and exertion: Some historical, theoretical and empirical aspects. In: Borg G, Ottoson D (eds), *The Perception of Exertion in Physical Work.* London: Macmillan, 1986, pp. 3–12.
4. Borg GAV. Psychophysical bases of perceived exertion. *Med Sci Sports* 1982; **14:** 377–381.
5. Pandolf KB. Advances in the study and application of perceived exertion. In: Terjung R (ed.), *Exercise and Sport Science Reviews*, Vol. 11. Philadephia: Franklin Institute Press, 1983, pp. 118–158.
6. Robertson RJ, Gillespie RL, McCarthy J, Rose KD. Differentiated perceptions of exertion: Part I. Mode of integration of regional signals. *Percept Motor Skills* 1979; **49:** 683–689.
7. Robertson RJ, Goss FL, Auble TE *et al.* Cross-modal exercise prescription at absolute and relative oxygen uptake using perceived exertion. *Med Sci Sports Exercise* 1990; **22:** 653–659.
8. Borg G, Karlsson J-G, Ekelund L-G. A comparison between two work tests controlled subjectively and by heart rate. In: Borg G (ed.) *Physical Work and Effort.* Oxford: Pergamon Press, 1977, pp. 239–254.
9. Borg G. Some studies of perceived exertion in sports. In: Borg G, Ottoson D (eds), *The Perception of Exertion in Physical Work.* London: Macmillan, 1986, pp. 293–302.
10. American College of Sports Medicine. *Guidelines for Graded Exercise Testing and Exercise Prescription*, 4th edn. Philadelphia: Lea and Febiger, 1991, pp. 97–105.
11. Sjostrand T. Changes in the respiratory organs of workmen at an ore smelting works. *Acta Med Scand* (Suppl.) 1947; **196:** 687–689.
12. Dunbar CC, Robertson RJ, Baun R *et al.* The validity of regulating exercise intensity by ratings of perceived exertion. *Med Sci Sports Exercise* 1992; **24:** 94–99.

V Ambulatory Monitoring in Rehabilitation

17 Precursors of Sudden Cardiac Death

Xavier Viñolas, Josep Guindo, Eduardo Homs, Miquel Dorado, Antonio Bayés de Luna*

Departamento de Cardiología y Cirugía Cardiovascular, Hospital de Sant Pau, Avd. S. Antonio Mª Claret, 167, 08025 Barcelona, Spain

Introduction

Of the different forms of cardiac death, sudden death stands out due to its dramatic presentation and its socio-economic implications. At present, the incidence of sudden death is decreasing in the USA and in other industrialized countries due to a progressive decline in the incidence of ischaemic heart disease, probably following changes in diet and lifestyle. Nevertheless, sudden cardiac death continues to be responsible for nearly 400,000 deaths per year in the USA and still represents a major challenge to contemporary cardiology.

There is no universally accepted definition of sudden death. The main difference between the different studies concerns the time determination between the initial symptoms and cardiac arrest, varying from 1 to 24 h after the onset of symptoms in the different studies. Ambulatory sudden cardiac death may be defined as death due to a natural cause (so excluding accidents, poisoning, etc.) occurring unexpectedly and instantaneously or within the first hour after the onset of premonitory symptoms.

Ischaemic heart disease is present in more than 80% of patients dying suddenly in the West [1]. Sudden death is the first manifestation of ischaemic heart disease in 20–25% of patients [2]. About 75% of those who die suddenly have an old myocardial infarction, and recent infarction is found in 20% of

*To whom all correspondence should be addressed.

Proceedings of the Vth World Congress on Cardiac Rehabilitation

patients [3]. Less frequently, sudden cardiac death occurs in patients with other heart diseases. The most frequent non-ischaemic aetiologies are: hypertrophic cardiomyopathy, valvular heart disease (aortic stenosis), long QT syndrome, Wolf-Parkinson-White, dilated cardiomyopathy, right ventricular dysplasia, congenital heart disease (after correction of Fallot's tetralogy, congenital coronary abnormalities, etc.), aortic dissecting aneurysm, etc. Only in a few cases is an underlying heart disease not present. Depending on the triggering mechanism, sudden death may be classified into two groups according to Hinkle and Thaler [4]: sudden death due to a primary arrhythmia and sudden death secondary to a haemodynamic catastrophe. In these latter cases, the terminal arrhythmia is only a manifestation of the circulatory catastrophe (cardiac tamponade, massive myocardial infarction, etc.). If the time interval between premonitory symptoms and cardiac arrest is 1 h, most out-of-hospital sudden deaths are due to a primary arrhythmia. For this reason, we prefer this short interval limit.

Sudden cardiac death: A multifactorial problem

Sudden cardiac death is a multifactorial problem, resulting from the interaction of multiple factors, some of which are well-known while others are only partially understood as yet. It is a multifactorial problem first of all because sudden death could be related to different terminal arrhythmias. In most cases, the final event is a ventricular tachycardia degenerating into ventricular fibrillation, but in other cases a bradyarrhythmia is responsible for the death. It is a multifactorial problem because it requires not only the presence of a vulnerable myocardium (e.g. a scar after myocardial infarction, left ventricular dysfunction, etc.), but also the presence of some triggering factors, as we will discuss later. The triggering mechanisms without a vulnerable myocardium, or a vulnerable myocardium without triggering mechanisms do not usually lead to a malignant arrhythmia. Finally, it is also a multifactorial problem from a physiopathological point of view. Really, we can consider that all the marker and trigger mechanisms depend upon three factors: left ventricular dysfunction, ischaemia

Table 1
Interactions between electrical instability and ischaemia

1. Ischaemia → electrical instability
   - (a) Slowing of conduction; prolonged recovery of excitability
   - (b) Changes in refractoriness (shorter than in normal myocytes)
   - (c) Refractoriness dispersion allowing re-entry
2. Electrical instability → ischaemia
   - (a) Decreased blood flow with rapid heart rate

Table 2
Interactions between left ventricular dysfunction and electrical instability

1. Left ventricular dysfunction → electrical instability
   (a) *Neurohumoral factors*
      - increased sympathetic activity
      - increase in epinephrine and norepinephrine levels
      - renin-angiotensin–aldosterone system activation
      - atrial natriuretic factor level increased
   (b) *Elecrolytic disturbances*
      - hypokalaemia
      - hyponatraemia
      - hypomagnesaemia
   (c) *Pro-arrhythmic effect of drugs*
      - anti-arrhythmic drugs
      - diuretics
      - digitalis
      - inotropics
   (d) *Morphofunctional factors*
      - anatomical block allowing re-entry
        – scar after myocardial infarction
        – left ventricular aneurysm
      - functional block
        – ischaemia and drugs
      - triggered activity
        – mechanical stretch of Purkinje and muscle fibres
2. Electrical instability → left ventricular dysfunction
   (a) haemodynamic disturbances with rapid heart rates
   (b) Loss of atrial activity

and electrical instability. Nevertheless, the importance of each factor differs depending on whether sudden death is related to a malignant ventricular arrhythmia or due to a bradyarrhythmia. As we can see in Tables 1–3, these three factors interact, and the modification of any one of them may alter the other two. Thus, sudden death seems to be the centre of an imaginary triangle where the three vertices are the previously described factors (Fig. 1).

We will discuss briefly the terminal events leading to sudden death as well as the mechanisms leading to a malignant ventricular arrhythmia or bradyarrhythmia.

Final events

Ventricular fibrillation (VF) is the event most frequently responsible for ambulatory sudden death. In the Miami Study of 352 patients who suffered an out-of-hospital cardiac arrest [5], 62% presented VF when first examined. Sustained ventricular tachycardia (VT) was found in 7% and bradyarrhythmias or asystole in 31% of cases.

Table 3
Interactions between left ventricular dysfunction and ischaemia

1. Left ventricular dysfunction → ischaemia	
(a)	Increased diastolic ventricular pressure produces reduced subendocardial coronary blood flow
(b)	Low cardiac output
(c)	Increased ischaemia during exercise
2. Ischaemia → left ventricular dysfunction	
(a)	Hibernating myocardium

Holter recordings have been particulary useful in providing information about the final event and the triggering mechanisms of ambulatory sudden death. In a study reviewing the Holter tapes of 233 patients who died suddenly while wearing a Holter device [1], we observed that approximately 80% of deaths were due to ventricular tachyarrhythmia (10% primary VF, 50% classical VT degenerating into VF, and 20% Torsades de Pointe) (Fig. 2). In the study of Adgey *et al.* [6], which reviewed the factors that predispose to VF in patients with acute ischaemic events, the incidence of primary VF was higher than in our study. This could be explained by the fact that in our study most patients did not present an acute ischaemic event preceding sudden death. The clinical characteristics of the group dying suddenly while wearing a Holter device [1] are shown in Table 4. In the group dying due to VT-VF, there was a high incidence of ischaemic heart disease and a low incidence of pro-arrhythmia. Before the final event, an increase in heart rate and supraventricular arrhythmias was observed. Evidence of ST alterations preceding the final event

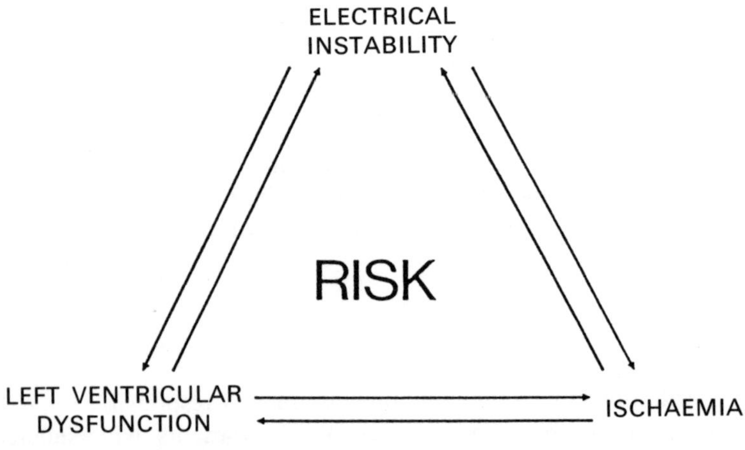

Fig. 1. Interactions between left ventricular dysfunction, electrical instability and ischaemia leading to sudden death. The interactions are bidirectional and can be direct or indirect via the other pathway.

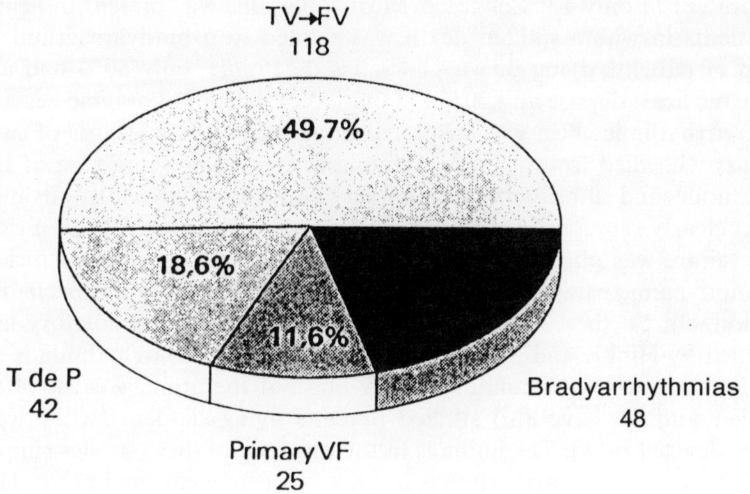

Fig. 2. Causes of ambulatory sudden death in patients dying while wearing a Holter device [1]. VT = ventricular tachycardia; VF = ventricular fibrillation; Primary VF = primitive ventricular fibrillation; T de P = Torsades de Pointe.

Table 4
Clinical characteristics of different groups of ambulatory sudden death

	Ventricular tachyarrhythmias		Bradyarrhythmias
	Group I (n = 143) VT-VF (%)	Group II (n = 42) T de P (%)	Group III (n = 48) (%)
Number of cases	61.3	18.6	20.1
Mean age (years)	70	60	70
Sex			
males	76	40	39
females	67	2	9
Coronary artery disease	84	50	70
No organic heart disease	4	22	10
Anti-arrhythmic treatment	63.8	76	?
ST modification	12	—	85
Pro-arrhythmia (probable)	10	66	20

Abbreviations: VT-VF = Classical ventricular tachycardia which triggers ventricular fibrillation, or primary ventricular fibrillation; T de P = Torsades de Pointe; ST modification = alterations of ST-segment suggesting an ischaemic event before the final event.

was present in only 12% of cases. Meanwhile, this was present in nearly 90% of patients in whom sudden death was related to a bradyarrhythmia. In the group of patients dying due to Torsades de Pointe, only 50% had a known ischaemic heart disease and 20% did not have evidence of organic heart disease. A pro-arrhythmic effect was suspected in as many as two-thirds of cases. The patients who died from a bradyarrhythmia (generally depression of the sino-atrial node and subsidiary automaticity, and less frequently advanced AV block) clearly represent a different sub-group of patients. A high incidence of heart failure was observed in this sub-group, as well as a higher incidence of "haemodynamic catastrophe" such as cardiac rupture, electromechanical dis-ociation, etc. So these cases correspond to death due to circulatory failure as classified by Hinkle and Thaler classification [4]. Bradyarrhythmia is only the manifestation of this circulatory failure and not the primary cause of death.

Other authors have also studied patients dying suddenly while wearing a Holter device [7–11]. The findings in the majority of these studies support also that ventricular tachyarrhythmias are the most frequent final event. However, in patients with advanced heart failure, as reported by Luu *et al.* [12], the incidence of bradyarrhythmia as the last cardiac rhythm before death is higher than in our study of ambulatory patients (61 *vs* 21%).

Sudden cardiac death due to ventricular arrhythmias

Concept of vulnerable myocardium and triggering factors

Sudden death related to malignant ventricular arrhythmias appears rarely in patients without underlying heart disease. Only 3.5% of patients dying suddenly present an ejection fraction >50% and non-significant coronary stenosis [13]. Nevertheless, 30% of these patients showed hypokinesia on left ventriculography, so patients with no evidence of cardiac abnormalities represent only 2%. Patients with wall motion or electrocardiographic abnormalities present a higher risk of recurrent cardiac arrest. The risk of recurrent cardiac arrest in a 5-year follow-up was 30% in patients with electrocardiographic abnormalities *vs* 5% in patients without. Thus, patients who present sudden death usually have a "vulnerable myocardium". If we speak about the most characteristic cases of sudden death, those related to the presence of ischaemic heart disease (especially post-myocardial infarction patients), this means a myocardium with different markers of vulnerability, that in the presence of some triggers may develop a ventricular tachycardia/ventricular fibrillation leading to sudden death.

Figure 3 shows the most important markers of a vulnerable myocardium and the most important triggers acting upon this vulnerable myocardium. The most important markers are represented by the presence of anatomic alterations (depressed left ventricular function), residual ischaemia and electrical instability. Electrical instability includes the presence of premature ventricular contractions, alterations to the autonomic nervous system (heart rate, heart rate

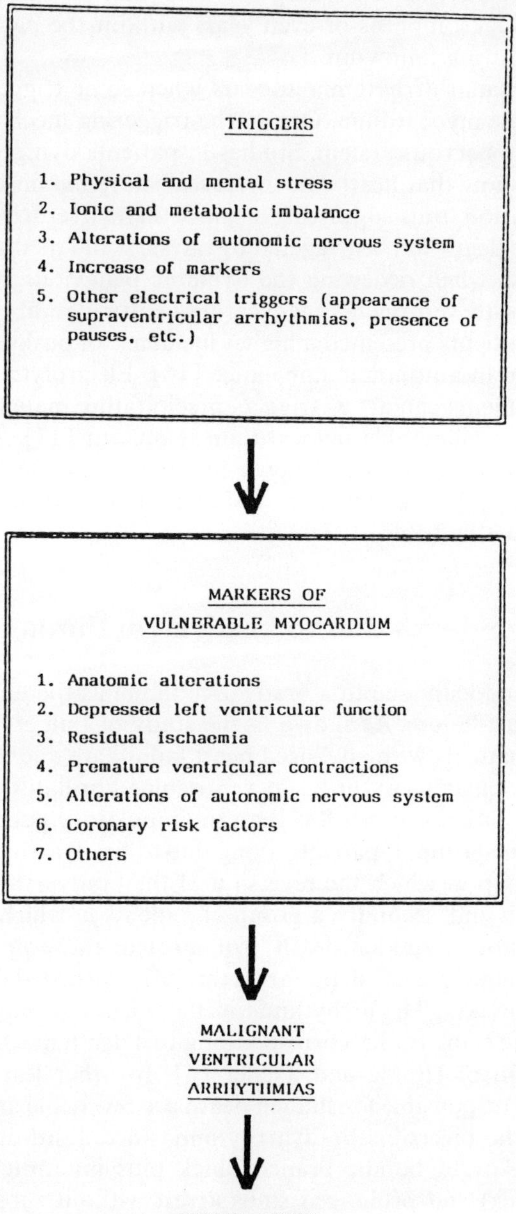

Fig. 3. The multifactorial problem of sudden cardiac death due to a malignant ventricular tachyarrhythmia in post-myocardial infarction patients. In the presence of a vulnerable myocardium, the triggering mechanisms lead to ventricular arrhythmias and sudden death.

variability, baroreflex sensitivity and QT interval) and changes in fibrillation threshold. Nevertheless, we must keep in mind that these markers may be present for days, weeks, months or even years without the patient having any arrhythmic event during follow-up.

Malignant ventricular arrhythmia appears when some triggering factor acts upon this vulnerable myocardium. One of the triggering mechanisms could be an alteration to the nervous system. Studies in patients dying while wearing a Holter device [1] show that heart rate increases before the onset of ventricular tachycardia/fibrillation, thus suggesting a sympathetic overdrive. It is also well known that sudden death can be triggered by physical and mental stress [14,15]. On the other hand, when reviewing the dynamic behaviour of QT in Holter tapes of patients with ventricular tachycardia/ventricular fibrillation, we observed that these patients presented a higher incidence of peaks of prolongation of QTc, suggesting an autonomic imbalance [16]. Electrolyte disturbances or metabolic derangements can act as triggers precipitating malignant ventricular arrhythmias when a vulnerable myocardium is present [17]. The significance of the other markers and triggers shown in Fig. 3 and the most important interactions between left ventricular dysfunction, electrical instability and ischaemia are shown in Tables 1–3.

Sudden cardiac death due to bradyarrhythmia

Patients who die suddenly due to a bradyarrhythmia as the final event usually have advanced heart failure. As shown in the study of Luu *et al.* [12], 61% of sudden deaths in patients with advanced heart failure are due to bradyarrhythmia (Fig. 4). Ventricular tachycardia or ventricular fibrillation represent 38% of deaths in these patients, much less than in ambulatory patients [1].

We can divide the group of patients dying due to bradyarrhythmias into two groups: first, a group in which the reversion of the bradyarrhythmia does not abort sudden death and, secondly, a group of patients in which recovery of the bradyarrhythmia aborts sudden death. For most of those in the first group, survival is very unlikely even if the arrhythmia is corrected, for example by implanting a pacemaker. The arrhythmia in these cases is only the expression of a haemodynamic catastrophe, corresponding to a death due to cardiac failure in the classification of Hinkle and Thaler [4]. In other less frequent cases, bradyarrhythmias responsible for sudden death are reversible and sudden death can be aborted. The reversible bradyarrhythmias are: third-degree AV block, trifascicular block (right bundle branch block plus intermitent anterior and posterior hemiblock) and prolonged sinus arrest without subsidiary rhythms. Vagal tone has a depressing effect on automaticity and/or conduction, leading to sinus arrest or AV block. All such situations could provoke syncope [18] and in some cases sudden death. Nevertheless, the patient usually is able to reach a hospital, the clinical situation is solved and sudden death may be aborted.

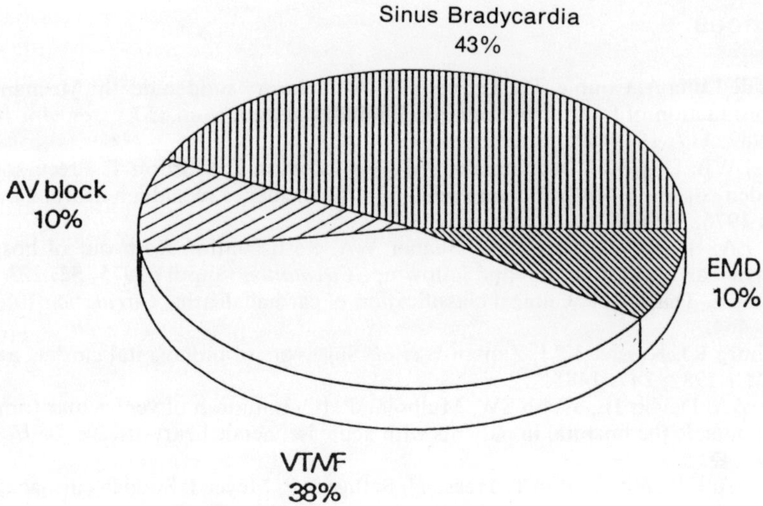

Fig. 4. Causes of sudden cardiac death in patients with advanced heart failure. EMD = electromechanical disociation; VT/VF = ventricular tachycardia/ventricular fibrillation; AV block = atrioventricular block. Adapted from Luu *et al.* [12].

Risk markers of ambulatory sudden death due to bradyarrhythmia differ from patient to patient. Left ventricular dysfunction and cardiac failure is the most important marker. Other factors such as ischaemia crises, extreme vagal tone and the administration of different drugs are particularly important as modulating and/or triggering mechanisms of malignant bradyarrhythmias. There is no doubt that acute myocardial ischaemia, when severe, transmural and prolonged, can induce slow rhythms, as seen in inferior myocardial infarction. Transient cardiac ischaemia (e.g. Prinzmetal's angina) may also trigger paroxysmal AV block and even sudden death. All anti-arrhythmic agents and some other cardiac drugs can also induce severe reversible bradyarrhythmias. In our experience, new ischaemic events are present in nearly 90% of patients dying due to a bradyarrhythmia.

We believe that malignant bradyarrhythmias could explain at least some of the cases of late pro-arrhythmia in the CAST study [19]. If all the deaths in the treated group of the CAST study were due to malignant ventricular arrhythmia, we would expect a greater incidence of hospital admittance due to sustained ventricular tachycardia in the flecainide/encainide group. We know now that this did not happen [20]. It would be also interesting to determine whether severe episodes of bradycardia or AV block were present in the last Holter recording in order to test this hypothesis. The occurrence of sudden death during the night would also suggest a bradycardia mechanism. We do not know how many of the CAST patients were admitted to hospital with sustained ventricular tachycardia [20], and many questions remain to be answered.

References

1. Bayés de Luna A, Coumel Ph, Leclercq JF. Ambulatory sudden death: Mechanisms of production of fatal arrhythmia on the basis of data from 157 cases. *Am Heart J* 1989; **117:** 151–159.
2. Kannel WB, Doyle JT, McNamara PM, Quinckenton P, Gordon T. Precursors of sudden coronary death: Factors related to the incidence of sudden death. *Circulation* 1975; **51:** 606.
3. Cobb LA, Baum RS, Alvarez H, Shaffer WA. Resuscitation from out of hospital ventricular fibrilation: 4 years' follow-up. *Circulation* (Suppl.) 1975; **52:** 223.
4. Hinkle LE, Thaler HT. Clinical classification of cardiac deaths. *Circulation* 1982; **3:** 457–464.
5. Myerburg RJ, Kessler KM, Zaman L *et al.* Survivors of prehospital cardiac arrest. *JAMA* 1982; **247:** 1485.
6. Adgey AA, Devlin JE, Webb SW, Mulholand HC. Initiation of ventricular fribrillation outside the hospital in patients with acute ischaemic heart disease. *Br Heart J* 1982; **47:** 55.
7. Olshausen KV, Witt T, Pop T, Treese N, Bethge KP, Meyer J. Sudden cardiac death while wearing a Holter monitor. *Am J Cardiol* 1991; **67:** 381.
8. Pepine CJ, Morganroth J, McDonald JT, Gottlieb SO. Sudden death during ambulatory monitoring. *Am J Cardiol* 1991; **68:** 785–788.
9. Gomes JA, Alexopulos D, Winters SL, Desmukh P, Fuster V, Suh K. The role of silent ischaemia, the arrhythmic substrate and the short long sequence in the genesis of sudden cardiac death. *J Am Coll Cardiol* 1989; **14:** 1618–1625.
10. Kempf FC, Josephson ME. Cardiac arrest recorded on ambulatory electrocardiograms. *Am J Cardiol* 1984; **53:** 1577–1582.
11. Leclerq JF, Coumel P, Maison-Blanche P *et al.* Mise en evidence des méchanismes déterminants de la mort subite. Enquete coopérative portant sur 69 cas enregistrés par la méthode de Holter. *Arch Mal Coeur* 1986; **79:** 1024–1033.
12. Luu M, Stevenson WG, Stevenson LW, Baron K, Walden J. Diverse mechanisms of unexpected cardiac arrest in advanced heart failure. *Circulation* 1989; **80:** 1675–1680.
13. Kudenchuk PJ, Cobb LA, Greene HL, Fahrenbruch CE, Sheehan FH. Late outcome of survivors of out-of-hospital cardiac arrest with left ventricular ejection fractions greater than or equal to 50% and without significant coronary artery narrowing. *Am J Cardiol* 1991; **67:** 704.
14. Lown B, Dasilva RA, Reich P, Murawsky B. Psychological factors in sudden cardiac death. *Am J Psych* 1980; **137;** 1325.
15. Carcía Sanchez S, Guindo J, Bayés de Luna A. Psychological stress and sudden cardiac death. In: Bayés de Luna A, Brugada P, Cosín J, Navarro Lopez F (eds.) *Sudden Cardiac Death.* Kluwer Academic: Dordrecht, 1990.
16. Martí V, Guindo J, Homs E, Viñolas X, Bayés de Luna A. Peaks of QTc lengthening measured in Holter recordings as a marker of life-threatening arrhythmias in post-myocardial infarction patients. *Am Heart J* (in press).
17. Hollenberg NK, Hollifield JW. Potassium magnesium depeletion: Is your patient at risk of sudden death? *Am J Med* 1987; **82:** 1.
18. Milstein S, Buetikofer J, Lesser J, Goldenberg IF, Benditt DG, Gornich C, Reyes WJ. Cardiac asystole: A manifestation of neurally mediated hypotension-bradycardia. *J Am Coll Cardiol* 1989; **14:** 1626.
19. Cardiac Arrhythmia Supression Trial (CAST) Investigators. Preliminary report: Effect of encainide and flecainide on mortality in a randomized trial of arrhythmia suppression after myocardial infarction. *N Engl J Med* 1989; **321:** 406–412.
20. Bigger JT. Implications of the Cardiac Arrhythmia Suppression Trial for anti-arrhythmic drug treatment. *Am J Cardiol* 1990; **65:** 3D.

18 The Use of Ambulatory ECG Monitoring in Cardiac Rehabilitation

Nanette K. Wenger

Department of Medicine, Division of Cardiology, Emory University School of Medicine, 69 Butler Street, SE, Atlanta, Georgia 30303 and Grady Memorial Hospital, Atlanta, Georgia, USA

Changes in the demographic characteristics of patients referred for rehabilitative care, as well as newly acquired information about exercise rehabilitation, have changed the role of ambulatory ECG monitoring in this setting. First, the widespread application of risk stratification procedures for coronary patients prior to discharge from the hospital has enabled the separation of high- and low-risk coronary patients. There has been consensus that low-risk patients do not require ECG monitoring during exercise training [2], and that most low-risk patients can safely exercise without supervision [1]. Second has been the documentation that modest-intensity exercise training can achieve comparable benefit to high-intensity physical activity. The lower exercise intensity engenders increased safety, particularly with unsupervised exercise, in that patients exercise farther from their ischaemic threshold; an increased exercise duration can compensate for the lowered intensity. The "Guidelines for Ambu latory Electrocardiography" [3], based on a Task Force Report of the American College of Cardiology and the American Heart Association, indicate that ambulatory electrocardiography is *not* indicated prior to enrollment in a cardiac rehabilitation programme. For most post-infarction or post-myocardial re vascularization patients entering an exercise training programme, 24 h electrocardiography appears to offer little or no information of value for clinical decision making.

However, concomitant expansion of the eligibility of patients for exercise rehabilitation has resulted in sizeable numbers of high-risk patients, previously excluded from exercise training, being enrolled in rehabilitative exercise training

Proceedings of the Vth World Congress on Cardiac Rehabilitation

regimens: elderly coronary patients and coronary patients with residual myocardial ischaemia, prior serious arrhythmias, and substantial ventricular dysfunction, albeit with compensated congestive cardiac failure. Ambulatory electrocardiography may provide particular benefit for these high-risk patients. Increasing numbers of patients with non-ischaemic ventricular dysfunction are also currently enrolled in exercise training programmes, owing to the demonstration that exercise training can improve their physical work capacity without associated deterioration of ventricular function. The optimal duration and intensity of their exercise surveillance (and ECG monitoring) has yet to be ascertained, although the occurrence of complications of exercise training has been surprisingly low. The same can be said for patients with prior serious arrhythmias unrelated to myocardial ischaemia.

The current major uses of ambulatory ECG recording in cardiac rehabilitation are (1) the evaluation of symptoms suggesting arrhythmia or myocardial ischaemia; (2) the evaluation of ECG-documentable therapeutic interventions in individual patients or groups of patients; (3) the evaluation of the ECG response to return to occupational or recreational activities, particularly after myocardial infarction, percutaneous transluminal coronary angioplasty or coronary artery bypass graft surgery; (4) the evaluation of clinical syndromes in situations where arrhythmia may increase the risk of sudden cardiac death; and (5) a variety of clinical and epidemiological research studies.

The major symptoms suggesting arrhythmia (palpitations; alterations of consciousness such as syncope, dizziness or lightheadedness; and less commonly atypical chest discomfort and/or dyspnoea) may have associated with them tachycardias, bradycardias, ectopic beats, or sinoatrial or atrioventricular conduction disturbances. Activity-precipitated arrhythmias are commonly detected with exercise testing, but the symptoms of arrhythmias precipitated by emotion or occurring at rest are more likely to be identified by ambulatory electrocardiography; the two methods of assessment are often complementary. Importantly, thc absence of concomitant arrhythmia requires evaluation for an alternative explanation for these symptons.

Increasing numbers of coronary patients with silent ischaemia [4] – which occurs more commonly in elderly patients, and in those with concomitant diabetes and hypertension – are now both identified and enrolled in exercise training regimens. In these coronary patients with asymptomatic ischaemia at exercise testing or with prior silent or unrecognized myocardial infarction, ambulatory ECG recording can evaluate the occurrence of silent ischaemia during exercise rehabilitation, suggest an intensity level of exercise training that can avoid this complication, and can guide the duration of required ECG surveillance. It can also document changes in the occurrence of silent ischaemia based on pharmacological and exercise interventions, as well as following myocardial revascularization. The occurrence of silent ischaemia at home, in the workplace or during recreational or leisure activities can be ascertained as patients resume their pre-illness lifestyles. Whereas exercise testing is superior to ambulatory ECG in documenting activity-precipitated ischaemia, ischaemic changes occurring at rest or precipitated by emotional factors are more likely to be identified by ambulatory electrocardiography; again, both studies are often complementary. Further, as patients improve their exercise tolerance with progressive exercise training, they may manifest myocardial ischaemia not evident at the low level of activity performed on their initial exercise test; ambulatory electrocardiography may help in the early detection of this problem.

To summarize, the identification of serious arrhythmias and/or silent ischaemia by ambulatory ECG recording, particularly in high-risk populations, can suggest the need for supervision and ECG monitoring of exercise rehabilitation, as well as suggest that interventions are warranted to prevent the occurrence of these complications during daily living, occupational or recreational activities. Serial ambulatory electrocardiography can define the response to therapeutic interventions, including the response to exercise training. The challenge to the clinician is to select those patients, typically at high risk and often symptomatic, likely to benefit from ambulatory ECG recording, given its costs and the requirements for trained personnel for its interpretation.

References

1. Van Camp FP, Peterson RA. Cardiovascular complications of outpatient cardiac rehabilitation programs. *JAMA* 1986; **256:** 1160–1163.
2. Williams RS, Miller H, Koisch FP Jr, Ribisl P, Graden H. Guidelines for unsupervised exercise in patients with ischemic heart disease. *J Card Rehab* 1981; **1:** 213–219.
3. ACC/AHA Task Force Report. Guidelines for Ambulatory Electrocardiography: A Report of the American College of Cardiology/American Heart Association Task Force on Assessment of Diagnostic and Therapeutic Cardiovascular Procedures (Subcommittee on Ambulatory Electrocardiography). *J Am Coll Cardiol* 1989; **13:** 249–258.
4. Rozanski A, Berman DS. Silent myocardial infarction. I. Pathophysiology, frequency of occurrences, and approaches toward detection. *Am Heart J* 1987; **114:** 615–638.

VI Silent Ischaemia

19 Long-Term Fate of Patients with Documented Myocardial Ischaemia and Total Occlusion of the Left Anterior Descending Coronary Artery

Yves Juillière[1], Nicolas Danchin*[1], Pierre-Yves Marie[1,2], Gilles Karcher[2], Alain Bertrand[2], François Cherrier[1]

[1]Department of Cardiology and [2]Department of Nuclear Medicine, CHU Nancy-Brabois, 54500 Vandoeuvre-lès-Nancy, France

Introduction

Numerous studies have shown that acute myocardial ischaemia results in severe left ventricular (LV) and right ventricular dysfunction [1–3]. Chronic myocardial ischaemia, whether symptomatic or clinically silent, can influence prognosis [3–6], but there is little information regarding its role in LV function. We studied a highly selected population of patients with total coronary occlusion and preserved left ventricular ejection fraction (LVEF) as a model of possible long-standing repeated myocardial ischaemia without interference of prior infarction or risk of subsequent infarction. The patients were followed for several years to determine by radionuclide studies (1) if myocardial ischaemia persisted at long-term follow-up and (2) what was the status of LV function after several years of persisting LV ischaemia.

Subjects and methods

Study patients

Of 7871 patients with coronary angiography between 1983 and 1987, a consecutive series of 24 with angina pectoris and no prior myocardial infarction

* To whom all correspondence should be addressed.

Proceedings of the Vth World Congress on Cardiac Rehabilitation

was selected because of the presence of a complete, isolated occlusion of the left anterior descending (LAD) coronary artery with collaterals from other coronary arteries. Of these 24 patients, 8 underwent myocardial revascularization (CABG 5 , PTCA 3) and were excluded from the study. Thus, the study population consisted of 16 medically treated patients (14 men, 2 women). At follow-up (December 1989), one patient had died (extracardiac cause) and one was lost to follow-up.

Initial cardiac catheterization

Left ventricular angiography was performed in the 30° right anterior oblique projection. Calculation of LVEF was based on the area–length method [7]. Collateral vessels visualized by selective coronary angiography with No 7 catheters, were scored by two independent observers according to the degree of opacification of the native vessel distal to its occlusion. Collateral vessels were assigned a numeric score between 0 and 3 according to the criteria of Cohen and Rentrop [8].

Follow-up stress tests protocol

Before stress tests were performed, all medications were stopped for 2 days. Upright cycle ergometer testing for exercise thallium-201 tomography and supine cycle ergometer testing for stress radionuclide LVEF were performed with 12-lead electrocardiographic monitoring at each minute of exercise and continuous monitoring of leads V1, V5 and aVF. The protocol started at 40 W and increased in increments of 30 W every 3 min. The exercise end-points were physical exhaustion, development of angina pectoris, sustained ventricular tachyarrhythmia or exertion hypotension. The stress ECG was considered positive if there was >2 mm ST-segment depression occurring 0.08 s after the J point on any of the surface electrocardiographic leads.

Thallium-201 imaging

At near maximal exercise, 1 mCi of thallium-201 per 25 kg body weight (without exceeding 3 mCi) was injected intravenously, and exercise was continued for an additional 1 min. The patients were imaged 10 min after stress; redistribution imaging was performed 4 h later and a second dose of 1 mCi of thallium-201 was reinjected to enhance detection of ischaemic viable myocardium [9]. Tomographic acquisition was performed using a rotating gamma camera equipped with a low-energy, general-purpose, parallel hole collimator. After reconstruction, the data were reorganized to contiguous short-axis, vertical long-axis and horizontal long-axis slices (8 mm thick) encompassing the left ventricle.

Analysis of thallium-201 tomograms

Stress and rest thallium-201 myocardial tomograms were divided into 20 sectors for each patient and assigned to five spaced regions. The anterior, septal, inferior and lateral regions were analysed in the apical, mid-ventricular and basal slices of the short-axis views; two apical sectors were studied on the mid-vertical long-axis slice [10]. All tomographic images were scored by two experienced observers [11].

Radionuclide LVEF

Multiple-gated equilibrium radionuclide studies were performed in the supine position using previously described techniques [12]. A dose of 20 mCi of technetium-99m was injected intravenously. The cardiac blood pool was imaged with a single crystal gamma camera interfaced to a computer system (Sopha-Medical). The camera head was oriented to maximize ventricular separation, usually with a 30–60° left anterior oblique orientation. The cardiac blood pool was imaged for 5 min at rest and during the last 2 mins of maximal exercise and 16 frames were obtained from the cardiac cycle.

Regions of interest and background regions were obtained using hand-drawn regions. Hand-drawn LVEF determinations were made by two independent observers who were blinded to each other's results as well as to the initial cine-angiographic results.

Statistical analysis

All values are presented as means ± standard deviations. The statistical analysis used Student's paired *t*-test for comparing resting radionuclide LVEF at baseline and follow-up. A p-value <0.05 was considered to be significant.

Results

Initial clinical and haemodynamic data

The mean age of the 14 patients was 59 ± 5 years at entry into the study. The mean duration of anginal symptoms was 27 ± 34 months. Except for the LAD occlusion, no patient had ≥50% stenosis in any of the other coronary vessels. Angiographic collateral circulation was well-developed in all patients. Mean cine-angiographic LVEF was 65 ± 6% (see Tables 1 and 2).

Follow-up and radionuclide data

The mean follow-up period was 48 ± 15 months. At follow-up, eight patients still had clinical chest pain. No Q-waves were present on resting ECGs. All but

Table 1
Individual clinical data at entry into the study (before catheterization) and at follow-up

Patient	Sex	Age (years)	Duration of AP before cath. (months)	Initial radio-nuclide LVEF	Follow-up (months)	CFC at follow-up	No. of anti-anginal medications at follow-up
1	F	57	3	—	78	atyp.	2
2	M	63	48	—	67	atyp.	2
3	M	59	19	64	65	I	2
4	M	58	12	—	64	0	0
5	M	65	3	60	57	0	1
6	M	54	7	—	47	0	0
7	M	55	1.5	66	46	II	2
8	M	54	108	56	42	I	2
9	M	62	12	—	39	atyp.	2
10	M	47	12	—	39	II	3
11	M	63	36	55	38	II	3
12	M	66	24	—	33	0	2
13	M	58	96	60	32	0	2
14	M	60	0.5	62	32	0	0

Abbreviations: AP, angina pectoris; atyp., atypical chest pain, LVEF, left ventricular ejection fraction; CFC, Canadian functional class of angina pectoris.

Table 2
Individual data for coronary angiography and left ventriculography at entry into the study

Patient	LAD segment	Collateral grading	No. of diseased LA wall segments (max. = 4)	LVEF (%)
1	distal	2	2	61
2	mid	2	0	55
3	proximal	2	2	73
4	proximal	2	1	59
5	mid	3	2	63
6	distal	2	1	60
7	mid	3	0	73
8	proximal	2	0	73
9	mid	3	0	69
10	distal	3	1	62
11	proximal	3	0	71
12	mid	3	1	68
13	mid	3	0	63
14	proximal	3	1	63

Abbreviations: LA, left anterior; LAD, left anterior descending coronary artery; LVEF, left ventricular ejection fraction.

Table 3
Individual data for exercise thallium-201 tomography and rest and stress radionuclide left ventricular ejection fraction

Patient	Stress test			No. of LA wall segments with stress defects (max. = 8)	Stress defects score	Reversibility (%)	Rest LVEF (%)	Stress LVEF (%)
	% TMHR	Pain	ECG					
1	91	−	−	0	0	—	61	64
2	75	−	−	1	2	100	58	—
3	75	−	−	0	0	—	61	65
4	87	−	−	0	0	—	61	58
5	100	−	−	0	0	—	56	60
6	96	−	−	1	3	100	61	67
7	77	+	+	2	3	100	65	59
8	77	+	+	1	2	100	63	57
9	100	−	−	1	2	100	62	57
10	78	+	+	4	3	50	61	57
11	67	+	+	3	2	100	60	—
12	66	−	−	1	3	0	57	57
13	97	−	−	3	3	100	55	60
14	75	−	−	0	0	—	60	74

Abbreviations: LA, left anterior; LVEF, left ventricular ejection fraction; % TMHR, % of theoretical maximal heart rate.

three patients were treated with anti-anginal medications. The exercise test was negative in 10 patients. However, thallium-201 tomography was normal in only five patients; it detected a moderate reversible anteroapical defect in seven cases and a mild persistent apical defect in two other cases (see Table 3). For technical reasons, two patients could not have radionuclide LVEF at stress. All patients had a normal LVEF at rest (mean 60 ± 3%) as well as a normal stress LVEF (mean 61 ± 5%). Resting regional wall motion was normal in all but three patients with a moderate anteroseptal hypokinesia without compensatory increase in wall motion in the non-ischaemic regions. No difference was seen in resting regional wall motion between baseline and follow-up in the seven patients who had two serial radionuclide studies. During exercise, six patients showed no increase in LVEF.

On the whole, at follow-up, four patients had no stress ischaemia, showing that the collateral circulation was sufficient to protect their myocardium. However, the remaining 10 patients had at least one sign of stress ischaemia and their resting LVEF at follow-up remained normal. Three of these patients were of particular interest: at follow-up, all three had unequivocal signs of persisting myocardial ischaemia despite which resting LVEF remained unchanged when compared with its baseline radionuclide value.

Discussion

Assessing the influence of repeated myocardial ischaemia on LV function in the long term is subject to several methodological difficulties, the most important of which is the possible occurrence of a myocardial infarction due to the acute closure of a coronary subtotal stenosis. To obtain a model of long-standing repeated myocardial ischaemia without the risk of subsequent myocardial infarction, we selected patients with isolated total LAD occlusion, who had not developed myocardial infarction at the time of occlusion.

Persistence of long-standing repeated myocardial ischaemia

In our patients, well-developed collateral vessels initially avoided the constitution of myocardial infarction at the time of occlusion and preserved LVEF [13–15]. It has been demonstrated by exercise thallium-201 tomography [16] that well-developed collateral vessels could provide at least relative protection from stress-induced ischaemia [17–19]. Our study showed that the functional significance of well-developed collaterals was different according to the individual patient, despite their similar angiographic appearance. Some patients still had angina pectoris; reversible myocardial defects were found in all but one of them; however, silent ischaemia was evidenced in three asymptomatic patients who also had reversible defects at stress [20]. Conversely, in four patients, collateral circulation was sufficient to avoid episodes of ischaemia.

Long-term evolution of LV function

Experimentally, Geft *et al.* [21] showed that repeated brief episodes of acute closure could cause myocardial necrosis in dogs. Schaper [22] performed myocardial biopsies during CABG in 40 patients with 75–100% occlusion of the LAD, no prior myocardial infarction and regional hypokinesia of the anterior wall. Compared with normal myocardium, the ischaemic areas showed ultrastructural alterations and more connective non-muscular tissue. Lastly, using biopsies during coronary artery bypass grafting, Hess *et al.* [23] studied 15 patients without prior myocardial infarction and normal resting LV function. In the areas exhibiting exercise-induced wall motion abnormalities before CABG, they noted muscle fibre hypertrophy and an increased mass of interstitial tissue. Interestingly, however, compensatory hypertrophy and increased interstitial tissue were also found in non-ischaemic areas, testifying to adaptive mechanisms in these segments [23].

Compared with these data, our study failed to show any deterioration in LVEF, even after several years. It seems quite probable, therefore, that ultrastructural alterations of ischaemic myocardium do not have any clinical relevance as regards LVEF.

Conclusion

Well-developed coronary collaterals may preserve LVEF both at the time of coronary occlusion and at long-term follow-up, despite the persistence of clinical ischaemia. These findings are observed both for silent and symptomatic myocardial ischaemia.

References

1. Iskandrian AS, Hakki AH. Left ventricular function in patients with coronary heart disease in the presence or absence of angina pectoris during exercise radionuclide ventriculography. *Am J Cardiol* 1984; **53:** 1239–1243.
2. Bertrand ME, Lablanche JM, Fourrier JL, Traisnel G, Mirsky I. Left ventricular systolic and diastolic function during acute coronary artery balloon occlusion in humans. *J Am Coll Cardiol* 1988; **12:** 341–347.
3. Danchin N, Juillière Y, Schrijen F, Cherrier F. Differential effects on right ventricular function of transient right, left anterior descending and left circumflex coronary occlusions during percutaneous transluminal coronary angioplasty. *J Am Coll Cardiol* 1991; **18:** 437–442.
4. Theroux P, Waters DD, Halphen C, Debaisieux JC, Mizgala HF. Prognostic value of exercise testing soon after myocardial infarction. *N Engl J Med* 1979; **301:** 341–345.
5. Deedwania PC, Carbajal EV. Silent ischaemia during daily life is an independent predictor of mortality in stable angina. *Circulation* 1990; **81:** 748–756.

6. Fleg JL, Gerstenblith G, Zonderman AB, *et al.* Prevalence and prognostic significance of exercise-induced silent myocardial ischaemia detected by thallium scintigraphy and electrocardiography in asymptomatic volunteers. *Circulation* 1990; **81:** 428–436.
7. Dodge HT, Sandler H, Baxley WA, Hawley RR. Usefulness and limitations of radiographic methods for determining left ventricular volumes. *Am J Cardiol* 1966; **18:** 10–24.
8. Cohen M, Rentrop KP. Limitations of myocardial ischaemia by collateral circulation during sudden controlled coronary occlusion in human subjects: A prospective study. *Circulation* 1986; **74:** 973–979.
9. Dilsizian V, Rocco TP, Freedman NMT, Leon MB, Bonow RO. Enhanced detection of ischaemic but viable myocardium by the reinjection of thallium after stress-redistribution imaging. *N Engl J Med* 1990; **323:** 141–146.
10. Yang LD, Berman DS, Kiat H, Resser KJ, Friedman JD, Rozanski A, Maddahi J. The frequency of late reversibility in SPECT thallium-201 stress-redistribution studies. *J Am Coll Cardiol* 1990; **15:** 334–340.
11. Kiat H, Berman DS, Maddahi J, Yang LD, Train K van, Rozanski A, Friedman J. Late reversibility of tomographic myocardial thallium-201 defects: An accurate marker of myocardial viability. *J Am Coll Cardiol* 1988; **12:** 1456–1463.
12. Pavel DG, Zimmer M, Patterson VN. *In vivo* labelling of red blood cells with Tc99m: A new approach to blood pool visualization. *J Nucl Med* 1977; **18:** 305–308.
13. Juillière Y, Danchin N, Grentzinger A, Suty-Selton C, Lethor JP, Courtalon T, Pernot C, Cherrier F. Role of previous angina pectoris and collateral flow to preserve left ventricular function in the presence or absence of myocardial infarction in isolated total occlusion of the left anterior descending coronary artery. *Am J Cardiol* 1990; **65:** 277–281.
14. Danchin N, Oswald T, Voiriot P, Juillière Y, Cherrier F. Significance of spontaneous obstruction of high degree coronary artery stenoses between diagnostic angiography and later percutaneous transluminal coronary angioplasty. *Am J Cardiol* 1989; **63:** 660–662.
15. Rentrop KP, Thornton JC, Feit F, Van Buskirk M. Determinants and protective potential of coronary arterial collaterals as assessed by an angiographic model. *Am J Cardiol* 1988; **61:** 677–684.
16. Berger BC, Watson VD, Taylor GJ, Burwell LR, Martin RP, Beller GA. Effect of coronary collateral circulation on regional myocardial perfusion assessed by quantitative thallium-201 scintigraphy. *Am J Cardiol* 1980; **46:** 365–370.
17. Rigo P, Becker LC, Griffith LSC, Alderson PO, Bailey IK, Pitt B, Burow RD, Wagner HN. Influence of coronary collateral vessels on the results of thallium-201 myocardial stress imaging. *Am J Cardiol* 1979; **44:** 452–458.
18. Tubau JF, Chaitman BR, Bourassa MG, Lesperance J, Dupras G. Importance of coronary collateral circulation in interpreting exercise test results. *Am J Cardiol* 1981; **47:** 27–32.
19. Blood DK, McCarthy DM, Sciacca RR, Cannon PJ. Single dose myocardial perfusion imaging with thallium-201: Application in patients with nondiagnostic electrocardiographic stress tests. *Am J Cardiol* 1979; **43:** 899–906.
20. Hecht HS, Shaw RE, Bruce T, Myler RK. Silent ischaemia: Evaluation by exercise and redistribution tomographic thallium-201 myocardial imaging. *J Am Coll Cardiol* 1989; **14:** 895–900.
21. Geft IL, Fishbein MC, Ninomiya K *et al.* Intermittent brief periods of ischaemia have a cumulative effect and may cause myocardial necrosis. *Circulation* 1982; **66:** 1150–1153.
22. Schaper J. Effects of multiple ischaemic events on human myocardium: An ultrastructural study. *Eur Heart J (Suppl.)* 1988; **9:** 141–149.
23. Hess OM, Schneider J, Nonogi H *et al.* Myocardial structure in patients with exercise-induced ischaemia. *Circulation* 1988; **77:** 967–977.

20 Regional Diastolic Dysfunction During Exercise-induced Ischaemia: Influence of Myocardial Structure

Otto M. Hess,* Juerg Traber, Otto N. Krogmann, Markus Jakob, Jakob Schneider, Marko Turina, Hans P. Krayenbuehl

Department of Internal Medicine, Cardiology, Institute of Pathology and Clinic of Cardiovascular Surgery, University Hospital, CH-8091 Zurich, Switzerland

Introduction

Left ventricular systolic dysfunction has been observed in patients with coronary artery disease during acute myocardial ischaemia. However, little is known about the influence of recurrent ischaemia on left ventricular (LV) diastolic function in the absence of acute myocardial infarction. Previous investigations [1–3] have shown that myocardial fibrosis is increased in permanently and transiently hypokinetic regions of the left ventricle. Thus, the purpose of the present study was (a) to evaluate the influence of exercise on regional diastolic function in patients with coronary artery disease (CAD) before and after successful revascularization and (b) to assess whether the structural alterations seen with recurrent myocardial ischaemia influence adversely the passive elastic properties of the left ventricle.

Subjects and methods

Twenty patients with either normal ($n = 7$) or stenotic coronary arteries ($n = 13$) were included in the present analysis. Patients with coronary artery disease who underwent an exercise test during cardiac catheterization were selected on a

* To whom all correspondence should be addressed.

Proceedings of the Vth World Congress on Cardiac Rehabilitation

Table 1
Haemodynamic data for controls and patients with coronary artery disease (CAD) at rest and during exercise[a]

		No. of subjects	LVEDP (mmHg)	LVSP (mmHg)	LVEF (%)	EDVI (ml/m^2)	Workload (W)	Duration (min)
Controls	Rest	7	20 ± 6	130 ± 29	61 ± 5	94 ± 5		
	Exercise	7	24 ± 7	154 ± 25**	68 ± 8*	97 ± 8	93 ± 37	2.0 ± 0.3
CAD[a]			*		**			
pre	Rest	13	23 ± 9	139 ± 29	58 ± 4	99 ± 17		
	Exercise	13	38 ± 15**	153 ± 22*	49 ± 10**	101 ± 24	88 ± 27	3.0 ± 0
post	Rest	7	19 ± 5	*131 ± 12	* 62 ± 11	99 ± 19		
	Exercise	7	30 ± 12**	173 ± 5 **	61 ± 9	112 ± 17	94 ± 29	3.0 ± 0

[a] Patients with CAD were studied before (pre-) and 7.7 months after (post-) successful bypass surgery.
Abbreviations: LVEDP, LV end-diastolic pressure; LVSP, LV peak systolic pressure; EDVI, LV end-diastolic volume.
* $P < 0.05$; ** $P < 0.01$.

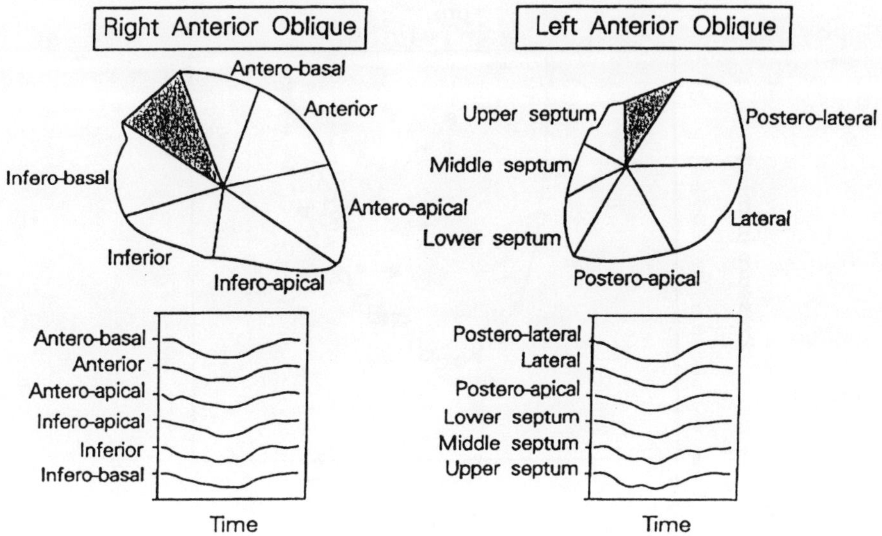

Fig. 1. Regional analysis of LV angiograms in the right and left anterior oblique projection. Six regions (excluding the aortic valve) are analysed for each projection on a frame-by-frame basis. The areas of these regions are determined quantitatively and plotted *vs* time (lower panels).

consecutive basis; patients with previous myocardial infarction were excluded from the study. LV function was evaluated from simultaneous high-fidelity pressure and biplane angiographic measurements at rest and during supine bicycle exercise. Mean workload and mean exercise duration were similar in controls and patients with coronary artery disease (Table 1). Seven of the 13 patients with coronary artery disease were restudied 7.7 ± 3.9 months after successful bypass grafting.

LV chamber volume was determined from biplane LV angiography using the "area–length" method. LV end-diastolic and end-systolic volume as well as LV ejection fraction (LVEF) were calculated at rest and during bicycle exercise. The time constant of relaxation (τ, ms) and the pressure intercept (Pb, mmHg) were calculated during isovolumic relaxation using a linear regression analysis between LV pressure and neg. dP/dt [4]. Early (PFR_1) and late (PFR_2) peak diastolic filling rates were measured from biplane LV angiography using a frame-by-frame analysis (20-ms intervals).

Regional chamber stiffness was determined in six regions of both the left and right anterior oblique (LAO and RAO) projections (Fig. 1) using the diastolic pressure–area relationship (Fig. 2). The constant of regional chamber stiffness (b^*) was calculated from a three-constant model with shifting asymptote:

$$P = ae^{b^*A} + c$$

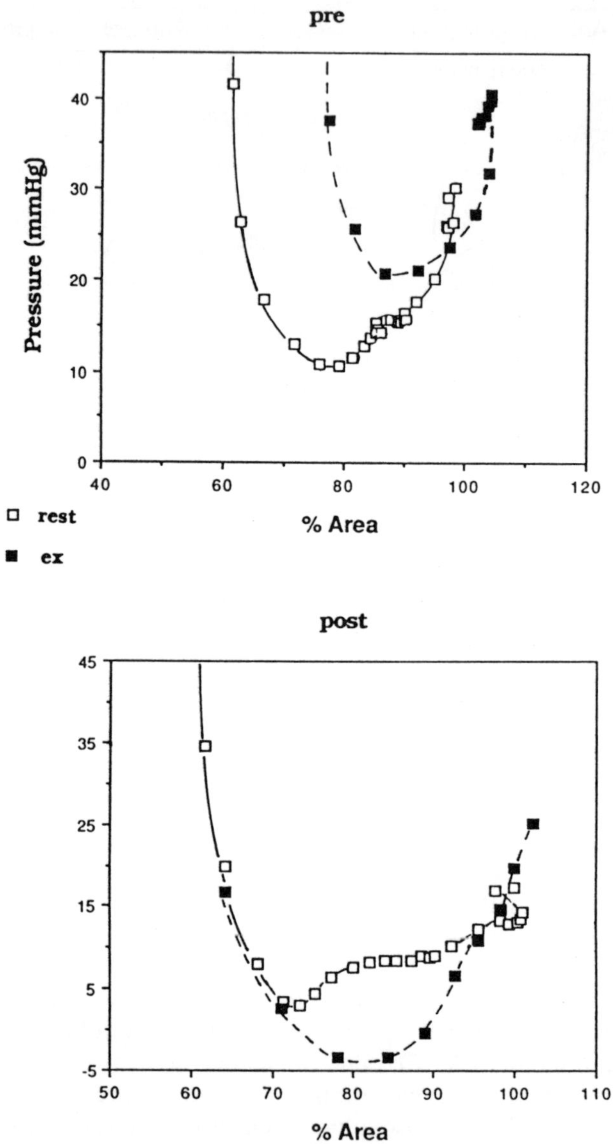

Fig. 2. LV pressure–area relationship of the hypokinetic region in a patient with coronary artery disease before (left) and after (right) bypass surgery. Please note that pre-operatively (pre) the curve is shifted upwards and to the right during exercise (closed squares) but shows a more complete relaxation with a decrease in the lowest diastolic pressure after surgery (post). Area is given in percent of end-diastolic area at rest. □, rest; ■, exercise.

where P = LV pressure (mmHg), a = intercept (mmHg), e = basis of the natural logarithm, b^* = slope of the pressure-area relationship (constant of regional chamber stiffness), A = area, (given as % of the end-diastolic area), and c = asymptote (mmHg). The three constants a, b^* and c were calculated using an iteration procedure [4]. A "normokinetic" zone was defined as region which showed an increase in regional ejection fraction during exercise or at least remained unchanged. A "hypokinetic" zone was defined as a region which showed a decrease in regional ejection fraction during exercise. The hypokinetic zone in CAD patients was usually located over the anterolateral (RAO projection) and the normokinetic zone over the posterolateral (LAO projection) region of the left ventricle (Fig. 1). The same regions were used for quantitative evaluation of regional chamber stiffness in control patients and in post-operative patients with CAD.

Transmural LV biopsies were taken during open heart surgery from the same two (normo- and hypokinetic) regions of the left ventricle using a schematic drawing as a guide for the surgeon. Quantitative evaluation of LV biopsies included determination of interstitial non-muscular tissue and LV muscle fibre diameter in the endo- and epicardial half of the biopsy whenever possible (10 of 13 samples).

Results

In CAD patients, LV end-diastolic pressure rose significantly from 23 to 38 mmHg during exercise, whereas LVEF fell from 58 to 49% ($P < 0.001$). LV peak systolic pressure increased during exercise in both the controls and CAD patients, whereas LV end-diastolic volume remained unchanged. After bypass surgery, LV end-diastolic pressure increased slightly but significantly during exercise, whereas LVEF remained unchanged (Table 1).

The time constant of relaxation (τ) decreased in both groups during exercise but was significantly larger during exercise in CAD patients than in controls (Table 2). Early (PFR_1) and late (PFR_2) peak filling rate increased in both groups during exercise but did not show any significant differences. Regional chamber stiffness increased significantly during exercise in controls in both evaluated regions. In CAD patients, regional stiffness increased significantly in the hypokinetic (from 0.07 to 0.21) but not in the normokinetic region (from 0.08 to 0.14). Moreover, regional chamber stiffness of the hypokinetic zone was significantly higher during exercise in the CAD patients than in the corresponding regions of the control patients (Fig. 3). Post-operatively, regional stiffness remained unchanged at rest and during exercise in both normo- and hypokinetic regions.

Interstitial fibrosis (Fig. 4) was significantly enhanced in the subendocardial layers of the transiently ischaemic myocardium (21 *vs* 16%, $P < 0.025$) but was not different in the epicardial layers. LV muscle fibre diameter was similar in the hypo- as well as normokinetic region of the left ventricle and did not show a difference between endo- and epicardial layers.

Table 2
Diastolic Function data for controls and patients with coronary artery disease (CAD) at rest and during supine bicycle exercise[a]

		No. of subjects	Relaxation τ (ms)	Relaxation P_b (mmHg)	Normokinetic region PFR_1 (cm^2/s)	Normokinetic region PFR_2 (cm^2/s)	Normokinetic region b^*	Normokinetic region c (mmHg)	Hypokinetic region PFR_1 (cm^2/s)	Hypokinetic region PFR_2 (cm^2/s)	Hypokinetic region b^*	Hypokinetic region c (mmHg)
Controls	Rest	7	52 ± 10	0.1 ± 8	16 ± 6	7 ± 4	0.04 ± 0.02	2.3 ± 8.4	10 ± 5	8 ± 1	0.04 ± 0.03	4 ± 8
	Exercise	7	30 ± 15**	14 ± 17	17 ± 7	12 ± 6	0.07 ± 0.03*	1.7 ± 6.2	18 ± 8	17 ± 6	0.09 ± 0.05*	5 ± 4
CAD[a]												
pre	Rest	13	58 ± 10	-4 ± 19	10 ± 6	5 ± 2	0.08 ± 0.06	3.0 ± 8.9	8 ± 5	7 ± 3	0.07 ± 0.05	2 ± 10
	Exercise	13	48 ± 12**	-4 ± 21	14 ± 8	8 ± 4	0.14 ± 0.10	$3.2 + 15.4$	14 ± 5	9 ± 4	0.21 ± 0.15**	9 ± 11
post	Rest	7	60 ± 12	1 ± 31	10 ± 5	7 ± 2	0.07 ± 0.03	2.7 ± 5.7	10 ± 6	7 ± 2	0.09 ± 0.05	1 ± 7
	Exercise	7	44 ± 20	10 ± 54	11 ± 8	8 ± 5	0.09 ± 0.06	-1.5 ± 8.2	14 ± 6	9 ± 3	0.13 ± 0.1	-3 ± 9

(Hypokinetic b^*: Controls Exercise vs CAD pre Exercise *)

[a] Patients with CAD were studied before (pre) and after (post) bypass surgery.
Abbreviations: τ, time constant of relaxation; P_b, pressure intercept; PFR_1, PFR_2, early and late peak diastolic filling rates; b^*, constant of regional chamber stiffness; c, asymptote.
*$P < 0.05$; **$P < 0.01$.

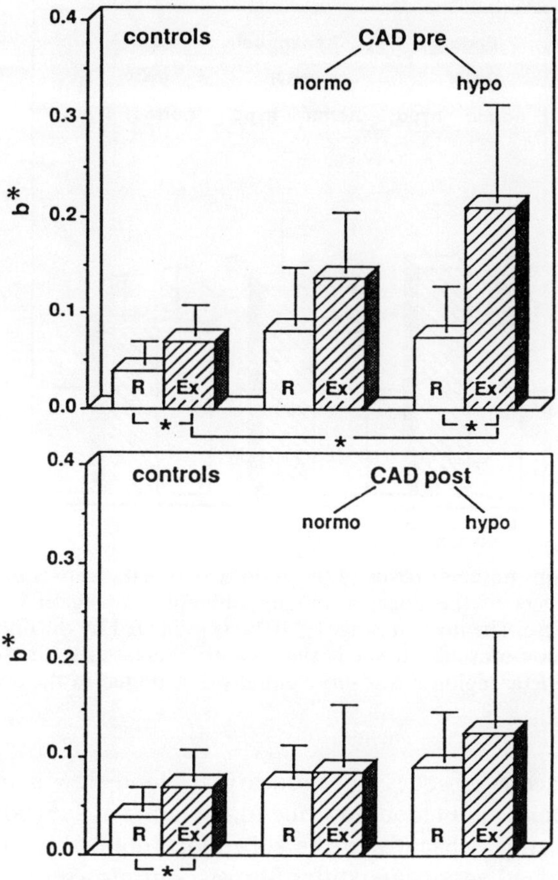

Fig. 3. Regional chamber stiffness (*b**) in controls and patients with coronary artery disease (CAD) at rest (R) and during bicycle exercise (Ex). CAD patients were studied before (pre; upper panel) and 7.7 months after (post; lower panel) successful bypass surgery. Data are given for the normokinetic and hypokinetic regions. Note that pre-operative patients with CAD show a significant increase in regional chamber stiffness of the hypokinetic but not of the normokinetic region. *: $P < 0.05$.

No correlations (linear regression analysis) between myocardial structure and diastolic function were observed.

Discussion

Recurrent myocardial ischaemia is associated with structural alterations of the left ventricle, which are especially pronounced in the subendocardium of the transiently ischaemic myocardium [3]. In the absence of myocardial infarction, these changes may result from repeated ischaemic injuries of the heart muscle

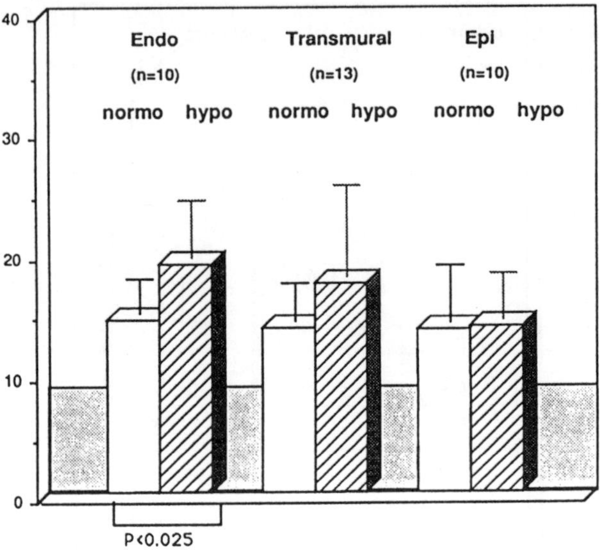

Fig. 4. Interstitial non-muscular tissue of the endocardial (left), transmural (middle) and epicardial (right) layers of the normo- and hypokinetic LV region in patients with coronary artery disease. The normal range ($\leq 10\%$) is indicated by the dotted area. Note that the interstitial non-muscular tissue is significantly increased in the subendocardial layers of the hypokinetic region but is more equally distributed in the epicardial layers of the left ventricle.

cells. During ischaemic episodes, subendocardial blood flow is more severely reduced than subepicardial blood flow due to the fact that subendocardial wall stress is higher during ischaemia in the subendocardium than in the subepicardium. Not only enhanced interstitial fibrosis, but also severe muscle fibre hypertrophy with a large scatter between normal, subnormal (atrophic) and hypertrophic fibres can be observed as a compensatory mechanism to sustain the increased wall stress during exercise-induced myocardial ischaemia [5]. These morphological changes are especially pronounced in the subendocardium of the hypokinetic zone, but are also seen in the normally perfused region of the myocardium, although less severe and without predilection for the subendocardial layers (Fig. 4).

Asynergy of the left ventricle can be found during exercise which is reversible after bypass surgery. Typically, a drop in the LVEF with an upward shift of the diastolic pressure–volume curve is observed during exercise-induced ischaemia [5]. However, little is known about regional diastolic function of the left ventricle during dynamic exercise in patients with coronary artery disease before and after successful bypass surgery although previous studies have focused on pre-/post-operative changes in global LV function [6].

Regional chamber stiffness was determined in 12 regions of the left ventricle (RAO and LAO projection) in 7 controls and 13 patients with coronary artery disease. An increase in regional chamber stiffness was observed during exercise in control patients which was small without a significant increase in LV end-diastolic pressure and volume (Table 2 and Fig. 3). A large increase in regional chamber stiffness was observed in the hypokinetic region of the left ventricle in CAD patients, which was no longer present after successful bypass surgery. In contrast, regional stiffness of the normokinetic zone increased only slightly during exercise both pre- and post-operatively. Thus, recurrent ischaemia in the absence of myocardial infarction is accompanied by changes in the passive elastic properties of the left ventricle which are no longer observed after successful bypass surgery. No correlation existed between passive elastic properties and myocardial fibrosis, suggesting that the observed changes in regional stiffness during exercise are ischaemia-induced and not dependent on the structural alterations of the subendocardium. Some sort of mild systolic dysfunction was observed after bypass surgery because LV end-diastolic pressure increased significantly and LV end-diastolic volume slightly during exercise, whereas LVEF remained essentially unchanged (Frank-Starling mechanism) which is not seen in normal subjects [3]. Thus, increased subendocardial fibrosis might act as an additional load on the muscle fibres by reducing the contractile material for a given wall segment. Post-operative function in the present study can then be characterized by the following four points:

1. No signs of persisting myocardial ischaemia were found because regional ejection did not fall during exercise.
2. LV pump function is not normal because global LVEF did not increase during exercise as in true normals.
3. The reduced contractile state of the myocardium requires the use of the Frank-Starling mechanism (preload reserve) to maintain cardiac output during exercise.
4. Although no exercise-induced increase in regional chamber stiffness was observed, baseline stiffness was twice as high as in controls.

In summary, diastolic dysfunction of transiently ischaemic segments of the left ventricle can be found during exercise in pre-operative patients with coronary artery disease. After coronary revascularization, diastolic function remains normal during exercise but systolic pump function cannot be kept within normal limits, probably due to increased subendocardial fibrosis which acts as an additional load on the muscle fibres. Thus, pre-operative alterations in regional LV diastolic function are caused by acute ischaemia, whereas the post-operative changes in systolic function are due to the structural alterations of the myocardium.

References

1. Bodenheimer MM, Banka VS, Hermann GA, Trout RG, Pasdar H, Helfant RH: Reversible asynergy: Histopathologic and electrocardiographic correlations in patients with coronary artery disease. *Circulation* 1976; **53:** 792–796.

2. Flameng W, Wouters L, Sargeant P, Lewi P, Borgers M, Thone F, Suy R. Multivariate analysis of angiographic, histologic, and electrocardiographic data in patients with coronary heart disease. *Circulation* 1984; **70:** 7–17.
3. Hess OM, Schneider J, Nonogi H, Carroll JD, Schneider K, Turina M, Krayenbuehl HP. Myocardial structure in patients with exercise-induced ischemia. *Circulation* 1988; **77:** 967–977.
4. Corin W, Murakami T, Monrad ES, Hess OM, Krayenbuehl HP. Left ventricular passive diastolic properties in chronic mitral regurgitation. *Circulation* 1991; **83:** 797–807.
5. Nonogi H, Hess OM, Bortone AS, Ritter M, Carroll JD, Krayenbuehl HP. Left ventricular pressure–length relation during exercise-induced ischemia. *J Am Coll Cardiol* 1989; **13:** 1062–1070.
6. Carroll JD, Hess OM, Hirzel HO, Turina M, Krayenbuehl HP. Left ventricular systolic and diastolic function in coronary artery disease: effects of revascularization on exercise-induced ischemia. *Circulation* 1985; **72**: 119–129.

21 Differential Enhancement of Post-ischaemic Segmental Systolic Thickening by Diltiazem

Anne L. Taylor[1], Paolo Golino[2], Robin Eckels[2], Patricia Pastor[2], L. Maximilian Buja[2], James T. Willerson[2]

[1]Division of Cardiology, University Hospital of Cleveland, 2074 Abington Road, Cleveland, OH 44106, USA and [2]Division of Cardiology, University of Texas Southwestern Medical Center, Dallas, Texas, USA

Introduction

The evolution of regional systolic function after transient myocardial ischaemia is a complex function of cellular events occurring during the ischaemic period, as well as events occurring at reperfusion. Despite the fact that timely reperfusion is essential for tissue survival [1], it provides the substrate for a new set of events, which themselves may superimpose a significant component of injury [2]. Thus, during coronary artery occlusion, the severity and duration of ischaemia importantly affect post-ischaemic myocardial function [3]. At reperfusion, factors such as cytosolic calcium overload [1], oxygen free radical generation [4] and leukocyte influx [5] may become critical determinants of post-ischaemic contractile behaviour.

With reperfusion of ischaemic myocardium, calcium accumulates both in the cytosol and in mitochondria of injured myocytes [2, 6–11]. Several mechanisms that contribute to cellular calcium overload may act singly or in concert. These include increased influx through membrane calcium channels [9–11] or as a result of membrane defects secondary to ischaemic membrane injury [12, 13]. Increased intracellular sodium concentrations occurring with ischaemia may promote increased sodium–calcium exchange and concurrent calcium accumulation [14–16]. Inappropriate intracellular compartmentalization of Ca^{2+} [13, 17] as a result of altered release or uptake of calcium by the sarcoplasmic reticulum may also contribute to abnormal calcium homeostasis.

Proceedings of the Vth World Congress on Cardiac Rehabilitation

Regardless of the mode of accumulation, increased cellular calcium adversely affects contractile behaviour. In contrast, if calcium accumulation during reperfusion of ischaemic myocardium is controlled, contractile function is significantly enhanced [7, 8, 13–15]. We tested the hypothesis that limitation of intracellular calcium by antagonism of calcium entry through membrane calcium channels would enhance recovery of segmental systolic function after 15 min of ischaemia and during 24 h of reperfusion in a canine model. Furthermore, we examined the relation between gradation of ischaemic segmental dysfunction and recovery of systolic thickening with and without diltiazem treatment.

Methods

This study was approved by the Institutional Review Board for Animal Experimentation. Care of the animals conformed to guidelines defined by the National Institutes of Health and the Food and Drug Administration.

Surgical preparation

Conditioned mongrel dogs weighing 25–35 kg were chronically instrumented with a Konigsberg catheter, intra-aortic and left atrial catheters, and an occluder secured around the left anterior descending (LAD) coronary artery. Four to five pairs of 5-MHz pulse transit piezoelectric crystals were distributed in the ischaemic and non-ischaemic regions of the left ventricle.

Measurement of segmental systolic wall thickening

Four to five pairs of 5-MHz ultrasonic crystals were placed in an endocardial to epicardial orientation within the cyanotic ischaemic zone, the border zone and non-ischaemic control regions [18]. For analysis of the signals, the transit time of ultrasound was converted to distance, assuming a velocity of sound in myocardium of 1.5 mm/μs [18]. Systolic wall thickening was measured as the difference in millimeters between the end-diastolic dimension (the dimension at the point just before the onset of the positive dP/dt signal) and that at end-systole (maximal systolic excursion occurring between peak positive and peak negative dP/dt).

Measurements of wall thickening were expressed as a percent of control values. Control values were those taken 30 min after drug or saline solution infusion, but *before* coronary artery occlusion. Segments were separated into functional classes according to the scheme described by Roan *et al.* [19]. Briefly, segments were classified according to percent of control systolic thickening retained at 15 min after occlusion. Class 1 segments were those retaining $>67\%$ of control thickening; class 2 segments were those retaining between 0 and 67% of control thickening; and class 3 segments were those retaining $<0\%$ thickening (that is, segments with systolic wall thinning).

Measurement of regional myocardial blood flow and determination of tissue necrosis

Regional myocardial blood flow was measured with radiolabelled 15 μm diameter carbonized microspheres [19]. Microspheres were suspended in a solution containing 10% dextran and 0.01% Tween 80, mechanically agitated and then injected into the left atrium. A simultaneous reference central arterial blood sample was withdrawn at a constant rate by pump from the aortic catheter.

Transmural tissue samples between crystal pairs and from a remote control region in the circumflex coronary artery distribution were divided into endocardial, mid-myocardial and epicardial segments, weighed and placed in formalin and then into a scintillation counter for determination of regional myocardial blood flow. Regional myocardial blood flow was calculated by a computer-assisted program in which flow is determined by the general formula:

$$Qm = Qr \times Cm/Cr$$

where Qm = myocardial flow (ml/min), Qr = reference blood flow (ml/min), Cm = counts/min in myocardium and Cr = counts/min in the reference blood sample. The tissue samples were then reassembled, embedded in paraffin, sectioned and stained with haematoxylin-eosin. After this, sections were carefully examined to confirm the *absence* of recent necrosis.

Experimental protocol

When the dogs had recovered from surgery for ≥ 7 days, they were taken to the laboratory and placed in a standing sling in the awake unsedated state.

Protocol 1

Thirteen dogs survived two coronary artery occlusions of 15 min each, followed by 24 h reperfusion. The occlusions were separated by at least 3 days. One occlusion was performed during infusion of diltiazem (Marion Laboratories) dissolved in normal saline solution at a dose of 15 μg/kg/min; the other occlusion was performed during infusion of an equal volume of saline solution. Infusions were begun 30 min before occlusion and continued over 3 h of reperfusion. The order of the infusion was alternated. Before each occlusion, dogs were pretreated with lidocaine, followed by intravenous infusions at a rate of 2 mg/min.

Protocol 2

Because diltiazem infusion was associated with mild but significant decreases in mean arterial pressures, an additional group of 10 dogs underwent a single 15-min coronary artery occlusion during infusion of sodium nitroprusside at a dose titrated to achieve a reduction in mean arterial blood pressure similar to that seen during diltiazem infusion.

Measurements

During the experimental period, the following haemodynamic measurements were recorded: heart rate, left ventricular pressure, the first derivative of left ventricular pressure (dP/dt), aortic pressure, mean left atrial pressure, electrocardiogram, and regional wall thickening from the four to five pairs of ultrasonic crystals. Recordings of haemodynamic variables and regional wall thickening were made in the control period (before coronary artery occlusion but after administration of diltiazem, saline solution or nitroprusside), immediately after occlusion and 15 min after occlusion, at reflow and at 10, 15, 30, 60, 120 and 180 min and 24 h of reflow.

Statistical analyses

A repeated-measures analysis of variance was performed to assess whether or not effects of time and individual variability among dogs were responsible for the changes in function during the experiment. For this analysis, we stratified our sample by treatment and level of function and looked at the effects of time and variation on regional cardiac function among individual dogs. Similarly, to assess the effect of treatment and variation on regional cardiac function among individual dogs, we stratified by time and functional level and performed a one-way analysis of variance. Variation among individual dogs was not sufficiently significant to explain differences between treatment groups; however, time and treatment did exert significant effects.

Segmental function, haemodynamic variable and regional myocardial blood flow over time for each treatment group were analysed by using multiple Student's t-tests, with a Bonferroni adjustment of the P-value based on the number of comparisons. Segmental function and regional myocardial blood flow at given time points among treatment groups were compared by unpaired t-tests, with a Bonferroni correction when more than a single comparison was made. Haemodynamic variables at given time points were compared among saline solution-, diltiazem- and nitroprusside-treated occlusions by t-tests, with corrections of the P-values based on three comparisons.

Results

Data from individual dogs were included in the final analysis if two criteria could be met: (1) the dog survived *both* coronary artery occlusions of protocol 1 or the single occlusion of protocol 2 and (2) regional blood blow and function analyses confirmed that effective occlusions and reperfusion occurred. The total number of animals in each protocol were as follows: protocol 1 (alternate infusion of diltiazem or saline solution), 13 dogs; protocol 2 (nitroprusside infusion), 10 dogs.

The number of left ventricular segments in each class and treatment group were as follows:

- Class 1: saline solution, 12 segments; diltiazem, 15 segments; nitroprusside, 12 segments.
- Class 2: saline solution, 20 segments; diltiazem, 20 segments; nitroprusside, 17 segments.
- Class 3: saline solution, 15 segments; diltiazem, 15 segments; nitroprusside, 6 segments.

Segmental systolic thickening

Control segmental wall thickening was measured at 30 min of drug or saline solution infusion, but immediately before coronary artery occlusion. Because of the concern that diltiazem or nitroprusside infusion may have significantly altered function before occlusion, thereby resulting in different absolute levels of control function in the two groups, we compared segmental systolic thickening before infusion with that at 30 min of infusion (but before coronary occlusion) by paired *t*-tests. Segmental systolic function was not significantly different at these two time points within groups treated with saline solution, diltiazem or nitroprusside.

The evolution of systolic segmental myocardial thickening (expressed as a percent on control values) for each class of crystal and each treatment group is summarized in Fig. 1. There were no significant differences in function at any time point among saline solution-, diltiazem- and nitroprusside-treated class 1 (Fig. 1A) or class 2 (Fig. 1B) segments. In contrast, significant functional differences evolved in class 3 segments (Fig. 1C), that is, those segments with $<0\%$ of control thickening (systolic wall thinning) at 15 min of coronary artery occlusion. At 15 min of occlusion, the degree of ischaemic dyskinesia was identical in the three treatment groups. On reperfusion, however, important functional divergences were observed. At all time points during reperfusion, segmental systolic thickening was better preserved in the diltiazem-treated segments than in saline solution-treated segments, with the differences achieving statistical significance compared with saline solution at immediate reflow and at 10, 30 and 120 min of reflow. In the nitroprusside-treated segments, function was not significantly better than that in segments treated with saline solution until 120 min of reflow, although there was a trend towards enhanced function at earlier time points. When diltiazem-treated segments were compared with nitroprusside-treated segments, the differences in segmental thickening were not significantly different at any time point. Thus, reduction in arterial pressure had an effect intermediate between that from treatment with saline solution or diltiazem (Fig. 1D).

When the time at which *sustained* return to control thickening was considered, class 3 segments in the diltiazem-treated group again fared better.

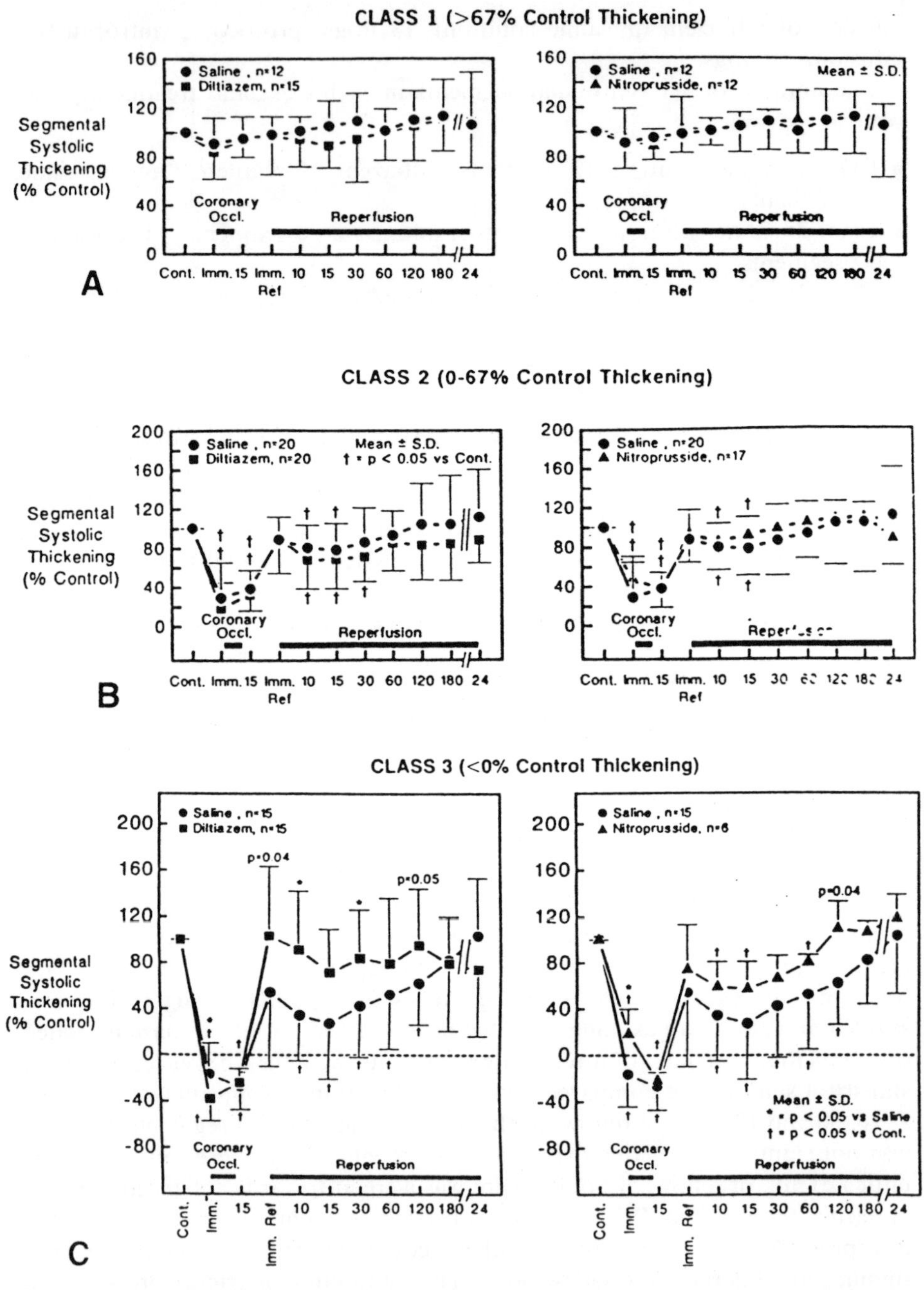

Fig. 1. Segmental systolic thickening (as a percent of control) over time comparing treatment with saline solution, diltiazem and nitroprusside in each class of ischaemic segments. (A) Class 1 (>76% of control thickening); (B) class 2 (0–67% of control thickening); and (C) class 3 (<0% thickening or systolic all thinning).

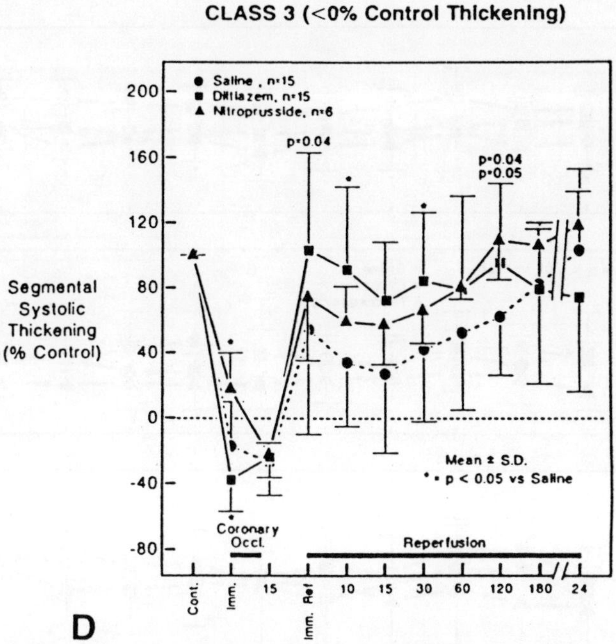

Panel (D) simultaneously displays class 3 segments for all three treatment groups. Treatment groups are shown compared separately with saline because of extensive overlap of points in class 1 and class 2 segments; however, statistical analysis was based on a three-way comparison. Cont., control study; Imm., immediately after coronary artery occlusion; Imm. Ref, at immediate reflow; Occl., occlusion.

Diltiazem-treated segments had *sustained* return to control thickening at immediate reperfusion compared with 120 min for nitroprusside-treated segments and 180 min for saline solution-treated segments.

Haemodynamics

When haemodynamic variables in the three treatment groups were compared (Fig. 2), significant differences were found only with respect to arterial pressure and left arterial mean pressure. Systolic, diastolic and mean arterial pressures were slightly but significantly reduced during both diltiazem and nitroprusside infusion. Despite an identical reduction in mean arterial pressure, only the diltiazem-treated class 3 segments showed significantly enhanced early recovery of segmental thickening compared with that in segments treated with saline solution.

Regional myocardial blood flow

In class 1 segments, blood flow during coronary artery occlusion and reperfusion was not different from control values in either the diltiazem- or saline

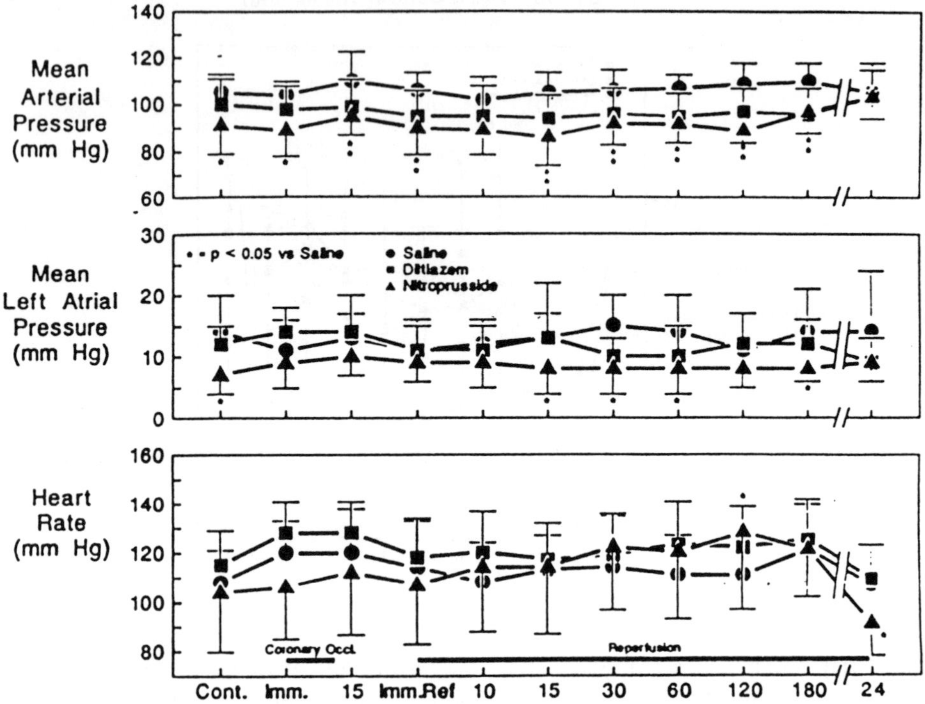

Fig. 2. Mean arterial pressure, mean left atrial pressure and heart rate during coronary occlusion (occl.) and reperfusion. Abbreviations as in Figure 1.

solution-treated occlusions. In class 2 and class 3 segments, regional myocardial blood flow was significantly reduced during coronary artery occlusion compared with control (Table 1). Importantly, when blood flow at each time point was compared, there were no differences in blood flow between saline solution- and diltiazem-treated groups during coronary occlusion and at reflow except in the epicardial portions of class 3 segments. The difference was small (0.3 ml/g tissue/min); however, statistical significance was achieved. Importantly, blood flow was not statistically different in this class of segments in the endocardial or mid-myocardial portions. Thus, diltiazem neither alleviated the severity of ischaemia nor improved blood flow at 30 min of reperfusion in class 2 or class 3 segments.

Discussion

Effect of diltiazem on segmental systolic thickening during reperfusion

Because the threshold for irreversible myocardial injury is reached at approximately 20 min of ischaemia [1], a coronary occlusion period of 15 min duration

Table 1
Mean (±SD) regional myocardial blood flow by class of ischaemic segment

Class	Level	No.	Treatment group	Control	Occlusion	Reflow
1	Epicardial	8	S	0.91 ± 0.28	1.04 ± 0.33	1.08 ± 0.18
		11	D	1.49 ± 0.75*	1.47 ± 0.44*	1.20 ± 0.19
	Mid-wall	8	S	1.20 ± 0.28	1.36 ± 0.32	1.47 ± 0.24**
		11	D	1.68 ± 0.95	1.72 ± 0.67	1.34 ± 0.28
	Endocardial	8	S	1.11 ± 0.26	1.25 ± 0.25	1.35 ± 0.24
		11	D	1.58 ± 0.82	1.61 ± 0.61	1.24 ± 0.32
2	Epicardial	15	S	1.04 ± 0.43	0.85 ± 0.49	1.10 ± 0.39
		15	D	1.86 ± 0.85	0.95 ± 0.55**	1.17 ± 0.26**
	Mid-wall	15	S	1.33 ± 0.56	0.88 ± 0.73	1.34 ± 0.50
		15	D	2.27 ± 1.21*	0.88 ± 0.57**	1.25 ± 0.34**
	Endocardial	15	S	1.40 ± 0.60	0.90 ± 0.80**	1.30 ± 0.50
		15	D	2.47 ± 1.43*	0.97 ± 0.72**	1.34 ± 0.30**
3	Epicardial	11	S	0.95 ± 0.30	0.51 ± 0.34**	0.86 ± 0.23
		7	D	1.37 ± 0.47	0.54 ± 0.41**	1.11 ± 0.22*
	Mid-wall	11	S	1.31 ± 0.45	0.56 ± 0.49**	1.10 ± 0.26
		7	D	1.73 ± 1.06	0.58 ± 0.69**	1.21 ± 0.32
	Endocardial	11	S	1.30 ± 0.41	0.63 ± 0.60**	1.07 ± 0.31**
		7	D	2.00 ± 2.00	0.68 ± 0.72	1.19 ± 0.31

* $P \leq 0.05$ saline solution (S) *vs* diltiazem (D); **$P \leq 0.05$ *vs* control within any treatment group.
Regional myocardial blood flow is expressed in ml/g myocardium/min.

results in structural and functional alterations that are fully reversible [1, 20]. Thus, the effect of calcium channel blockade on post-ischaemic systolic function could be evaluated in this experiment without differences in the amount of tissue necrosis as a factor in functional recovery. The principal finding of this study using a model of brief coronary occlusion was that diltiazem infusion (15 μg/kg/min) significantly enhanced recovery of segmental systolic thickening during reperfusion after 15 min of ischaemia in the absence of improved function during ischaemia. Improvement in contractile function was seen only in those segments with systolic thinning during ischaemia; thus, segments with the most severe ischaemic dysfunction benefited most. Although regional myocardial blood flow was enhanced before coronary occlusion, there were no important differences in regional myocardial blood flow between diltiazem- and saline solution-treated occlusions during ischaemia and at 30 min of reperfusion. Diltiazem, therefore, did not exert a beneficial effect by alleviating the intensity of ischaemia nor by augmenting blood flow during reperfusion. Arterial pressures were slightly but significantly reduced by diltiazem; an identical reduction in mean arterial pressure by nitroprusside infusion resulted in functional recovery intermediated between that occurring with infusion of saline solution and diltiazem, suggesting that afterload reduction by diltiazem only partially accounted for the early enhancement in functional recovery seen in this treatment group.

Myocardial consequences of reperfusion

Myocardium that has undergone ischaemia followed by reperfusion differs from permanently ischaemic myocardium biochemically, ultrastructurally and functionally [21, 26]. Prominent biochemical features of reperfused myocardium include increases in cell water, sodium and chloride [21], as well as prolonged but reversible depression in high-energy phosphate concentration [1]. Severely injured myocytes also show evidence of contraction bands and prominent electron-dense mitochondrial granules consisting of calcium phosphate precipitates [1]. Functionally, systolic thickening recovers slowly over a period of time usually substantially longer than the ischaemic interval [3, 20]. Thus, both the severity of biochemical, ultrastructural and functional impairment and the time course of recovery are linearly related to the intensity and duration of ischaemia. The final extent of segmental functional recovery is inversely related to these factors. Although many factors undoubtedly influence recovery of segmental function after transient ischaemia, maintenance of calcium homeostasis may be particularly important.

In reperfused myocardium, calcium overload is prominent ultrastructurally [1, 11] and has adverse consequences functionally [7–9]. The most extensive calcium accumulation, which has been found in irreversibly injured cells, is thought to occur as a consequence of loss of membrane integrity, with diffusion of calcium down an electrochemical gradient or as the result of an inability of intracellular calcium storage sites to sequester calcium normally, or both. In reversibly injured cells, however, lesser amounts of calcium accumulate with ischaemia and reperfusion; importantly, calcium may accumulate in the *absence* of morphological alteration in membrane integrity [9, 11, 16, 22], and thus may enter by physiological pathways that may have been altered by ischaemia. The mechanism or mechanisms that might singly, simultaneously or sequentially facilitate entry or accumulation, or both, of excessive amounts of calcium in reversibly injured cells include the membrane slow inward calcium current, the sodium–calcium exchanger or the altered release or uptake of intracellular calcium stores by the sarcoplasmic reticulum.

Mechanisms of protective effect of calcium channel blockers on ischaemic myocardium

One potential physiological route of calcium entry during ischaemia as well as at reperfusion may be through membrane calcium channels. Diltiazem is a calcium channel antagonist that inhibits myocardial calcium entry by blockade of voltage-dependent membrane calcium channels [23, 24] in both myocardium and vascular smooth muscle [24].

Although regional myocardial blood flow tended to be somewhat enhanced before coronary artery occlusion during diltiazem infusion, flow during ischaemia and at 30 min of reperfusion was not significantly different in the saline solution- and diltiazem-treated groups. The only exception was a small increase in blood flow to the epicardial third of the class 3 segments. Although this difference was significant, it was small (0.3 ml/g tissue/min) and of questionable physiological importance because segmental function is far more sensitive to changes in endocardial blood flow [19]. We therefore could not conclude that the beneficial effect of diltiazem was based on alleviation of ischaemia or enhanced regional blood flow during the reperfusion period. Despite equal reductions in blood flow and function during ischaemia in diltiazem- and saline solution-treated groups, we cannot, however, exclude the possibility that diltiazem's beneficial effect did not result from protection from the effects of ischaemia.

Treatment of ischaemic myocardium with calcium channel blockers before coronary artery occlusion has been found to decrease ultrastructural evidence of injury [11, 26], decrease calcium influx [11, 28] and improve post-ischaemic left ventricular segmental function [25, 27, 28]. When given after occlusion but before reperfusion, calcium channel blockers may still be protective [11, 27, 29]. Because most studies have shown that calcium channel blockers provide benefit when given before ischaemia or before but *not at* reperfusion, it has been postulated that benefit is due to protection from the effects of ischaemia rather than from decreases in reperfusion-related calcium influx. An alternative hypothesis to explain why calcium channel blockers provide benefit when given before reperfusion may be that the time required for drug binding and action may be longer than the time required for calcium influx at reperfusion.

Several authors have shown preserved levels of ATP associated with pretreatment with verapamil [26, 30] and diltiazem [26]. However, functional recovery was not well correlated with the degree of ATP preservation. Thus, even though preservation of ATP may be an important contributor to ultimate cell survival, it may not be the principal determinant of functional recovery after brief coronary artery occlusion.

Role of afterload reduction

We considered that the mild decrease in blood pressure afforded by diltiazem in our study may have been the important determinant of enhanced recovery of segmental thickening by diltiazem; however, identical reductions in mean arterial pressure in the nitroprusside-treated group did not result in equivalent improvements in function (Fig. 1C, D). The fact that the nitroprusside-treated class 3 segments had functional recovery intermediate between that of saline solution- and diltiazem-treated segments can best be interpreted as showing that afterload reduction may be responsible for part, but not all, of the beneficial effect of diltiazem in reperfused myocardium.

Finally, diltiazem has been found to decrease intracellular calcium accumulation at reperfusion [11, 28]. Decreases in calcium accumulation have been reported to correlate with decreased histologic injury [11] and improved function [28]. Green *et al.* [31] observed that in isolated myocytes, binding sites of nitrendipine, a dihydropyridine calcium antagonist, reversibly increased by 115% as a function of increasing membrane depolarization. Thus, ischaemia may modify calcium channel conductance, such that entry of calcium may be facilitated.

Irrespective of the modes of calcium entry, limitation of calcium entry during reperfusion has been shown to be functionally and ultrastructurally beneficial [7, 11]. Conversely, Kitakaze *et al.* [32] reported that both contractile function and ATP were transiently depressed in isolated hearts by exposure to 10 mM calcium solution in the absence of ischaemia.

Conclusion

Using an awake, unsedated, chronically instrumented canine model undergoing brief coronary artery occlusion, we found that treatment with diltiazem resulted in significantly improved recovery of regional systolic thickening in segments with the most severe ischaemic dysfunction. Improvement occurred independently of the reduction in mean arterial pressure by diltiazem and in the absence of alteration in heart rate–blood pressure product or left ventricular dP/dt. Benefit also occurred in the absence of enhanced regional myocardial blood flow during ischaemia and reperfusion.

References

1. Schaper J, Mulch J, Winkler B, Schaper W. Ultrastructural, functional, and biochemical criteria for estimation of reversibility of ischaemic injury: A study on the effects of global ischaemia on the isolated dog heart. *J Mol Cell Cardiol* 1979; **11:** 521–541.
2. Braunwald E, Kloner RA. Myocardial reperfusion: A double-edged sword? *J Clin Invest* 1985; **76:** 1713–1719.
3. Theroux P, Ross J Jr, Franklin D, Kemper WS, Sasayama S. Coronary arterial reperfusion. III. Early and late effects on regional myocardial function and dimensions in conscious dogs. *Am J Cardiol* 1976; **38:** 599–606.
4. Jolly SR, Kane WJ, Bailie MB, Abrams GD, Lucchesi BR. Canine myocardial reperfusion injury: Its reduction by the combined administration of superoxide dismutase and catalase. *Circ Res* 1984; **54:** 277–285.
5. Engler RL, Dahlgren MD, Morris DD, Peterson MA, Schmid-Schonbein GW. Role of leukocytes in response to acute myocardial ischaemia and reflow in dogs. *Am J Physiol* 1986; **251:** H93–100.
6. Kloner RA, Ganote CE, Whalen DA Jr, Jennings RB. Effect of a transient period of ischaemia on myocardial cells. II. Fine structure during the first few minutes of reflow. *Am J Pathol* 1974; **74:** 399–422.

7. Shine KI, Douglas AM. Low calcium reperfusion of ischaemic myocardium. *J Mol Cell Cardiol* 1983; **15:** 251–260.
8. Shine KI, Douglas AM, Ricchiuti NV. Calcium, strontium, and barium movements during ischaemia and reperfusion in rabbit and ventricle. Implications for myocardial preservation. *Circ Res* 1978; **43:** 712–720.
9. Bourdillon PDV, Poole-Wilson PA. Effects of ischaemia and reperfusion on calcium exchange and mechanical function in isolated rabbit myocardium. *Cardiovasc Res* 1981; **15:** 121–130.
10. Murphy JG, Marsh JD, Smith TW. The role of calcium in ischaemic myocardial injury. *Circulation* (Suppl. V) 1987; **75:** 15–24.
11. Ashraf M, Rahamathulla PM. Cardiac injury in short duration anoxia and modification by diltiazem, a calcium channel blocking agent. *J Am Col Cardiol* 1984; **3:** 1237–1244.
12. Chien KR, Han A, Sen A, Buja LM, Willerson JT. Accumulation of unesterified arachidonic acid in ischaemic canine myocardium: Relationship to a phosphatidylcholine decylation–recylation cycle and the depletion of membrane phospholipids. *Circ Res* 1984; **54:** 313–322.
13. Poole-Wilson PA, Harding DP, Bourdillon PDV, Tones MA. Calcium out of control. *J Mol Cell Cardiol* 1984; **16:** 175–187.
14. Murphy JG, Smith TW, Marsh JD. Mechanisms of reoxygenation-induced calcium overload in cultured chick embryo heart cells. *Am J Physiol* 1988; **254** (*Heart Circ Physiol*): H133–141.
15. Renlund DG, Gerstenblith G, Lakatta EG, Jacobus WE, Kallman CH, Weisfeldt ML. Perfusate sodium during ischaemia modifies post-ischaemic functional and metabolic recovery in the rabbit heart. *J Mol Cell Cardiol* 1984; **16:** 795–801.
16. Pike M, Kitakaze M, Chacko VP, Marban E. Lidocaine prevents the increase in myocardial free calcium during ischaemia and reperfusion: an antiarrhythmic mechanism? *Circulation* (Suppl. IV, abstr.) 1987; **76:** 16.
17. Nayler WG, Dresel PE. Ca^{2+} and the sarcoplasmic reticulum. *J Mol Cell Cardiol* 1984; **16:** 165–174.
18. Sasayama A, Franklin D, Ross J, Kemper WS, McKown D. Dynamic changes in left ventricular wall thickness and their use in analyzing cardiac function in the conscious dog: A study based on a modified ultrasonic technique. *Am J Cardiol* 1976; **38:** 870–879.
19. Roan PG, Buja LM, Isquierdo C, Hashimi H, Saffer S, Willerson JT. Interrelationships between regional left ventricular function, coronary blood flow, and myocellular necrosis during the initial 24 hours and 1 week after experimental coronary occlusion in awake, unsedated dogs. *Circ Res* 1981; **49:** 31–40.
20. Heyndrickx GR, Millard RW, McRitchie RJ, Maroko PR, Vatner SF. Regional myocardial functional and electrophysiological alterations after brief coronary artery occlusion in conscious dogs. *J Clin Invest* 1975; **56:** 978–985.
21. Jennings RB, Schaper J, Hill ML, Steenbergen C Jr, Reimer KA. Effect of reperfusion late in the phase of reversible ischaemic injury: Changes in cell volume, electrolytes, metabolites, and ultrastructure. *Circ Res* 1985; **56:** 262–278.
22. Steenbergen C, Murphy E, Levy L, London RE. Elevation in cytosolic free calcium concentration early in myocardial ischaemia in perfused rat heart. *Circ Res* 1987; **60:** 700–707.
23. Triggle DJ, Swamy VC. Calcium antagonists: some chemical-pharmacologic aspects. *Circ Res* (Suppl. I) 1983; **52:** 17–28.
24. Millard RW, Grupp G, Gupp IL, DiSalvo J, DePover A, Schwartz A. Chronotropic, inotropic, and vasodilator actions of diltiazem, nifedipine, and verapamil: A comparative study of physiological responses and membrane receptor activity. *Circ Res* (Suppl. I) 1983; **52:** 29–39.

25. Clozel J-P, Theroux P, Bourassa MG. Effects of diltiazem on experimental myocardial ischaemia and on left ventricular performance. *Circ Res* (Suppl. I) 1983; **52:** 120–128.
26. Hamm CW, Opie LH. Protection of infarcting myocardium by slow channel inhibitors: comparative effects of verapamil, nifedipine, and diltiazem in the coronary-ligated, isolated working rat heart. *Circ Res* (Suppl. I) 1983; **52:** 129–138.
27. Bush LR, Buja LM, Tilton G. Effects of propranolol and diltiazem alone and in combination on the recovery of left ventricular segmental function after temporary coronary occlusion and long-term reperfusion in conscious dogs. *Circulation* 1985; **72:** 413–430.
28. Higgins AJ, Blackburn KJ. Prevention of reperfusion damage in working rat hearts by calcium antagonists and calmodulin antagonists. *J Mol Cell Cardiol* 1984; **16:** 427–438.
29. Knabb RM, Rosamond TL, Fox KAA, Sobel BE, Bergmann SR. Enhancement of salvage of reperfused ischaemic myocardium by diltiazem. *J Am Coll Cardiol* 1986; **8:** 861–871.
30. Watts JA, Maiorano LJ, Maiorano PC. Protections by verapamil of globally ischaemic rat hearts: Energy preservation, a partial explanation. *J Mol Cell Cardiol* 1985; **17:** 797–804.
31. Green FJ, Framer BB, Wiseman GL, Jose MJL, Watanabe AM. Effect of membrane depolarization on binding of [^{3}H]nitrendipine to rat cardiac myocytes. *Circ Res* 1985; **56:** 576–585.
32. Kitakaze M, Weisman HF, Marban E. Contractile dysfunction and ATP depletion after transient calcium overload in perfused ferret hearts. *Circulation* 1988; **77:** 685–695.

22 A Review of Myocardial Stunning in Coronary Artery Patients Following Treadmill Exercise Testing

John W. Allen*, Timothy A. Cox, Robert A. Kloner, Carlos E. Ruiz

Hospital of the Good Samaritan and University of Southern California, Los Angeles, CA, USA

Total occlusion of a coronary artery followed by reperfusion in animal models resulted in prolonged left ventricular dysfunction [1]. This response to ischaemia has been termed myocardial stunning. Further study in dogs with partial coronary artery stenosis who were exercised to induce myocardial ischaemia had delay in recovery of function for up to 1 hour [2]. Thus, myocardial stunning was demonstrated in animal models post-exercise. Several published studies address the issue of myocardial stunning in humans following exercise treadmill testing [3–7]. From these studies, we will review the evidence, clinical features and implications of post-exercise stunning in humans.

In discussing the clinical evidence of myocardial stunning, we will review two of our studies and then review studies from other laboratories. Details of our studies are published elsewhere [6, 8].

We have identified stunning in 31 patients referred for exercise testing. Our patients exercised on a treadmill following the Bruce or Modified Bruce Protocol. Two-dimensional echocardiograms from four standard views (parasternal long, short, apical 2- and 4-chambers) were attempted before, immediately after, and 15 or 30 mins post-exercise or both. Studies in 22 patients were evaluated by a semi-quantitative technique that graded left ventricular wall motion using a previously published scoring system: grade 1 = normal contractions, grade 2 = hypokinesis, grade 3 = akinesis, and grade 4 = dyskinesis [9].

* Address all correspondence to John W. Allen, 616 South Witmer Street, Los Angeles, CA 90017, USA.

Proceedings of the Vth World Congress on Cardiac Rehabilitation

Mean segment grade was determined by totalling each segment score and dividing it by the number of patients with a scored segment.

From the 31 patients we selected 9 with high-quality echograms for evaluation with a quantitative technique. Using this technique, a centre-line method adapted from Dodge and Sheehan was used to obtain 100 chord measurements for apical 2- and 4-chamber views [9]. The chord measurements were constructed by the computer perpendicular to a centre-line and extended from the diastolic to the systolic tracings. The chord length measured in centimetres represented systolic endocardial motion. The computer printed out a measurement of 10 chords from the 2- and 4-chamber views that were used in our studies.

Nine patients free from chest pain, ST-segment abnormalities or history of coronary disease were selected as a control group for obtaining quantitative measurements. The changes in the 20 chord segments from rest to 30 min post-exercise were used to identify significant differences in chord segments between the patients and the control group. The findings from our studies are summarized first from the semi-quantitative approach and then from the quantitative approach. All 31 patients used in the studies had angiographic evidence of coronary artery disease.

Figure 1 outlines the 16 segments of the heart scored by our semi-quantitative technique. Only walls that moved normally at rest were assessed. No wall motion abnormalities were observed in the nine control patients. In our patient group, several ventricular walls showed significant wall motion abnormalities immediately post-exercise, and 15 and 30 min post-exercise when compared to rest. Data from three of these walls are illustrated in Tables 1, 2, and 3. From these tables we documented persistent wall motion abnormalities in selected patients using a semi-quantitative technique. Figure 2 shows an illustrative echogram of a patient with stunning.

To further evaluate this process, we used the quantitative assessment in a group of nine patients. Twenty chords from two views were available for analysis. Upon comparing the chords from rest to 30 min post-exercise, we determined that in the control subjects, most chords showed an increase in endocardial motion at 30 min compared to rest. However, in the coronary artery disease patients, most chords showed a decrease in length. Five chord measurements from the 2-chamber view showed significant differences when coronary artery disease patients were compared to controls. Figure 3 illustrates quantitative measurements at rest and 30 min following exercise in a patient with myocardial stunning. From these studies, we have evidence in our patient groups of myocardial stunning using both quantitative and semi-quantitative techniques.

Next we turn to other evidence in the literature of post-exercise stunning using three techniques: (1) echographic, (2) radionuclide and (3) positron emission tomography. Using echographic techniques, Robertson *et al.* [7] found regional wall motion abnormalities that persisted for 30 min post-exercise in 7 of 20 patients studied. All of these patients had multi-vessel coronary disease.

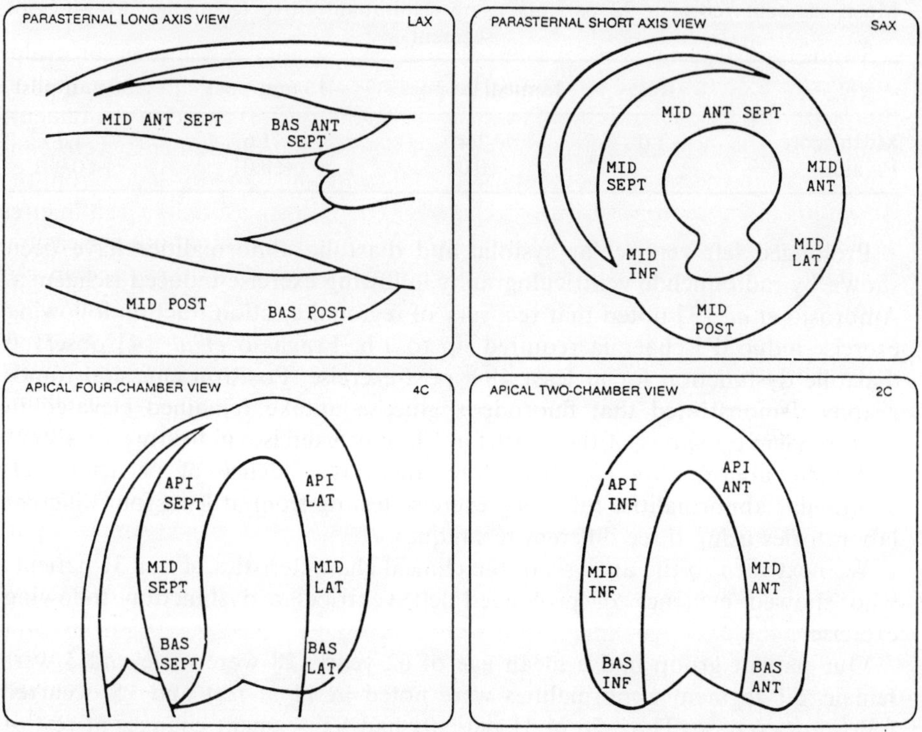

Fig. 1. Location of the 16 segments graded for the semi-quantitative assessment of wall motion at rest and during recovery.

Table 1

Mean segment score in 22 patients using semi-quantitative technique: Mid-septal segment

	Rest	Immediate post	15 min post	30 min post
Mean score	1.0	1.4	1.6	1.6
P-value	—	<0.02	<0.01	<0.004

Table 2

Mean segment score in 22 patients using semi-quantitative technique: Basilar inferior segment

	Rest	Immediate post	15 min post	30 min post
Mean score	1.0	2.0	2.0	1.9
P-value	—	<0.01	<0.03	<0.01

Table 3
Mean segment score in 22 patients using semi-quantitative technique: Mid-inferior segment

	Rest	Immediate post	15 min post	30 min post
Mean score	1.0	1.4	1.6	1.7
P-value	—	<0.02	<0.01	<0.001

Prolonged left ventricular systolic and diastolic abnormalities have been shown by radionuclide ventriculography following exercise-induced ischaemia. Ambrosio *et al.* [3] noted that recovery of regional ejection fraction following exercise-induced ischaemia required up to 1 h. Fragasso *et al.* [4] observed diastolic dysfunction for at least 48 h post-exercise. Positron emission tomography demonstrated that fluorodeoxyglucose uptake remained elevated in post-ischaemic regions of the heart for 1 h after exercise, indicating persistent metabolic abnormality [5]. Therefore, there is evidence of persistent left ventricular abnormalities following exercise testing from at least four different laboratories using three different techniques.

We next turn to the analysis of the clinical characteristics of our 31 patients who showed evidence of prolonged left ventricular dysfunction following exercise.

Our patient group had a mean age of 62 years; 28 were male and 3 were female. ST-segment abnormalities were noted in 11 at rest and 15 occurred following exercise. Thus, 26 of 31 patients had ST-segment changes at rest or with exercise. Coronary angiographic studies showed single vessel disease in 6 patients, double vessel disease in 7 patients and triple vessel disease in 18 patients. Thus, 25 of 31 patients had multi-vessel disease. The functional capacity in our patients varied from 2 to 11 METs. Nine patients exercised

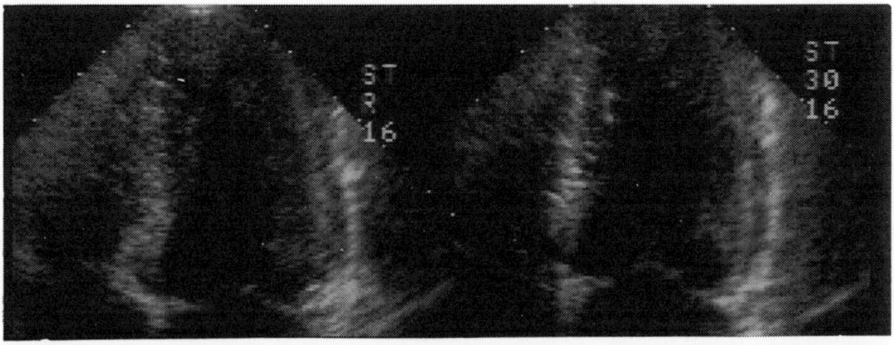

Fig. 2. Two echograms showing end-systolic frames taken at rest (R) and 30 min post-exercise (30). In this 4-chamber view, the mid-portion of the ventricle shows a greater end-systolic dimension that identifies a regional wall motion abnormality consistent with stunning. Dots represent centimetre marker.

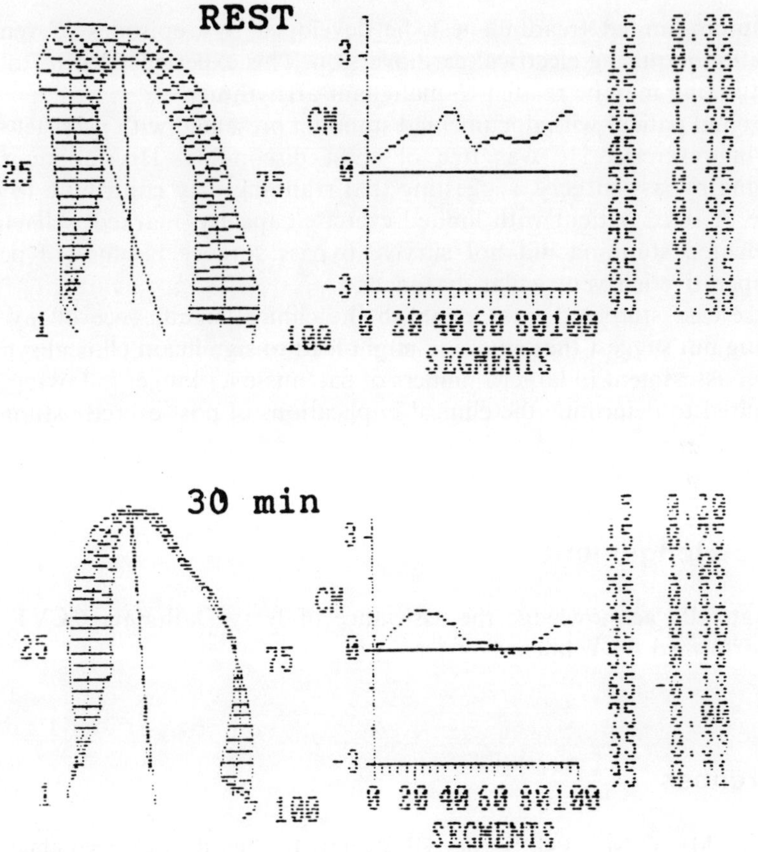

Fig. 3. A 4-chamber view shows a quantitative assessment of two tracings, one taken pre-exercise (rest) and the other taken 30 min post-exercise (30 min). These tracings quantitate systolic motion. Note the diminished motion in chords 35–95, 30 min post-exercise. The measurements are plotted on a graph and 10 chords measured are displayed (5–95).

from 2 to 5 METs, 12 patients 6 to 8 METs, and 10 patients 9 to 11 METs. Thirteen of our patients suffered angina, while 18 had silent ischaemia.

Our experience suggests that stunning is most likely to occur in older males who have multi-vessel coronary disease and ST-segment abnormalities at rest or with exercise. These patients have a variable exercise capacity and may have angina or silent ischaemia.

Finally, we will focus on the implications of our findings. If stunning occurs, does it have clinical significance? Recently, we evaluated a 51-year-old male with multi-vessel coronary artery disease, ST-segment depression and high echographic scores following exercise. These findings were similar to our patients who developed myocardial stunning. Twenty minutes after performing a symptom-limited treadmill test, he developed two episodes of ventricular fibrillation requiring electrical cardioversion. This experience led us to suspect that stunning may be related to malignant arrhythmia.

A second patient with documented stunning presented with persistent fatigue following exercise. He was free of chest discomfort. His fatigue resolved following bypass surgery, suggesting that stunning may contribute to chronic fatigue. A third patient with limited exercise capacity, marked ischaemia and documented stunning did not survive bypass surgery because of persistent post-operative left ventricular dysfunction.

These case studies do not establish the clinical significance of myocardial stunning but suggest that stunning might lead to significant clinical symptoms. Further assessment in larger numbers of patients over longer follow-up periods is required to determine the clinical implications of post-exercise stunning.

Acknowledgement

We gratefully acknowledge the assistance of Jerry Dalhman, CCVT, ROCS who performed the echocardiograms.

References

1. Charlat ML, O'Neill PG, Hartley CJ, Roberts R, Bolli R. Prolonged abnormalities of left ventricular diastolic wall thinning in the 'stunned' myocardium in conscious dogs: Time course and relation to systolic function. *J Am Coll Cardiol* 1989; **13:** 185–194.
2. Homans DC, Sublett E, Dai X-Z, Bache RJ. Persistence of regional left ventricular dysfunction after exercise-induced myocardial ischaemia. *J Clin Invest* 1986; **77:** 66–73.
3. Ambrosio G, Betocchi S, Pace L, Ciarmeiello A, Salvatore C, Salvatore M, Chiariello M. Prolonged impairment of regional left ventricular systolic function after exercise in patients with stable angina. *Circulation* (Suppl. II) 1991; **84:** 475.
4. Fragasso G, Benti R, Sciammarella M, Rossetti E, Savi A, Gerundini P, Chierchia SL. Symptom-limited exercise testing causes sustained diastolic dysfunction in patients with coronary disease and low effort tolerance. *J Am Coll Cardiol* 1991; **17:** 1251–1255.
5. Camici P, Arajuo LI, Spinks T, Lammertsma AA, Kaski JC, Shea MJ, Selwyn AP, Jones TJ, Maseri A. Increased uptake of 18-F fluorodeoxy-glucose in postischemic myocardium in patients with exercise-induced angina. *Circulation* 1986; **74:** 81–88.
6. Kloner RA, Allen J, Cox TA, Zheng Y, Ruiz CE. Stunned left ventricular myocardium after exercise treadmill testing in coronary artery disease. *Am J Cardiol* 1991 **68:** 329–334.
7. Robertson WS, Feigenbaum H, Armstrong WF, Dillon JC, O'Donnell J, McHenry PW. Exercise echocardiography: A clinically practical addition in the evaluation of coronary artery disease. *J Am Coll Cardiol* 1983; **2:** 1085–1091.

8. Cox TA, Kloner RA, Ruiz CE, Allen J. Quantitative echocardiography in assessing myocardial stunning in humans following exercise testing. *Am J Cardiac Imaging* 1992; **6**: 208–213.
9. Sheehan FH, Bolson EL, Dodge HT, Mathey DG, Schofer J, Woo HW. Advantages and applications of the centerline method for characterizing regional ventricular function. *Circulation* 1986; **74:** 293–305.

VII Rehabilitation in Chronic Heart Failure

23 Structural and Vascular Alterations Within Skeletal Muscle of Patients with Chronic Heart Failure

Helmut Drexler

Medical Clinic III, University of Freiburg, Hugstetterstrasse 55, 7800 Freiburg, Germany

Introduction

Numerous studies have documented that the degree of ventricular dysfunction in chronic heart failure (CHF) does not correlate with the severity of clinical CHF, that is, indices of left ventricular dysfunction do not predict and correlate with the functional status of patients with CHF as assessed by exercise testing [1]. There is evidence, however, that impaired perfusion of skeletal muscle during exercise is one important factor determining exercise performance in patients with chronic heart failure. Almost 20 years ago, Zelis *et al.* [2] reported that in patients with chronic heart failure, the increase in blood flow to working muscle with exercise is attenuated for each given workload compared with that in normal persons. This observation was confirmed more recently for large muscle mass by Sullivan *et al.* [3]. Oxygen consumption at each level of work is lower in patients with chronic heart failure and is accompanied by an early increase in plasma lactate concentration [2]. The reduced maximal blood flow to working muscle during exercise appears to be confined to oxidative working muscle [4]. This impaired metabolic vasodilatory capacity within skeletal muscle in patients with chronic heart failure during exercise has often been attributed to excessive sympathetically mediated vasoconstriction, activation of the plasma renin–angiotensin system and, more recently, to increased levels of endothelin [5]. Although these neurohumoral factors exert potent systemic and regional vasoconstriction, they do not completely explain the impaired vasodi-

Proceedings of the Vth World Congress on Cardiac Rehabilitation

lating capacity within skeletal muscle in patients with chronic heart failure. Impaired metabolic vasodilatation during exercise cannot be restored by alpha blockade with phentolamine [6, 7]. Similarly, angiotensin-converting enzyme (ACE) inhibition does not restore impaired metabolic vasodilatation after acute administration, despite a substantial reduction of plasma angiotensin II and norepinephrine levels [8]. This indicates that blockade of the plasma renin–angiotensin system by ACE inhibitors does not interfere with blood flow to working muscle during exercise in patients with CHF [8, 9]. However, after chronic treatment with an ACE inhibitor over 3 months, a significant increase in femoral blood flow was noted during exercise and was accompanied by improved peak oxygen consumption [8]. Thus, chronic ACE inhibitor therapy reversed the inability of peripheral vessels to dilate. These findings are consistent with previous observations of the delayed beneficial effect of ACE inhibitor therapy in large-scale trials [10], indicating that the full beneficial effect of ACE inhibitors emerges slowly over time.

What is the explanation of the temporal dissociation between the rapid improvement in haemodynamics and gradual improvement in exercise performance? Obviously, exercise tolerance in patients with heart failure appears not solely to be determined by central haemodynamics. One possible explanation could be that the delayed effect of ACE inhibitors may be, in part, due to interference with the vascular tissue renin–angiotensin system, thereby reversing chronic structural alteration of the vessel. Experimental evidence indicates that angiotensin II induces hypertrophy of cultured rat aortic smooth muscle cells [11]. Angiotensin II and possibly endothelin and norepinephrine appear to be involved in the activation of proto-oncogenes [12]. This suggests that angiotensin II may be involved in the proliferative process of tissues during growth ('endogenous growth factor'). Recent observations indicate that ACE inhibition can reverse structural vascular alteration in a rat model of hypertension [13] and that these beneficial vascular effects appear to be more prominent with ACE inhibitors than other anti-hypertensive drugs [14].

Endothelial dysfunction

Recent data from our laboratory and others demonstrated that endothelium-dependent relaxation of the skeletal muscle microcirculation in response to acetylcholine is impaired in chronic heart failure, whereas the vasodilating effect of nitroglycerin is preserved [15–17]. There is experimental evidence that long-term treatment with ACE inhibitors restores endothelial dysfunction in experimental heart failure [18]. This beneficial effect of ACE inhibitors on endothelial function might be due to the inhibition of the breakdown of bradykinin, which is degraded by the angiotensin-converting enzyme [19]. Inhibition of the angiotensin-converting enzyme mechanism may increase local tissue levels of bradykinin, which, in turn, stimulates the release of nitric oxide (which accounts for the biological activity of the endothelium-derived relaxing factor EDRF) and vasodilating prostaglandins [19, 20]. Other potential mechanisms involved in impaired metabolic peripheral dilation in chronic heart failure include a vascular stiffness component owing to the increased vascular sodium content, which in part can be reduced with diuretic therapy in decompensated heart failure [21]. Whereas it remains controversial whether structural changes occur in the microcirculation of skeletal muscle, changes in compliance suggest that structural alterations emerge in large conduit vessels [22]. Moreover, flow-dependent dilation and nitroglycerin-induced dilation of large conduit vessels are impaired in patients with heart failure, indicating that relaxation of vascular smooth muscle is impaired in patients with chronic heart failure [23].

Intrinsic alterations of skeletal muscle in chronic heart failure

Although some vasodilators or positive inotropes have been shown to improve blood flow to skeletal muscle during exercise after acute administration, exercise duration and maximal oxygen consumption did not increase immediately after administration of these drugs [24]. This indicates that oxygen uptake of skeletal muscle during exercise cannot be improved during short-term intervention in patients with chronic heart failure even when oxygen delivery is enhanced. This observation suggests shunting of blood flow away from active muscle or intrinsic alterations of skeletal muscle in chronic heart failure, or both. We have noted previously that there may be a shift from oxidative skeletal muscle to activation of more glycolytic working muscle fibres [4], again indicating a change in the properties of the skeletal muscle itself. Muscle biopsies taken from patients with chronic heart failure revealed moderate atrophy (reduced muscle mass) and biochemical alterations including a shift in fibre type distribution of skeletal muscle (Fig. 1) [25, 26]. Ultrastructural analysis of skeletal muscle biopsy specimens has shown a reduced oxidative capacity of the muscle as indicated by a reduced volume density and reduced surface area of the cristae of mitochondria [27]. Cytochrome *c* oxidase staining of ultrastructural and biochemical quantification of citrate synthase demonstrated a significantly reduced concentration of these oxidative enzymes [27, 28], suggesting that the oxidative capacity of skeletal muscle is diminished in severe chronic heart failure. In fact, a close relation has been found between the oxidative capacity of working muscle as assessed by cytochrome *c* oxidase or cristae surface density of mitochondria within the skeletal muscle and the peak oxygen consumption during exercise (see Fig. 2) [27, 29]. Thus, exercise capacity appears to be, in part, determined by the condition of the working muscle [30]. The pattern obtained by nuclear magnetic resonance (NMR) spectroscopy revealed abnormal metabolism of skeletal muscle [31], supporting the ultrastructural and biochemical observations. Using NMR, it was demonstrated that the intracellular pH values during exercise are much lower for a given workload in

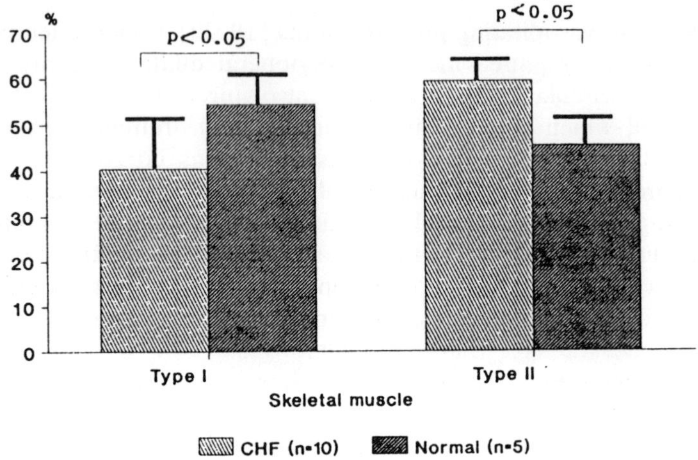

Fig. 1. Fibre type distribution in skeletal muscle in normal individuals (darker right bars) and patients with chronic heart failure (left bars). Fibre types I and II were determined by myofibrillar ATPase staining. Compiled from data published previously in Drexler *et al.* [27].

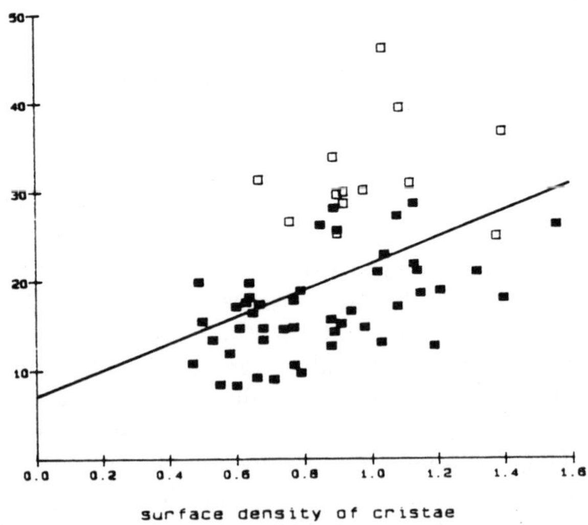

Fig. 2. Relationship between surface density of cristae of mitochondria (structural membranes on which oxidatives enzymes are located) and oxygen consumption at anaerobic threshold in patients with heart failure (■) and normal individuals (□). $P < 0.001$; $r = 0.46$; $n = 60$. Compiled from data published previously in Drexler *et al.* [27].

patients with severe heart failure. Moreover, during exercise, the concentrations of plasma inorganic phosphate and phosphocreatinine decreased much faster in patients with heart failure than in normal persons [31, 32].

The impact of impaired blood flow during exercise on these skeletal muscle alterations remains controversial. Subsequent studies utilizing NMR spectroscopy as well as skeletal muscle function tests in patients with chronic heart failure demonstrated these abnormalities under ischaemic conditions, unrelated to different rates of blood flow to working muscle during exercise [33–35]. This does not exclude, however, that repeated episodes of reduced blood flow within skeletal muscle may be involved in the development of skeletal muscle alterations, despite the fact that these alterations, once developed, can be demonstrated regardless of measured flow during the assessment of muscle function [35] or metabolism [33, 34].

β-Adrenergic receptors in skeletal muscle

There is experimental and clinical evidence that the properties of skeletal muscle can be modulated by hormones such as thyroxine or catecholamines acting via β-receptors [36, 37]. Since cardiac β-receptors are downregulated in patients with chronic heart failure [38, 39], we reasoned that downregulation of β-receptors could be involved in the alterations of skeletal muscle in patients with chronic heart failure. However, the β-receptor density was not reduced and, if anything, slightly increased [40]. β_2-Receptors of vascular tissue predominantly account for the β-receptor density measured in skeletal muscle tissue [41]. Therefore, our results suggest that β_2-receptors are not downregulated in the peripheral circulation in chronic heart failure. This is consistent with the recent findings of Creager *et al.* [42], who demonstrated a normal response of β_2-agonists in the peripheral circulation. Interestingly, Bristow *et al.* [38] have shown that even in cardiac muscle, downregulation was predominantly observed for β_1-adrenergic receptors.

In chronic heart failure, plasma levels of norepinephrine rather than epinephrine are increased. Since norepinephrine is a β_1-adrenergic receptor selective agonist [43], it predominantly exerts a subtype selective downregulation of β_1-receptors in chronic heart failure; the latter would not affect the β_2-receptor density of skeletal muscle.

Acknowledgement

This study was supported in part by Deutsche Forschungsgemeinschaft (Dr 148/3–4, 4–1, 4–2).

References

1. Franciosa JA, Park M, Levine B. Lack of relation between exercise capacity and indices of resting left ventricular performance in heart failure. *Am J Cardiol* 1981; **47:** 33–39.

2. Zelis R, Longhurst J, Capone RJ, Mason DT. A comparison of regional blood flow and oxygen utilization during dynamic forearm exercise in normal subjects and patients with congestive heart failure. *Circulation* 1974; **50:** 137–143.
3. Sullivan MJ, Knight JD, Higginbotham MB, Cobb FR. Relationship between central and peripheral haemodynamics during exercise in patients with chronic heart failure. Muscle blood flow is reduced with maintenance of arterial perfusion pressure. *Circulation* 1989; **80:** 769–781.
4. Drexler H, Faude F, Höing S, Just H. Blood flow distribution within skeletal muscle during exercise in the presence of chronic heart failure: effect of milrinone. *Circulation* 1987; **76:** 1344–1352.
5. McMurray JJ, Ray SG, Abdullah I, Dargie HJ, Morton JJ. Plasma endothelin in chronic heart failure. *Circulation* 1992; **85:** 1374–1379.
6. Zelis R, Mason DT, Braunwald E. A comparison of the effects of vasodilator stimuli on peripheral resistance vessels in normal subjects and patients with congestive heart failure. *J Clin Invest* 1968; **47:** 960–970.
7. Le Jemtel TH, Maskin CS, Lucido D, Chadwick BJ. Failure to augment maximal limb blood flow in response to one leg versus two-leg exercise in patients with severe heart failure. *Circulation* 1986; **74:** 245–251.
8. Drexler H, Banhardt U, Meinertz T, Wollschläger H, Lehmann M, Just H. Contrasting peripheral short-term and long-term effects of converting enzyme inhibition in patients with congestive heart failure: A double-blind, placebo-controlled trial. *Circulation* 1989; **79:** 491–502.
9. Wilson JR, Ferraro N. Effect of renin–angiotensin system on limb circulation and metabolism during exercise in patients with heart failure. *J Am Coll Cardiol* 1985; **6:** 556–563.
10. Captopril Multicenter Research Group: A placebo-controlled trial of captopril in refractory chronic congestive heart failure. *J Am Coll Cardiol* 1983; **2:** 755–763.
11. Geisterfer AAT, Peach MJ, Owens GK. Angiotensin II induces hypertrophy not hyperplasia, of cultured rat aortic smooth muscle cells. *Circ Res* 1988; **62:** 749–756.
12. Naftilan AJ, Pratt RE, Eldridge CS, Lin HL, Dzau VJ. Angiotensin II induces c-fos expression in smooth muscle via transcriptional control. *Hypertension* 1989; **13:** 706–711.
13. Levy BI, Michel JB, Salzmann J-L, Azizi M, Poitevin P, Safar M, Camilleri JP. Effects of chronic inhibition of converting enzyme on mechanical and structural properties of arteries in rat renovascular hypertension. *Circ Res* 1988; **63:** 227–239.
14. Sano T, Tarazi RC. Differential structural responses of small resistance vessels to antihypertensive therapy. *Circulation* 1987; **75:** 618–626.
15. Drexler H, Lu W. Endothelial dysfunction of hindquarter resistance vessels in experimental heart failure. *Am J Physiol* 1992; **262:** H1640–1645.
16. Drexler H, Hayoz D, Münzel T, Hornig B, Just H, Brunner HR, Zelis R. Endothelial function in chronic congestive heart failure. *Am J Cardiol* 1992; **69:** 1596–1601.
17. Kubo SH, Rector TS, Bank AJ, Williams RE, Heifetz SM. Endothelium-dependent vasodilation is attenuated in patients with heart failure. *Circulation* 1991; **84:** 1589–1596.
18. Ontkean MT, Gay R, Greenberg B. Effects of chronic captopril therapy on endothelium-derived relaxing factor activity in heart failure. *J Am Coll Cardiol* (Abstr.) 1992; **19:** 207A.
19. Wiemer G, Schölkens BA, Becker RHA, Busse R. Ramiprilat enhances endothelial autacoid formation by inhibiting breakdown of endothelium-derived bradykinin. *Hypertension* 1991; **18:** 558–563.
20. Mombouli J-V, Naphtali M, Vanhoutte PM. Effects of the converting enzyme inhibitor cilazaprilat on endothelium-dependent responses. *Hypertension* (Suppl. II) 1991; **18:** 22–29.

21. Sinoway LI, Minotti J, Musch T, Goldner D, Davis D, Leaman D, Zelis R. Enhanced metabolic vasodilation secondary to diuretic therapy in decompensated congestive heart failure secondary to coronary artery disease. *Am J Cardiol* 1987; **60:** 107–111.
22. Arnold JMO, Marchiori GE, Imrie JR, Burton GL, Pflugfelder PW, Kostuk WJ. Large artery function in patients with chronic heart failure: Studies of brachial artery diameter and haemodynamics. *Circulation* 1991; **84:** 2418–2425.
23. Hayoz D, Drexler H, Münzel T, Hornig B, Zeiher AM, Just H, Brunner HR, Zelis R. Flow mediated arterial dilation is abnormal in congestive heart failure. *Circulation* (in press).
24. Wilson JR, Martin JL, Ferraro N, Weber KT. Effect of hydralazine on perfusion and metabolism in the leg during upright bicycle exercise in patients with heart failure. *Circulation* 1983; **68:** 425–432.
25. Mancini DM, Walter G, Reichek N, Lenkinski R, McCully KK, Mullen JL, Wilson JR. Contribution of skeletal muscle atrophy to exercise intolerance and altered muscle metabolism in heart failure. *Circulation* 1992; **85:** 1364–1373.
26. Lipkin DP, Jones DA, Round JM, Poole-Wilson PA. Abnormalities of skeletal muscle in patients with chronic heart failure. *Int J Cardiol* 1988; **18:** 187–195.
27. Drexler H, Riede U, Münzel T, König H, Funke E, Just H. Alterations of skeletal muscle in chronic heart failure. *Circulation* 1992; **85:** 1751–1759.
28. Sullivan MJ, Green HJ, Cobb FR. Skeletal muscle biochemistry and histology in ambulatory patients with long-term heart failure. *Circulation* 1990; **81:** 518–527.
29. Drexler H. The effect of ace-inhibitors on the peripheral circulation in heart failure. *Am J Cardiol* 1992; **70**: 50C–54C.
30. Drexler H. Skeletal muscle failure in heart failure. *Circulation* 1992; **85:** 1621–1623.
31. Wilson JR, Fink L, Maris J, Ferraro N, Power-Vanwart J, Eleff S, Chance B. Evaluation of energy metabolism in skeletal muscle of patients with heart failure with gated phosphorus-31 nuclear magnetic resonance. *Circulation* 1985; **71:** 57–62.
32. Massie BM, Conway M, Yonge R, Frostick S, Sleight P, Ledingham J, Radda G, Rajagopalan B. ^{31}P nuclear magnetic resonance evidence of abnormal skeletal muscle metabolism in patients with congestive heart failure. *Am J Cardiol* 1987; **60:** 309–315.
33. Wiener DH, Fink LI, Maris J, Jones RA, Chance B, Wilson JR. Abnormal skeletal muscle bioenergetics during exercise in patients with heart failure: Role of reduced muscle blood flow. *Circulation* 1986; **73:** 1127–1136.
34. Massie BM, Conway M, Rajagopalan B, Yonge R, Frostick S, Ledingham J, Sleight P, Radda G. Skeletal muscle metabolism during exercise under ischemic conditions in congestive heart failure: Evidence for abnormalities unrelated to blood flow. *Circulation* 1988; **78:** 320–326.
35. Minotti JR, Christoph I, Oka R, Weiner MW, Wells L, Massie BM. Impaired skeletal muscle function in patients with congestive heart failure: Relationship to systemic exercise performance. *J Clin Invest* 1991; **88:** 2077–2082.
36. Meiler SEL, Leier CV. Effects of beta-adrenergic stimulation on skeletal-muscle conditioning. *Heart Failure* 1986; June/July: 128–137.
37. Liggett SB, Shah SD, Cryer PE. Increased fat and skeletal muscle β-adrenergic receptors but unaltered metabolic and haemodynamic sensitivity to epinephrine *in vivo* in experimental human thyrotoxicosis. *J Clin Invest* 1989; **83:** 803–809.
38. Bristow MR, Ginsburg R, Minobe W *et al.* Decreased catecholamine sensitivity and β-adrenergic-receptor density in failing human hearts. *N Engl J Med* 1982; **307:** 205–211.
39. Brodde OE, Schüler S, Kretsch R *et al.* Regional distribution of β-adrenoceptors in the human heart: Coexistence of functional β_1- and β_2-adrenoceptors in both atria and ventricles in severe congestive cardiomyopathy. *J Cardiovasc Pharmacol* 1986; **8:** 1235–1242.

40. Drexler H, Brodde OE, Münzel T, Riede U, Wirth P, König H. Characterization of skeletal muscle β-adrenergic receptors in patients with chronic heart failure. *Circulation* (Abstr.) 1989; **80:** 116.
41. Liggett SB, Shah SD, Cryer PE. Characterization of β-adrenergic receptors of human skeletal muscle obtained by needle biopsy. *Am J Physiol* 1988; **254:** E795–798.
42. Creager MA, Quigg RJ, Ren CJ, Roddy M-A, Colucci WS. Limb vascular responsiveness to β-adrenergic receptor stimulation in patients with congestive heart failure. *Circulation* 1991; **83:** 1873–1879.
43. Lands AM, Arnold A, McAuliff JP, Luduena FP, Brown TG Jr. Differentiation of receptor systems activated by sympathomimetic amines. *Nature* 1967; **214:** 597–598.

24 Endothelium-dependent Vasodilatation is Improved by Physical Training in Normal Subjects

Stuart D. Katz, Marc Klapholz, Guillaume Jondeau, Marie Galvao, Paola Levato, Steven Solomon, Thierry H. LeJemtel*

Department of Medicine, Division of Cardiology, Albert Einstein College of Medicine, 1300 Morris Park Avenue, Forchheimer G-42, Bronx, New York, NY 10461, USA

Introduction

In normal subjects, the cardiac responses to physical training have included an increase in maximal oxygen uptake ($\dot{V}O_2$ max), stroke volume and cardiac output, without overt change in maximal heart rate [1, 2]. Physical training also induces alterations in skeletal muscles, which include a shift to fat muscle metabolism during sub-maximal exercise, an increase in oxidative capacity in mitochondrial proteins, and an increase in capillary density [3–9]. Lastly, physical training substantially increases maximal vascular conductance in the trained skeletal muscle vasculature. Increased vascular conductance appears to be mediated by local rather than systemic mechanisms [10, 11].

Recently, Furchgott and Zawadzki [12] discovered that acetylcholine-mediated relaxation of isolated arterial preparations is dependent on the presence of endothelium. Acetylcholine interacts with muscarinic receptors on endothelial cells to stimulate the release of a substance that induces relaxation of the underlying vascular smooth muscle, i.e. nitric oxide (NO) [13–16]. In view of the role played by the endothelium in regulating vascular smooth muscle tone, improved vascular endothelial function may contribute to the increase in maximal vascular conductance induced by training [17]. Accordingly, the

* To whom all correspondence should be addressed.

Proceedings of the Vth World Congress on Cardiac Rehabilitation

vasodilatory responses to acetylcholine, an endothelium-dependent stimulus, and nitroglycerin, an endothelium-independent stimulus, were evaluated in the lower limbs of normal subjects before and after intense physical training involving treadmill or bicycle exercise.

Methods

Maximal exercise testing protocol

Three women and three men (aged 34 ± 6 years) leading sedentary lifestyles, performed symptom-limited, upright bicycle or treadmill maximal exercise before and after 4 and 8 weeks of intense physical training. For each bicycle ergometer test, exercise work rate was increased from 0 W continuously at the onset of exercise to a rate of 25 W/min, until the subjects were unable to continue. Treadmill exercise tests were performed according to the Bruce Protocol. Expired gases were measured as previously described.

Physical training programme

The programme consisted of 4 weekly 45-min sessions of lower extremity exercise for 8 weeks. According to individual preference, four subjects performed training sessions on the bicycle ergometer and two subjects on the motorized treadmill. Maximal exercise testing was concordant with the training modality for each subject. Training was performed at workloads corresponding to 70–80% of pre-training maximal oxygen uptake.

Doppler ultrasonography

The regional vascular effects of physical training were assessed in the lower limb by determining the mean blood flow velocity in the superficial femoral artery (cm/s) by transcutaneous duplex Doppler ultrasonography [18, 19]. Measurements of superficial femoral artery blood flow velocity correlate significantly with venous occlusion plethysmography measurements of blood flow in the calf [19]. Superficial femoral artery blood flow velocity was determined by integrating the mean Doppler spectral display throughout systole and diastole and dividing by the RR interval. Five consecutive beats were averaged for each determination.

Forearm blood flow measurements

The regional vascular effects of lower limb physical training were assessed in the upper limb by determining forearm blood flow (ml/min/100 ml of forearm volume) with strain gauge venous occlusion plethysmography as previously described [20]. Doppler ultrasonography in the upper limb is not feasible because of the difficulty of maintaining the Doppler sample volume within the small calibre of the brachial artery. Five plethysmographic tracings were averaged for each blood flow determination. During each blood flow measurement, mean arterial pressure was determined in the contralateral arm at 15-s intervals by the cuff method with an automated blood pressure measurement device (Dinamapp, Model 1846).

Drug administration

All drugs were administered directly into the brachial and femoral arteries through small-gauge infusion catheters; infusion rates were adjusted according to the resting basal limb blood flows measured prior to each infusion to achieve final regional blood concentrations as stated. Graded concentrations of acetylcholine (10^{-7}, 10^{-6} and 10^{-5} M), an endothelium-dependent vasodilator, and nitroglycerin (10^{-8}, 10^{-7} and 10^{-6} M), an endothelium-independent vasodilator, were administered in the brachial and femoral arteries as a 2-min continuous infusion in a randomized order. Serial infusions were administered at 5- to 10-min intervals when forearm blood flow and superficial femoral artery mean blood flow velocity had returned to basal values.

Determination of regional vascular responses

The regional vascular responses to intra-arterial administration of endothelium-dependent and -independent vasodilators were determined in the upper and lower limbs before and after 8 weeks of physical training. Small-gauge catheters were placed in the brachial and superficial femoral arteries for regional drug administration under local anaesthesia. Thirty minutes after catheter placement, baseline measurements of forearm blood flow and superficial femoral artery blood flow velocity were obtained. Graded concentrations of acetylcholine and nitroglycerin were then administered sequentially in the brachial and superficial femoral arteries. Regional vascular responses in the upper and lower limbs were determined during the last minute of each 2-min drug infusion.

Data analysis

All values are stated as mean $\pm$ SEM. Maximal oxygen uptake and regional vascular responses to administration of graded concentrations of acetylcholine and nitroglycerin were compared before and after training with paired Student's *t*-tests. A two-tailed *P*-value <0.05 was considered statistically significant.

Results

Maximal oxygen uptake

Physical training increased maximal oxygen uptake in all six subjects (Table 1).

Table 1
Maximal oxygen uptake before and after physical training

			Before training		After training	
Patient	Age (yrs) (years)	Sex	Weight (kg)	$\dot{V}O_2$ max (ml/kg/min)	Weight (kg)	$\dot{V}O_2$ max (ml/kg/min)
1	30	F	56.0	38.0	55.0	55.0
2	34	M	94.5	38.7	91.8	46.3
3	47	M	70.0	47.0	71.0	57.0
4	32	F	52.0	40.0	53.0	55.0
5	32	M	62.0	40.0	64.2	48.0
6	31	F	59.5	30.0	57.5	33.0
Mean ± SEM	34 ± 3		65.7 ± 6.3	39.0 ± 2.2	65.4 ± 5.9	49.1 ± 3.7*

* $P < 0.01$ before *vs* after training.

Regional vascular effects of physical training

Lower limb

Before physical training, intra-arterial administration of acetylcholine 10^{-7}, 10^{-6} and 10^{-5} M in the superficial femoral artery increased superficial femoral artery blood flow velocity to 10.2 ± 0.9, 21.5 ± 5.9, and 32.8 ± 6.3 cm/s, respectively. After physical training, increases in superficial femoral artery blood flow velocity were 15.5 ± 2.4, 34.1 ± 3.5 and 47.6 ± 4.5 cm/s, respectively. The increases in superficial femoral artery blood flow velocity in response to administration of acetylcholine were significantly greater after physical training when compared to those observed before physical training (Fig. 1A).

Before physical training, intra-arterial administration of nitroglycerin 10^{-8}, 10^{-7} and 10^{-6} M in the superficial femoral artery increased superficial femoral artery blood flow velocity to 11.8 ± 1.3, 18.4 ± 2.1 and 26.3 ± 1.9 cm/s, respectively. After physical training, the increase in superficial femoral artery blood flow velocity in response to administration of nitroglycerin was unchanged (Fig. 1B).

Mean systemic arterial pressure was unchanged by intraarterial drug administrations in the lower limb: 86.3 ± 3.8 *vs* 83.0 ± 1.7 mmHg ($P = 0.5$).

Upper limb

Before physical training, intra-arterial administration of acetylcholine 10^{-7}, 10^{-6} and 10^{-5} M in the brachial artery increased mean forearm blood flow to 5.9 ± 2.1, 12.7 ± 3.3 and 33.5 ± 2.8 ml/min/100 ml, respectively. After physical training, the increase in forearm blood flow in response to administration of acetylcholine was unchanged (Fig. 2A).

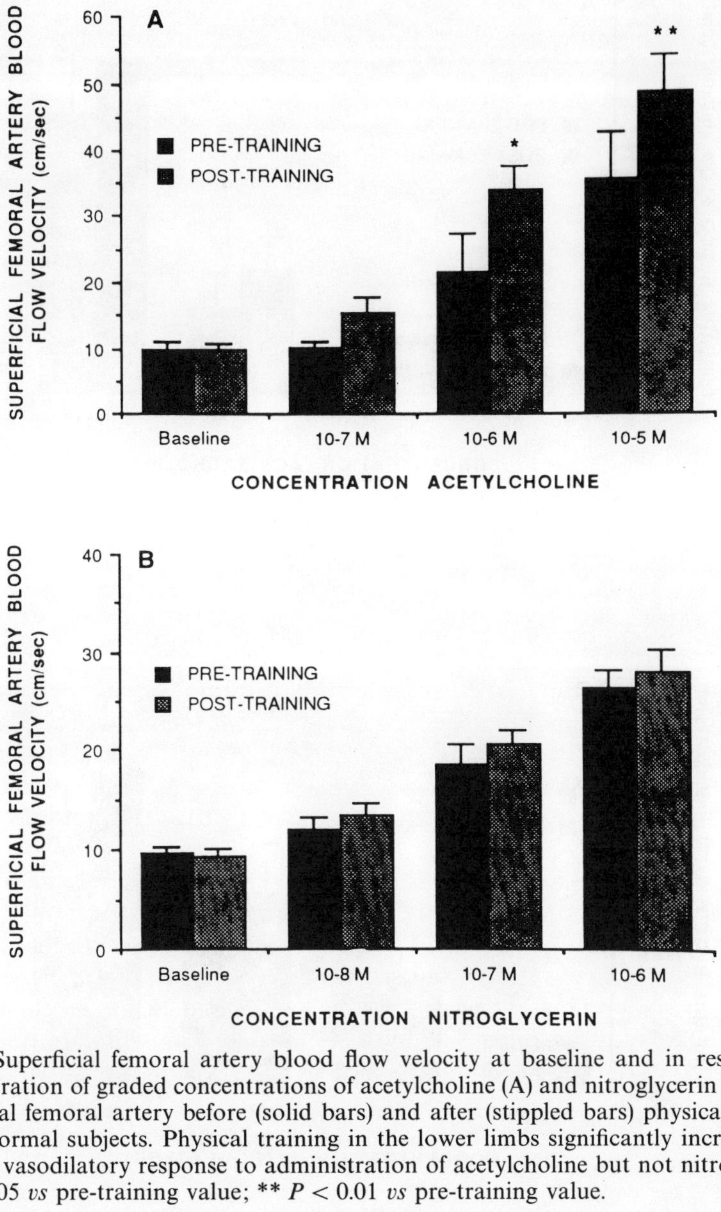

Fig. 1: Superficial femoral artery blood flow velocity at baseline and in response to administration of graded concentrations of acetylcholine (A) and nitroglycerin (B) in the superficial femoral artery before (solid bars) and after (stippled bars) physical training in five normal subjects. Physical training in the lower limbs significantly increased the regional vasodilatory response to administration of acetylcholine but not nitroglycerin. * $P < 0.05$ *vs* pre-training value; ** $P < 0.01$ *vs* pre-training value.

Before physical training, intra-arterial administration of nitroglycerin 10^{-8}, 10^{-7} and 10^{-6} M in the brachial artery increased mean forearm blood flow to 8.2 ± 3.1, 14.5 ± 3.6 and 23.6 ± 3.3 ml/min/100 ml, respectively. After physical training, the increase in forearm blood flow in response to administration of nitroglycerin was unchanged (Fig. 2B).

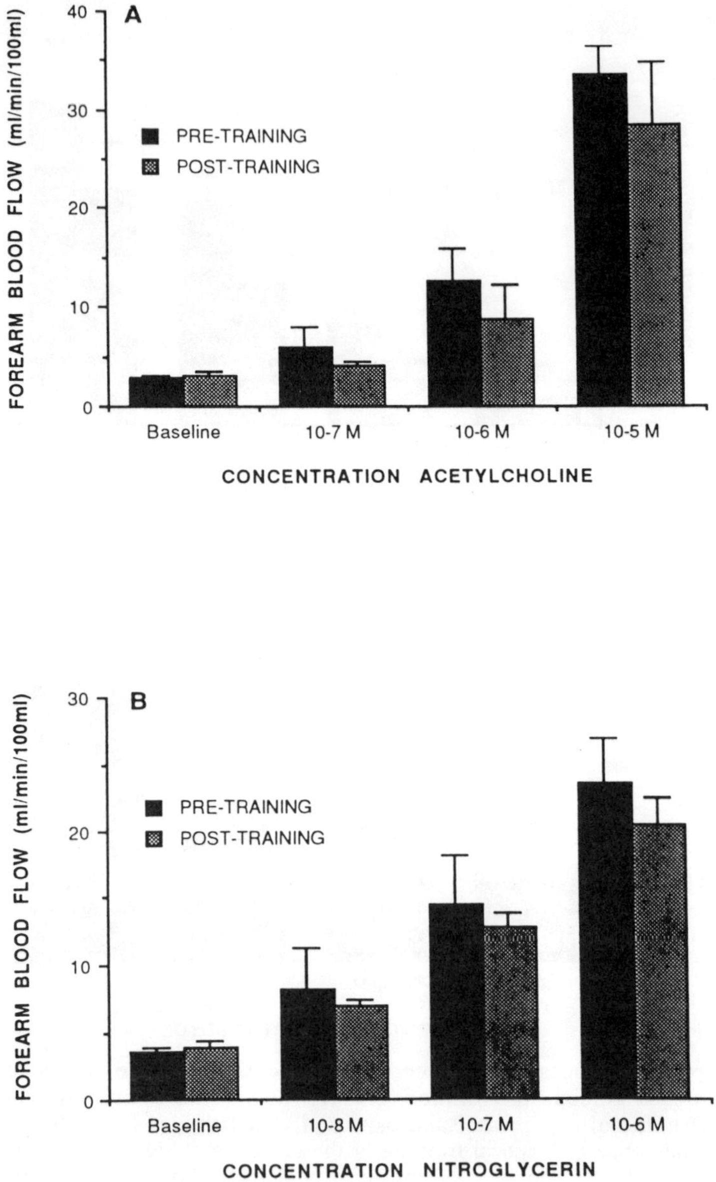

Fig. 2: Forearm blood flow at baseline and in response to administration of graded concentrations of acetylcholine (A) and nitroglycerin (B) in the brachial artery before (solid bars) and after (stippled bars) physical training in six normal subjects. Physical training of the lower limbs did not change the regional vasodilatory response to acetylcholine or nitroglycerin in the upper limb.

Mean systemic arterial pressure was unchanged by drug administrations in the upper limb.

Discussion

The present data clearly indicate that intense physical training resulting in an average increase of 26% in maximal oxygen uptake is associated with an enhanced vasodilatory response to intra-arterial administration of acetylcholine (an endothelium-dependent vasodilator) but not to intra-arterial administration of nitroglycerin (an endothelium-independent vasodilator). The enhanced vasodilatory response to acetylcholine is specifically limited to the trained skeletal muscle vasculature of the lower limb and is not observed in the untrained skeletal muscle vasculature of the upper limb.

The enhanced vasodilatory response to acetylcholine suggests that physical training improves endothelium function in the trained skeletal muscle vasculature. The vascular endothelium released NO, a potent vasodilating agent, in response to increased shear stress at the endothelial cell surface, and thereby plays an important role in mediating flow-dependent vasodilation and co-ordinating the behaviour of conduit and resistance blood vessels [21, 22]. Whether improved endothelium function contributes to an increase in skeletal muscle blood flow during maximal exercise cannot be ascertained from the present study. Few investigators have documented the effects of physical training on blood flow to the trained skeletal muscle during exercise. Varnauskas and colleagues [3] have reported that physical training reduces skeletal muscle blood flow at constant sub-maximal workloads corresponding to 60% of maximal oxygen uptake. Several investigators have observed that maximal skeletal muscle blood flow significantly increases after one-legged but not two-legged training [23–25]. During two-legged maximal exercise, when active skeletal muscle mass oxygen requirements exceed cardiac output reserve, potent vasoconstricting mechanisms are activated which oppose regional skeletal muscle vasodilatation to maintain adequate perfusion pressure [26]. This balance between vasodilatory and vasoconstricting forces makes it difficult to detect change in the maximal vasodilatory capacity of the trained skeletal muscle vasculature.

The increased maximal arteriovenous oxygen difference observed after physical training has been attributed to vascular adaptations which lead to more efficient oxygen extraction by the active skeletal muscle [1]. Endothelial release of NO, which may be viewed as a local feedback mechanism for the skeletal muscle circulation, may play an important role in the regional vascular adaptations to physical training which promote efficient skeletal muscle oxygen utilization.

References

1. Blomqvist CG. Cardiovascular adaptations to physical training. *Ann Rev Physiol* 1983; **45:** 169–189.
2. Scheuer J, Tipton CM. Cardiovascular adaptations to physical training. *Ann Rev Physiol* 1977; **39:** 221–251.
3. Varnauskas E, Bjorntorp P, Fahlen M, Prerovsky I, Stenberg J. Effects of physical training on exercise blood flow and enzymatic activity in skeletal muscle. *Cardiovasc Res* 1970; **4:** 418–422.
4. Gollnick PD, Armstrong RB, Saltin B, Saubert IV CW, Sembrowich WL, Sepherd RE. Effect of training on enzymatic activity and fibre composition of human skeletal muscle. *J Appl Physiol* 1973; **34:** 107–111.
5. Gollnick PD. Metabolism of substrates: energy substrate metabolism during exercise and as modified by training. *Fed Proc* 1985; **44:** 353–357.
6. Gollnick PD, Armstrong RB, Saubert IV CW, Piehl K, Saltin B. Enzyme activity and fibre composition in skeletal muscle of untrained and trained men. *J Appl Physiol* 1972; **343:** 312–319.
7. Brodal P, Ingger F, Hermansen L. Capillary supply of skeletal muscle fibers in untrained and endurance trained men. *Am J Physiol* 1977; **232:** H705–712.
8. Andersen P, Henriksson J. Capillary supply of the quadriceps femoris muscle of man: adaptive response to exercise. *J Physiol* 1977; **270:** 677–690.
9. Clausen JP. Effect of physical training on cardiovascular adjustments to exercise in man. *Physiol Rev* 1977; **57:** 779–815.
10. Clausen JP, Klausen K, Rasmusson B, Trap Jonsen J. Central and peripheral circulatory changes after training of the arm or legs. *Am J Physiol* 1973; **225:** 675–682.
11. Clausen JP, Trap Jensen J, Lassen NA. The effects of training on heart rate during arm and leg exercise. *Scand J Clin Lab Invest* 1970; **26:** 295–301.
12. Furchgott RF, Zawadzki JV. The obligatory role of endothelial cells in the relaxation of arterial smooth muscle by acetylcholine. *Nature* 1980; **288:** 373–376.
13. Furchgott RF. Role of endothelium in responses of vascular smooth muscle. *Circ Res* 1983; **53:** 557–573.
14. Furchgott RF. The role of endothelium in the responses of the vascular smooth muscle to drugs. *Ann Rev Pharmacol Toxicol* 1984; **24:** 175–197.
15. Palmer RMJ, Ferrige AG, Moncada S. Nitric oxide release accounts for the biological activity of endothelium derived factor. *Nature* 1987; **327:** 524–526.
16. Moncada S, Palmer RM, Higgs AE. The discovery of nitric oxide as the endogenous nitrovasodilator. *Hypertension* 1988; **12:** 365–372.
17. Ignaro LJ. Biological actions and properties of endothelium-derived nitric oxide formed and released from artery and vein. *Circ Res* 1989; **65:** 1–21.
18. Katz SD, Biasucci L, Sabba C *et al.* Impaired endothelium-mediated vasodilation in the peripheral vasculature of patients with congestive heart failure. *J Am Coll Cardiol* 1992; **19:** 918–925.
19. Jondeau G, Klapholz M, Katz SD, Maher M, Galvao M, Levato P, LeJemtel TH. Control of arteriolar resistance in heart failure: Partial attenuation of specific phosphodiesterase inhibitor-mediated vasodilation by digitalis glycosides. *Circulation* 1992; **85:** 54–60.
20. Greenfield ADM, Whitney RJ, Mowbray JF. Methods for the investigation of peripheral blood flow. *Br Med Bull* 1963; **19:** 101–109.
21. Vane JR, Anggard EE, Botting RM. Regulatory functions of the vascular endothelium. *N Engl J Med* 1990; **323:** 27–37.
22. Griffith TM, Edwards DH, Davies RLI, Harrison TJ, Evans KT. EDRF coordinates the behavior of vascular resistance vessels. **Nature** 1987; **329:** 442–445.

23. Davies CTM, Sargeant AJ. Effects of training on the physiological responses to one- and two-leg work. *J Appl Physiol* 1975; **38:** 377–381.
24. Gleser MA. Effects of hypoxia and physical training on haemodynamic adjustments to one-legged exercise. *J Appl Physiol* 1973; **34:** 655–659.
25. Saltin B, Nazar K, Costill DL *et al.* The nature of the training response: Peripheral and central adaptations to one-legged exercise. *Acta Physiol Scand* 1976; **96:** 289–305.
26. Sinoway L, Prophet S. Skeletal muscle metabaroreceptor stimulation opposes peak metabolic vasodilatation in humans. *Circ Res* 1990; **66:** 1576–1584.

25 Mechanism of Increased Vascular Resistance in Heart Failure

P. A. Poole-Wilson

Department of Cardiology, National Heart and Lung Institute, Dovehouse Street, London SW3 6LY, UK

Introduction

The last decade has seen major advances in the treatment of heart failure [1]. The most dramatic has been the success achieved by transplantation of the human heart; the most important has been the demonstration that new forms of therapy can not only improve the symptoms of patients with heart failure, but also prolong life [2–4]. Both surgical and medical strategies add years of active life to patients with heart failure. At the same time and partly inspired by the availability of these new treatments, there has been a vast increase in research directed towards understanding the pathophysiology of heart failure. This has led to several new concepts which may provide further opportunities in the future [1]. A major question at the moment, for example, is how angiotensin-converting enzyme (ACE) inhibitors bring about benefit in heart failure so as to improve symptoms, reduce mortality, reduce hospital admissions and most surprisingly prevent the recurrence of acute coronary events. Possible mechanisms include vasodilatation, a renal action, a synergistic action with diuretics, effects on peptides other than angiotensin, interactions with other hormonal systems and an effect of angiotensin II on cell growth within the myocardium and the vascular wall.

Proceedings of the Vth World Congress on Cardiac Rehabilitation

Termination of exercise

The major symptoms of heart failure are shortness of breath and fatigue [5–7]. In the past, conventional thinking has been that fatigue was related to a low cardiac output and shortness of breath on exercise to an elevated left ventricular end diastolic pressure. Little is known about the causes of fatigue in any cardiac syndrome. How fatigue might be limited by a transient or maintained reduction in cardiac output is unclear. Fatigue can often masquerade as tiredness, exhaustion, muscle weakness or even depression. Cardiologists are familiar with a similar symptom of fatigue in patients with angina pectoris, particularly when treated with beta-blockers, and in patients with transient arrhythmias. In this latter group, the fatigue may persist for the remainder of the day after a transient arrhythmia.

More is known about the relationship between the left ventricular end-diastolic pressure and shortness of breath. In acute heart failure there is a link, presumably due to the retention of fluid in the lung leading to increased stiffness and pulmonary oedema [8]. Treatments which lower the left ventricular end-diastolic pressure acutely, such as the nitrates [9] and vasodilators [10], lead fairly quickly to symptomatic improvement. This idea has been transferred inappropriately to patients with treated chronic heart failure. Much research has now indicated that the concept is invalid in patients with chronic heart failure [1, 5, 11]. At the end of exercise in such patients, there is no correlation between the left ventricular end-diastolic pressure and the duration of exercise [11]. Were the end-diastolic pressure to be the limiting factor, then it would be expected that all patients would terminate exercise when that pressure was substantially elevated.

A further and fundamental problem is what body system is responsible for the termination of exercise. The answer may be different in trained athletes, normal persons and those with heart failure [12]. Measurement of gas exchange [13, 14] during exercise has led to the concept that there is a peak oxygen consumption which can be achieved by any person and that this is determined by the function of the cardiovascular system. That may be true in some athletes and in occasional normal persons, but it is probably untrue in most healthy individuals and in many patients with heart failure [12]. In heart failure and many other situations, it may not be the function of the cardiovascular system, but the function of the muscle itself, which finally leads to the signals which cause a person to terminate exercise.

Termination of exercise in patients with heart failure

There are several physiological reasons why the patient with heart failure may not be able to continue to exercise (Table 1). The left atrial pressure does increase on exercise and subtle signals within the lung, particularly ventilation perfusion mismatch [15], may give rise to signals contributing to the patient's

Table 1
Origin of symptoms on exercise in chronic heart failure

1. Lung abnormalities	Increased stiffness due to raised venous pressure and lymphatic distension Increased left atrial pressure Increased physiological dead space Increased respiratory rate
2. Circulation	Reduced blood flow to skeletal muscle Increased production of metabolites
3. Skeletal muscle	Rest atrophy Ischaemic atrophy Specific abnormality

symptoms. This mismatch may be at the level of the microcirculation and could be similar to changes which occur in the systemic circulation. On exercise when flow increases this abnormality might contribute to the sensation of breathlessness.

Recent work has indicated that at peak exercise in patients with heart failure the oxygen content of the femoral vein is almost zero [16]. There is, therefore, no shunting of blood in the peripheral limbs and the muscles are extracting virtually all the oxygen that is available. Furthermore, in patients with severe heart failure undertaking bicycle exercise, the perfusion pressure in the limbs is not greatly increased. Since flow is reduced up to five-fold, that means there is an increase in the peripheral resistance [16]. The ability to increase flow to skeletal muscle is not therefore directly related to the function of the heart, but is a long-term adaptation to ventricular dysfunction. A consequence is that unless the peripheral vasoconstriction is reversed, the supply of oxygen to skeletal muscle cannot be increased and there would be a substantial limitation to the ability to increase the exercise capacity in such patients. The only possibility would be to alter the efficiency or the nature of the muscle in the limbs and such a change could only lead to a limited improvement in exercise capacity.

Two lines of evidence provide some support for this hypothesis. First, the maximal effect of angiotensin-converting enzyme inhibitors is not reached for at least 4 weeks. Where there is benefit with these drugs the increase in exercise capacity is related to the increase in blood flow to the exercising limbs [17]. Secondly, studies in patients who have undergone transplantation show that blood flow and the resistance does not improve immediately but only after a period of 4–5 weeks [18]. This crucial experiment provides almost overwhelming evidence for the idea that there is a limitation of blood flow in patients with heart failure caused by changes in the peripheral circulation.

The final cause for symptoms in heart failure is atrophy of the muscle itself [19]. Merely reducing the muscle mass will, of course, increase the peripheral resistance and can mimic the changes in gas exchange seen in patients with heart failure [20]. To demonstrate a true increase of resistance attributable to the vasculature requires that the resistance is measured per unit weight or volume of muscle. Even then small changes could occur if the muscle type were to alter. There is weak evidence for alteration of muscle type in heart failure [19, 21]. Furthermore, there are histological [19], metabolic [22] and functional [23] changes which occur in the muscles of patients with heart failure. The mechanisms limiting muscle function and possibly contributing to fatigue are complex [24].

Causes of increased resistance in heart failure

The body responds to heart failure in several different ways (Table 2). Harris [25] has argued that these changes are part of a reflex response of the body and that the primary purpose of this reflex was to maintain the blood pressure. A major response is an increase in the systemic resistance. Although some of the increase in resistance can be accounted for by a reduction of muscle mass, this cannot account for the whole fall in resistance. A large number of mechanisms have been proposed and are shown in Table 3. The only anatomical change reported is a thickening of the basement membrane of arterioles [26]. There are no major anatomical changes in blood vessels nor is there a major change in the capillary density. Biopsies allow only assessment of small vessels and angiography permits study of large vessels. Between these are vessels (diameter 100–300 μm) which have not been studied. The increase in resistance is not explained by activation of the sympathetic and renin–angiotensin systems, since the resistance remains abnormally high after these systems have been blocked acutely by appropriate pharmaceutical agents. Arteriolar constriction has been attributed to the retention of sodium in the vessel wall [27]. Presumably, if there were an increase of intracellular sodium, then via a calcium–sodium exchange mechanism, cytosolic calcium would be increased causing constriction of smooth muscle.

Table 2
Body responses to heart failure

1. Heart	Structure	Loss of cells, fibre orientation, size, shape, fibrosis, hypertrophy
	Function	Systolic and/or diastolic
2. Circulation	Increased resistance	1. Anatomical abnormality
		2. Neuroendocrine response sympathetic system and renin–angiotensin
		3. Functional abnormality
3. Skeletal muscle	Atrophy	
	Function	Abnormal biochemistry

Table 3
Causes of increased peripheral resistance in chronic heart failure

1. Tissue oedema
2. Anatomical abnormality
3. Endothelial cell oedema
4. Arteriolar constriction
sodium–calcium exchange
unknown peptide
5. Neuroendocrine-induced vasoconstriction
6. Endothelial cell relaxing factor
7. Microvascular infarction

By far the most popular current hypothesis is that the function of the endothelium is abnormal. In animal models of heart failure, dilation of the isolated aorta in response to acetylcholine has been shown to be reduced suggesting endothelial dysfunction [28]. In humans, there is no flow-induced vasodilation of the femoral arteries [29], but possibly a limitation of vasodilator reserve both in coronary blood vessels [30, 31] and in systemic vessels. There are, however, major problems in accepting these conclusions. Coronary reserve is calculated from the flow at rest compared to that after a vasodilator. Common vasodilators such as adenosine, papaverine and dipyridamole do not always give the same answers and may not maximally vasodilate the coronary circulation. For example, the conclusion that endothelial function is abnormal, based on a similar response to adenosine but a reduced response to acetylcholine, is not well-founded [30]. Results are expressed as percentages, baseline differences may exist, the response to adenosine appeared less in heart failure and there are several reasons for a reduced response to acetylcholine. These include a vasodilatory action due to activation of receptors on the endothelium, constriction due to a direct action on smooth muscle, variable penetrance of the drug into the extracellular space, different effects in large and small vessels, different initial coronary flow, extracellular influences on coronary flow such as ventricular geometry and haemodynamics, and altered neurohumoral mechanisms. The demonstration of abnormal endothelial cell function in the peripheral circulation is even more complex. Most pharmaceutical agents do not cause maximal vasodilatation. In the lower limb, flow can increase after ischaemia and exercise (probably maximal stimuli) by more than ten-fold compared to a maximum of four-fold in the heart. Initial data are difficult to interpret.

In heart failure a primary reduction in cardiac function is accompanied by changes in the peripheral circulation which bring about an increase of systemic resistance. This increased resistance limits blood flow to the exercising limbs and is a major cause of the reduced exercise capacity and symptoms. The mechanism for the increased resistance remains unclear.

References

1. Poole-Wilson PA. Future perspectives in the management of congestive heart failure. *Am J Cardiol* 1990; **66:** 462–467.
2. The SOLVD Investigators. Effect of enalapril on survival in patients with reduced left ventricular ejection fractions and congestive heart failure. *N Engl J Med* 1991; **325:** 293–302.
3. Cohn JN, Johnson G, Ziesche S, Cobb F, Francis GS, Tristani F, Smith R, Dunkman WB, Loeb H, Wong M, Bhat G, Goldman S, Fletcher RD, Doherty J, Hughes CV, Carson P, Cintron G, Shabetai R, Haakenson C. A comparison of enalapril with hydralazine-isosorbide dinitrate in the treatment of chronic congestive heart failure. *N Engl J Med* 1991; **325:** 302–310.
4. Poole-Wilson PA, Lindsay D. Advances in the treatment of chronic heart failure: Two steps forward, one step back. *Br Med J* 1992; **304:** 1069–1070.
5. Lipkin DP, Poole-Wilson PA. Symptoms limiting exercise in chronic heart failure (editorial). *Br Med J* 1986; **292:** 1030–1031.
6. Poole-Wilson PA. The origin of symptoms in patients with chronic heart failure. *Eur Heart J* (Suppl.) 1988; **9:** H49–53.
7. Poole-Wilson PA, Buller NP. Causes of symptoms in chronic congestive heart failure and implications for treatment. *Am J Cardiol* 1988; **62:** 31A–34A.
8. Guyton AC, Lindsey AW. Effect of left atrial pressure and decreased plasma protein concentration on the development of pulmonary oedema. *Circ Res* 1959; **7:** 649–657.
9. Nelson GI, Silke B, Ahuja RC, Hussain M, Taylor SH. Haemodynamic advantages of isosorbide dinitrate over frusemide in acute heart-failure following myocardial infarction. *Lancet* 1983; **i:** 730–733.
10. Taylor SH, Silke B, Nelson GI. Principles of treatment of left ventricular failure. *Eur Heart J* (Suppl.) 1982; **3:** D19–43.
11. Lipkin DP, Canepa-Anson R, Stephens MR, Poole-Wilson PA. Factors determining symptoms in heart failure: comparison of fast and slow exercise tests. *Br Heart J* 1986; **55:** 439–445.
12. Noakes TD. Implications of exercise testing for prediction of athletic performance: a contemporary perspective. *Med Sci Sports Exercise* 1988; **20:** 319–330.
13. Lipkin DP, Perrins J, Poole-Wilson PA. Respiratory gas exchange in the assessment of patients with impaired ventricular function. *Br Heart J* 1985; **54:** 321–328.
14. Buller NB, Poole-Wilson PA. Extrapolated maximum oxygen consumption: a new method for the objective analysis of respiratory gas exchange during exercise. *Br Heart J* 1988; **59:** 212–217.
15. Buller NB, Poole-Wilson PA. Mechanism of the increased ventilatory response to exercise in patients with chronic heart failure. *Br Heart J* 1990; **63:** 281–283.
16. LeJemtel TH, Maskin CS, Lucido D, Chadwick BJ. Failure to augment maximal limb blood flow in response to one-leg versus two-leg exercise in patients with severe heart failure. *Circulation* 1986; **74:** 245–251.
17. Mancini DM, Davis L, Wexler JP, Chadwick B, LeJemtel TH. Dependence of enhanced maximal exercise performance on increased peak skeletal muscle perfusion during long-term captopril therapy in heart failure. *J Am Coll Cardiol* 1987; **10:** 845–850.
18. Sinoway LI, Minotti JR, Davis D, Pennock JL, Burg JE, Musch TI, Zelis R. Delayed reversal of impaired vasodilation in congestive heart failure after heart transplantation. *Am J Cardiol* 1988; **61:** 1076–1079.
19. Lipkin DP, Jones DA, Round JM, Poole-Wilson PA. Abnormalities of skeletal muscle in patients with chronic heart failure [published errata appear in *Int J Cardiol* **19**: 396 and *Int J Cardiol* **20**: 161]. *Int J Cardiol* 1988; **18:** 187–195.

20. Poole-Wilson PA, Buller NP, Lindsay DC. Blood flow and skeletal muscle in patients with heart failure. *Chest* 1992; **101:** 330S–332S.
21. Sullivan MJ, Green HJ, Cobb FR. Skeletal muscle biochemistry and histology in ambulatory patients with long-term heart failure. *Circulation* 1990; **81:** 518–527.
22. Loesser KE, Kukreja RC, Kazziha SY, Jesse RL, Hess ML. Oxidative damage to the myocardium: A fundamental mechanism of myocardial injury. *Cardioscience* 1991; **2:** 199–216.
23. Buller NP, Jones D, Poole-Wilson PA. Direct measurement of skeletal muscle fatigue in patients with chronic heart failure. *Br Heart J* 1991; **65:** 20–24.
24. Westerblad H, Lee JA, Lannergren J, Allen DG. Cellular mechanisms of fatigue in skeletal muscle. *Am J Physiol* 1991; **261:** C195–209.
25. Harris P. Congestive cardiac failure: Central role of the arterial blood pressure. *Br Heart J* 1987; **58:** 190–203.
26. Longhurst J, Capone RJ, Zelis R. Evaluation of skeletal muscle capillary basement membrane thickness in congestive heart failure. *Chest* 1975; **67:** 195–198.
27. Zelis R, Delea CS, Coleman HN, Mason DT. Arterial sodium content in experimental congestive heart failure. *Circulation* 1970; **41:** 213–216.
28. Lindsay D, Jiang C, Brunotte F, Adamopoulos S, Coats A, Rajagopolan B, Poole-Wilson PA, Collins P. Endothelium-dependent relaxation is impaired in aortic rings from a rat model of heart failure. *Eur Heart J* (Suppl., abstr.) 1991; **12:** 4.
29. Lindsay D, Clarke D, Holdwright D, McNeill J, Anand I, Poole-Wilson P, Collins P. Lack of flow-dependent dilatation of the human femoral artery. *Eur Heart J* (Suppl., abstr.) 1991; **12:** 84.
30. Treasure CB, Vita JA, Cox DA, Fish D, Gordon JB, Mudge GH, Colucci WS, St John Sutton MG, Selwyn AP, Alexander RW, Ganz P. Endothelium-dependent dilation of the coronary microvasculature is impaired in dilated cardiomyopathy. *Circulation* 1990; **81:** 772–779.
31. Cannon RO, Cunnion RE, Parrillo JE, Palmeri ST, Tucker EE, Schenke WH, Epstein SE. Dynamic limitation of coronary vasodilator reserve in patients with dilated cardiomyopathy and chest pain. *J Am Coll Cardiol* 1987; **10:** 1190–1200.

26 Exercise Rehabilitation in Chronic Heart Failure

Andrew J. S. Coats*[1,2], Stamatis Adamopoulos[1,2], Alberto Radaelli[2,3], Theo E. Meyer[2], Massimo Piepoli[1,2], Patrick Davey[2], Peter Sleight[2]

[1]Department of Cardiac Medicine, National Heart and Lung Institute, Dovehouse Street, London, SW3 6LY UK, [2]Department of Cardiovascular Medicine, John Radcliffe Hospital, Oxford, OX3 9DU, UK, and [3]Department of Internal Medicine, First Medical Clinic, University of Pavia, Pavia, Italy

Introduction

Chronic heart failure is a multisystem syndrome in which the initiating cause is a reduction in cardiovascular functional reserve, but in which also a variety of pathophysiological abnormalities develop in other organ systems [1]. These changes are poorly understood, but look likely to reduce exercise tolerance in their own right, and may also contribute to the symptoms suffered by patients with this condition.

Developments in the pharmacological treatment of heart failure have led to an increasingly common clinical syndrome of chronic non-oedematous heart failure. Patients with this condition can live for many months and years. Improved survival and exercise tolerance has been shown in this group of patients by vasodilators and in particular angiotensin-converting enzyme (ACE) inhibitors [2–5]. Their ability to exercise, however, remains extremely limited and they suffer the cardinal symptoms of dyspnoea and fatigue. The cause of exercise limitation in CHF was traditionally thought to be related to cardiac dysfunction, but attempts to predict the degree of symptomatic limitation from parameters of left ventricular functional impairment have proved disappointing. The search for other factors which may be limiting exercise has uncovered abnormalities in many disparate organ systems.

* To whom all correspondence should be addressed.

Proceedings of the Vth World Congress on Cardiac Rehabilitation

Peripheral circulation

Heart failure is associated with a reduced maximal blood flow to exercising limbs [6, 7]. The mechanisms of this is uncertain but it may involve any or all of the following: reduced skeletal muscle mass, reduced capillary density, thickened resistance vessel endothelial wall, persistent vasoconstrictor drive, or impaired endothelial-dependent vasodilator function or enhanced endothelial-dependent constrictor release. The enhancement of limb blood flow by inotropic support or peripheral vasodilators infused during exercise does not acutely increase exercise performance [8], so it may be either that the blood flow so enhanced does not go to the exercising muscles or that compensatory mechanisms prevent appropriate redistribution within the exercising muscle. Training may increase both peripheral arterial size and function and so may benefit this particular abnormality in heart failure. In one study, peak leg blood flow was increased by exercise training in chronic heart failure [9].

Skeletal muscle function

Some of the symptoms of muscular fatigue of chronic heart failure have been attributed to an inherent defect in oxidative metabolism in skeletal muscle in this condition [10]. Abnormalities have been described in oxidative phosphorylation, enzymatic content, mitochondrial structure, fibre type distribution, strength, fatiguability and mass. Some of these abnormalities can be corrected by single limb [11] or endurance training regimes [12] in chronic heart failure. In an animal model of heart failure, we have also confirmed that training can partially prevent or ameliorate abnormalities of oxidative phosphorylation and enzymic alterations [13]. These results are consistent with the known effects of training on skeletal muscle in normals [14].

Respiratory muscle function

Alterations occur in heart failure in respiratory muscle fatiguability and strength and in diaphragmatic muscle histology. It is not known to what extent these can be reversed by training, but respiratory muscle training can reduce respiratory muscle fatigue in other conditions, so it may be of benefit in CHF.

Ventilatory control

Chronic heart failure is associated with an increased ventilation at matched workloads and an increase in the ventilatory equivalent for carbon dioxide throughout exercise [15]. In other words, a greater minute ventilation is needed to excrete a given amount of carbon dioxide in heart failure. The mechanisms of this are not known, but this abnormality is probably a significant component in the sensation of breathlessness that patients complain of even at sub-maximal exercise workloads. Training in chronic heart failure has been shown to reduce ventilation at matched workloads [16] and to be associated with a delay in lactate release [16] and a decrease in the respiratory exchange ratio and ventilatory equivalent for carbon dioxide during incremental exercise [17]. The slope relating minute ventilation to the rate of carbon dioxide production (which has been shown to reflect the severity of heart failure [15]) was also reduced [17]. Such improvements may be related to a lessening of ventilation/perfusion mismatch in the lung or, alternatively, to a reduction in an alternative respiratory stimulus which is activated in chronic heart failure

Autonomic balance and neurohormonal activation

Chronic heart failure is associated with activation of the sympathetic nervous system, the renin–angiotensin system, and the arginino–vasopressin system as well as reduced vagal tone and impairment of arterial baroreflex activity. In addition, atrial natriuretic peptide levels are increased. Although initially helping maintain the circulation, with chronic activation these changes may lead to further left ventricular dilatation and dysfunction and may even predispose to sudden cardiac death and poor prognosis. It is known that training can reduce sympathetic activity and improve baroreflex gain, and we have shown that training in chronic heart failure can increase indices of vagal activity and reduce indices of sympathetic activation including noradrenaline spillover [18].

Exercise training prescriptions in chronic heart failure

It is too early to say how much exercise patients with heart failure should undertake, nor which is the best from of exercise – dynamic, isometric or a combination. Patients with moderate or even severe left ventricular dysfunction without clinical heart failure achieved significant improvements in exercise tolerance after participation in a rehabilitation exercise programme [19–21]. Patients with well-controlled mild to moderate heart failure also show improvements in exercise tolerance, leg blood flow and parameters of ventilatory function [9,16]. Such changes were seen after many months of exercise training. We have confirmed these findings in patients with stable class II and III heart failure in a controlled comparison of training *vs* rest [22]. We obtain significant benefits in patients after 6–8 weeks of training, exercising at 60–80% of peak heart rate for 20–60 min 3–5 days per week.

No trial to date has looked at exercise training for patients with oedematous or unstable heart failure, nor has any study recruited significant numbers of subjects with greater than class III heart failure. It is unlikely that exercise

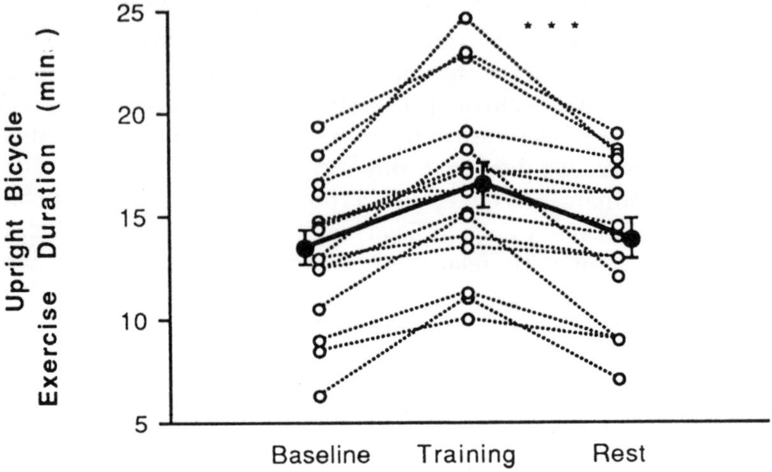

Fig. 1. Individual and mean (±SEM) patient upright exercise durations for baseline, training and detraining periods in 17 patients with stable chronic heart failure. *** $P < 0.001$ for the comparison between training and detraining periods ($n = 17$). Reproduced from Coats *et al.* [18] with the permission of the American Heart Association, Inc.

training would be feasible for class IV subjects with maximal oxygen uptakes less than 10 ml/kg/min. Left ventricular ejection fraction *per se* does not appear to be a reason to prohibit exercise training, as the majority of the benefits are probably mediated via training effects in the periphery, and no trial to date has shown any change in ejection fraction, either beneficial or detrimental. Our patients had a mean ejection fraction less than 20%, with a range down to 9% [18, 22]. Sullivan *et al.* [9] reported patients with a similar range of ejection fractions (mean 24%, range 9–33%).

Aetiology of heart failure

It remains possible that some rare forms of cardiomyopathy may show a paradoxical adverse response to exercise training, but the studies of Sullivan and colleagues appear to show similar benefits in ischaemic *vs* dilated cardiomyopathic patients. Specific exceptions include obstructive valvular disease (especially aortic stenosis), obstructive hypertrophic cardiomyopathy or active myocarditis, either viral or auto-immune. These conditions should remain contraindications to exercise therapy.

Selection of patients

Patients to undergo exercise training should be very carefully assessed prior to exercise therapy. A full cardiological examination is necessary including tests for the aetiology of heart failure, and the exclusion of active myocarditis or obstructive cardiomyopathy. Any patient exhibiting decompensation of their heart failure should reduce exercise activity and exercise should cease during intercurrent viral or febrile illnesses. Any patient exhibiting exercise-induced serious ventricular arrhythmias should only exercise under supervision and monitoring, although the situation with patients with asymptomatic non-sustained ventricular tachycardias not specifically exercise-induced is unclear. It may be that the reduction in sympathetic tone produced by training may be beneficial in these patients, but the safety of exercise in this group of patients has not been determined.

In exercise testing in heart failure, serious ventricular arrhythmias are not common events [23]. Exercise rehabilitation in coronary patients is associated with an extremely low incidence of cardiac arrests (less than 1 in 110,000 patient-hours of exercise [24]). None of the studies of training in heart failure reported so far have detected any serious ventricular arrhythmias during exercise, but these have so far only been small studies with careful entry criteria.

Conclusions

Physical exercise prescription as part of a comprehensive cardiac rehabilitation programme may be of benefit in patients with compensated stable non-oedematous chronic heart failure. Exercise training can improve peripheral vascular, muscular and metabolic function. Indices of sympatho-vagal balance may be improved and this suggests a potential protective role of training on the susceptibility to ventricular arrhythmias in this group, or the progression of their left ventricular dysfunction. These latter points should be the subject of future trials.

Acknowledgements

This work was supported by the British Heart Foundation, a Squibb Cardiovascular Fellowship and an ICI Research Fellowship at Pembroke College, Oxford.

References

1. Poole-Wilson PA. Chronic heart failure: Causes, pathophysiology, prognosis, clinical manifestations, investigations. In: Poole-Wilson PA (ed), *Diseases of the Heart*. London: Balliere Tindall, 1989, pp. 48–57.
2. Cohn JN, Archibald DG, Ziesche S *et al.* Effect of vasodilator therapy on mortality in chronic congestive heart failure. *New Engl J Med* 1986; **314:** 1547–1552.
3. The CONSENSUS Trial Study Group. Effects of enalapril on mortality in severe congestive heart failure: Results of the Cooperative North Scandinavian Enalapril Survival Study. *New Engl J Med* 1987; **316:** 1429–1435.

4. Cohn JN, Johnson G, Ziesche S *et al.* A comparison of enalapril with hydralazine-isosorbide dinitrate in the treatment of chronic congestive heart failure. *New Engl J Med* 1991; **325:** 303–310.
5. The SOLVD Investigators. Effect of enalapril on survival in patients with reduced left ventricular ejection fractions and congestive heart failure. *New Engl J Med* 1991; **325:** 293–302.
6. Wilson JR, Martin JL, Schwartz D, Ferraro N. Exercise intolerance in patients with chronic heart failure: Role of impaired nutritive flow to skeletal muscle. *Circulation* 1984; **69:** 1079–1087.
7. Zelis R, Nellis SH, Longhurst J, Lee G, Mason DT. Abnormalities in the regional circulations accompanying congestive heart failure. *Prog Cardiovasc Dis* 1975; **18:** 181–199.
8. Wilson JR, Martin JL, Ferraro N. Impaired skeletal muscle nutritive flow during exercise in patients with congestive heart failure: Role of cardiac pump dysfunction as determined by the effect of dobutamine. *Am J Cardiol* 1984; **53:** 1308–1315.
9. Sullivan MJ, Higginbotham MB, Cobb FR. Exercise training in patients with severe left ventricular dysfunction: Hemodynamic and metabolic effects. *Circulation* 1988; **78:** 506–515.
10. Massie BM, Conway M, Yonge R *et al.* ^{31}P nuclear magnetic resonance evidence of abnormal skeletal muscle metabolism in patients with congestive heart failure. *Am J Cardiol* 1987; **60:** 309–315.
11. Minotti JR, Johnson EC, Hudson TH *et al.* Skeletal muscle response to exercise training in congestive heart failure. *J Clin Invest* 1990; **86:** 751–758.
12. Adamopoulos S, Coats AJS, Arnolda L *et al.* Effects of physical training on skeletal muscle metabolism in chronic heart failure: 31-P NMR spectroscopy study. *Circulation* (Suppl. II, abstr.) 1992; **84:** 74.
13. Adamopoulos S, Brunotte F, Coats A *et al.* Skeletal muscle metabolism in experimental heart failure: Effects of infarct size and physical training. *J Am Coll Cardiol* (Suppl., abstr.) 1992; **17:** 158A.
14. Holloszy JO. Adaptations of muscular tissue to training. *Prog Cardiovasc Dis* 1976; **18:** 445–458.
15. Buller NP, Poole-Wilson PA. Mechanism of the increased ventilatory response to exercise in patients with chronic heart failure. *Br Heart J* 1990; **63:** 281–283.
16. Sullivan MJ, Higginbotham MB, Cobb FR. Exercise training in patients with chronic heart failure delays ventilatory anaerobic threshold and improves sub-maximal exercise performance. *Circulation* 1989; **79:** 324–329.
17. Davey P, Meyer T, Coats A *et al.* Ventilation in chronic heart failure: Effects of physical training. *Br Heart J* 1992; **68:** 473–477.
18. Coats AJS, Adamopoulos S, Radaelli A *et al.* Controlled trial of physical training in chronic heart failure: Exercise performance, hemodynamics, ventilation and autonomic function. *Circulation* 1992; **85:** 2119–2131.
19. Williams RS. Exercise training of patients with ventricular dysfunction and heart failure. *Cardiovasc Clin* 1985; **15:** 218–231.
20. Letac B, Cribier A, Desplanches JF. A study of left ventricular function in coronary patients before and after physical training. *Circulation* 1977; **56:** 375–378.
21. Conn EH, Williams RS, Wallace AG. Exercise responses before and after physical conditioning in patients with severely depressed left ventricular function. *Am J Cardiol* 1982; **49:** 296–300.
22. Coats AJS, Adamopoulos S, Meyer TE, Conway J, Sleight P. Effects of physical training in chronic heart failure. *Lancet* 1990; **335:** 63–66.
23. Tristani FE, Hughes CV, Archibald DG *et al.* Safety of graded symptom-limited exercise testing in patients with congestive heart failure. *Circulation* (Suppl. VI) 1987; **76:** 54–58.
24. Von Camp SP, Peterson RA. Cardiovascular complications of outpatient cardiac rehabilitation programs. *JAMA* 1986; **256:** 1160–1163.

27 Exercise Conditioning in Patients with Left Ventricular Dysfunction

Martin J. Sullivan

Department of Medicine, Division of Cardiology and Center for Living, Duke University Medical Center and Durham Veterans Administration Medical Center, Durham, NC 27710, USA

Introduction

In patients with coronary artery disease and preserved left ventricular (LV) function, exercise conditioning leads to an increased work rate at the angina threshold [1, 2], favourable alterations in blood lipids [1, 3], improved peak oxygen uptake ($\dot{V}O_2$) [4–7] and, although studies are not conclusive, a potential decrease in mortality and reinfarction rates [8]. Although patients with preserved LV function have been participating in exercise conditioning programmes for decades, it has been traditionally held that exercise was contraindicated in patients with severe left ventricular systolic dysfunction and chronic heart failure. Only in the last decade have the effects of exercise training been examined in these patients. The results of numerous studies now indicate that stable patients with chronic heart failure due to systolic LV dysfunction can safely participate in cardiac rehabilitation programmes and can improve peak $\dot{V}O_2$ and symptoms after exercise training [9–16]. This paper will focus on discussing the physiology of exercise training in patients with severe systolic LV dysfunction and will examine current issues in clinical application of cardiac rehabilitation in this high-risk subset of patients.

Proceedings of the Vth World Congress on Cardiac Rehabilitation

Training in patients with severe systolic LV dysfunction

Recent studies in patients with severe systolic LV dysfunction have indicated that exercise intolerance is due primarily to the early onset of anaerobic metabolism in skeletal muscle [17–20]. Two factors have been identified which may contribute to this response in patients: reduced muscle perfusion during exercise and reduced aerobic enzyme content in skeletal muscle [17–20]. Although increased intra-pulmonary pressures may be important in producing dyspnoea in acute heart failure, several lines of evidence indicate that this is not the primary factor limiting exercise in stable ambulatory patients with chronic heart failure. Massie *et al.* [18] have demonstrated no relationship between peak exercise pulmonary capillary wedge pressure and peak $\dot{V}O_2$ in patients with chronic heart failure. In examining ventilatory control in this disorder [21], we have demonstrated in patients with heart failure that during short-term maximal exercise: (1) 70% are limited by leg fatigue; (2) pulmonary wedge pressures are not higher in patients limited by dyspnoea *vs* those limited by fatigue; and (3) pulmonary dead space and ventilation are related to decreased cardiac output and not increased pulmonary wedge pressures. The concept that the skeletal muscle metabolic response to exercise plays the primary role in determining exercise tolerance in this disorder provides a physiological rationale for utilizing exercise training as a potential means to improve exertional symptoms in patients with chronic heart failure.

Although a small number of patients with severe systolic LV dysfunction have been included in earlier training studies [10, 12], it has only been in the last 10 years that research has been directed specifically at examining the training response in this group of patients. Lee *et al.* [11] were the first to report the effects of exercise training in patients with impaired LV dysfunction due to coronary artery disease. Eighteen patients with left ventricular ejection fractions (LVEFs) less than 0.40 underwent exercise testing and cardiac catheterization before and after 12–42 months of physical conditioning. Peak exercise capacity increased significantly, and there were no changes in LV dimensions or intra-cardiac pressures after exercise training. Studies from our institution by Conn *et al.* [13] demonstrated an increase in peak exercise capacity in patients with LVEFs of 13–25% after 4–37 months of exercise conditioning, which was accompanied by an increase in peak exercise oxygen pulse with no exercise-related complications.

An important recent study by Coats *et al.* [14] has also examined exercise training in patients with chronic heart failure (LVEF 16 ± 8%) employing a crossover design with the investigators blinded to training status. The patients demonstrated a significant improvement in peak $\dot{V}O_2$ and a decrease in heart rate during sub-maximal exercise after training. Symptom scores, assessed by a modified Likert questionnaire, were also improved in patients after training. These authors also demonstrated a decrease in sympathetic activation after training as indicated by power spectral analysis of heart rate variability and a decrease in resting norepinephrine spillover, suggesting that chronic exercise may act to decrease neurohumoral activation and therefore possibly delay progressive LV dysfunction in this disorder. In addition, these authors demonstrated a decrease in peak $\dot{V}O_2$ back to baseline after a period of detraining indicating that improved peak $\dot{V}O_2$ was not due solely to familiarization with the exercise protocol. Studies by Kellerman *et al.* [22] and Hoffman *et al.* [23] have also demonstrated an increase in peak exercise performance after training in patients with LV dysfunction and have noted no change in LVEF or wall abnormalities.

Studies in our laboratory [15, 16] have examined the effects of 4–6 months of exercise conditioning in patients with class I–III chronic heart failure due to systolic LV dysfunction (LVEF 24 ± 10%). Before and after training, patients underwent maximal graded bicycle exercise testing with measurement of expired gases and central and leg haemodynamics. At rest and at each workload, blood was drawn for determination of oxygen content and lactate. Haemodynamic measurements included right atrial pressure, pulmonary and pulmonary wedge pressures, leg blood flow by thermodilution, and cardiac output by the direct Fick technique. Radionuclide angiography was performed at rest and at each workload using a gated equilibrium technique to determine the LVEF. Left ventricular end-diastolic volume (LVEDV) and end-systolic volume (LVESV) were calculated from the Fick stroke volume and the radionuclide ejection fraction.

Patients exercised for 4.1 ± 0.6 h per week and improved both functional class from 2.4 ± 0.6 to 1.3 ± 0.7 ($P < 0.01$) and peak exercise workload from 520 ± 105 to 613 ± 119 kgm/min (100 ± 19 *W*; $P = 0.02$). Peak $\dot{V}O_2$ (Fig. 1A) increased from 1.11 ± 0.33 l/min (16.8 ± 3.7 ml/kg/min) to 1.40 ± 0.40 l/min (20.6 ± 4.7 ml/kg/min) after training (both $P < 0.01$). Cardiac output was unchanged during sub-maximal exercise (Fig. 1B) but demonstrated a tendency to increase at maximal exercise from 8.9 ± 2.9 to 9.9 ± 3.2 l/min ($P = 0.13$). Heart rate (Fig. 1C) was reduced at rest and during sub-maximal exercise but did not change at maximal exercise. The systemic arteriovenous oxygen ($A\dot{V}O_2$) difference (Fig. 1D) was increased at rest, unchanged during sub-maximal exercise and increased at peak exercise from 13.1 ± 1.4 to 14.6 ± 2.3 ml/dl ($P < 0.05$). Resting and exercise arterial, right atrial, pulmonary capillary wedge and pulmonary artery pressures were unchanged after training. Stroke volume was unchanged at rest but tended to increase during exercise, although these changes did not reach statistical significance ($P = 0.12$). Resting and exercise LVEF, LVESV and LVEDV were not significantly altered by training, and there were no changes in rest or exercise wall motion abnormalities.

Leg blood flow, leg oxygen delivery, leg vascular resistance and leg $A\dot{V}O_2$ difference (Fig. 2A–D) did not change at rest or during sub-maximal exercise after training. Blood flow to the single leg (Fig. 2A) increased at peak exercise from 2.5 ± 0.7 to 3.0 ± 0.8 l/min ($P < 0.01$), as did leg oxygen delivery (Fig. 2B). There was a tendency for leg vascular resistance (Fig. 2C) to decrease ($P = 0.06$) and leg $A\dot{V}O_2$ difference (Fig. 2D) to increase at peak exercise

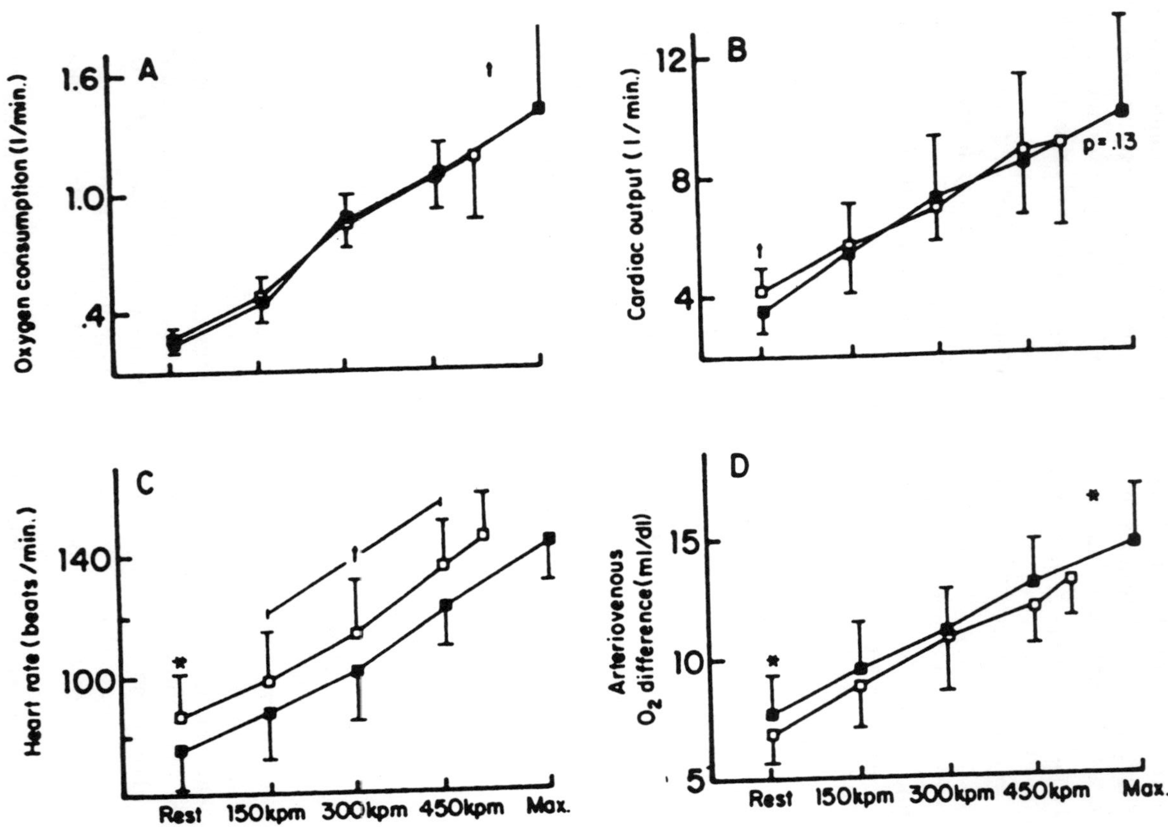

Fig. 1. Plots of resting and exercise oxygen consumption, cardiac output, heart rate and systemic arteriovenous oxygen difference in patients before (□) and after (■) training. * $P < 0.05$, $^+P < 0.01$ by Wilcoxon signed-rank test. Reprinted from Sullivan *et al.* [15] with the permission of the American Heart Association, Inc.

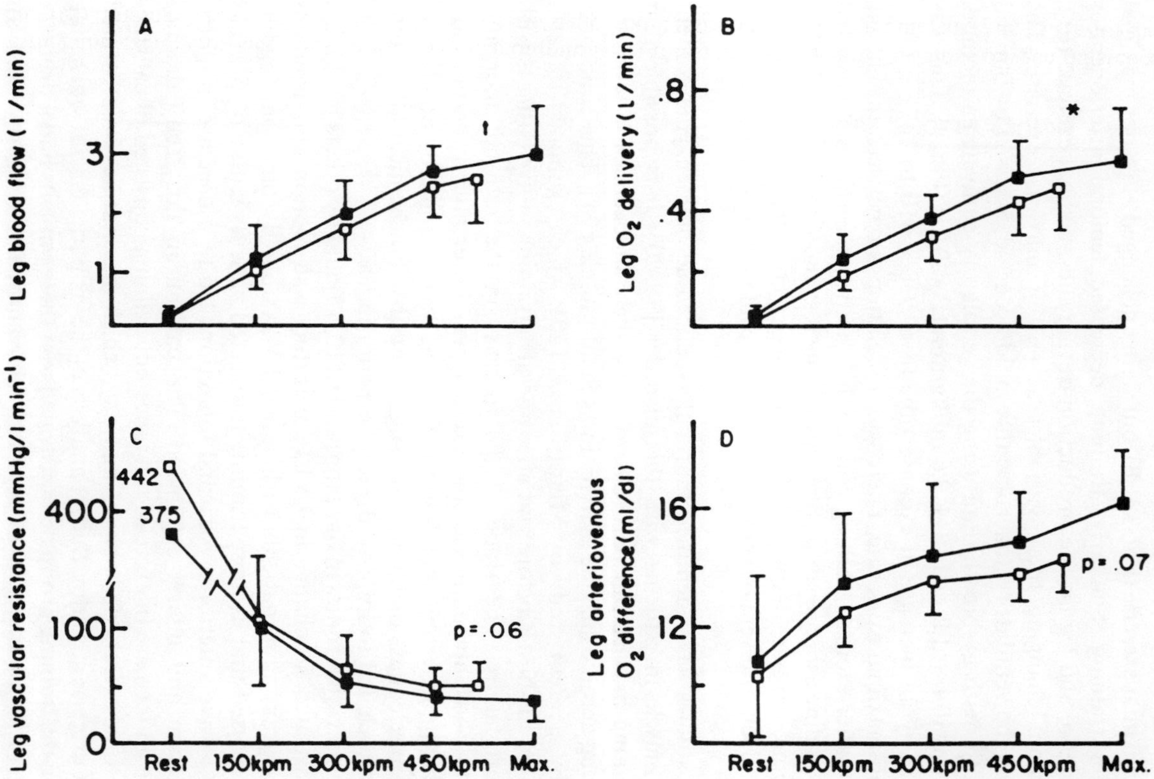

Fig. 2. Plots of resting and exercise single leg blood flow, leg oxygen delivery, leg vascular resistance and leg $A\dot{V}O_2$ difference in patients before (□) and after (■) training. * $P < 0.05$; $^{+}P < 0.01$ by Wilcoxon signed rank test. Reprinted from Sullivan *et al.* [15] with the permission of the American Heart Association, Inc.

(14.5 ± 1.3 *vs* 16.1 ± 1.9 ml/dl, $P = 0.07$). Thus, single-leg $\dot{V}O_2$, determined using the Fick principle, increased from 0.36 ± 0.11 to 0.47 ± 0.13 l/min ($P < 0.01$) at peak exercise.

Arterial and femoral venous lactate concentrations were markedly reduced during submaximal exercise (Fig. 3A, B), but were unchanged at rest or maximal exercise after training. Similarly, training decreased femoral arteriovenous lactate difference and leg lactate production during sub-maximal exercise (Fig. 3C, D) without changing these variables at rest or maximal exercise. The $\dot{V}O_2$ at which the ventilatory anaerobic threshold occurred, assessed by blinded inspection of breath-by-breath data using the ventilatory equivalents method, increased from 10.1 ± 1.2 to 12.1 ± 2.6 ml/kg/min ($P < 0.01$) (Fig. 4). This was accompanied by an increase in exercise time from 938 ± 410 to 1429 ± 691 s at a fixed sub-maximal work rate. There was no relationship between the change in peak $\dot{V}O_2$ after exercise training and any haemodynamic variable measured during the baseline exercise study. Specifically, the rest and peak exercise LVEF, stroke volume, cardiac output, $\dot{V}O_2$, systemic $A\dot{V}O_2$ difference, leg $A\dot{V}O_2$ difference and femoral vein oxygen saturation were all unrelated to the response to training.

Previous studies have identified markedly reduced aerobic enzyme content in skeletal muscle in patients with this disorder [19, 20]; it is possible that exercise training may act, in part, by reversing these biochemical alterations and increasing aerobic enzyme activity in skeletal muscle [24]. This concept is supported by a recent study by Minotti *et al.* [25], which examined forearm metabolism by ^{31}P-NMR before and after one-arm training in five patients with chronic heart failure. The slope of the increase in the ratio of inorganic phosphate to phosphocreatine during exercise was lower after training, indicating a delay in anaerobic metabolism. This was accompanied by no changes in forearm muscle mass or blood flow, suggesting that biochemical alterations in skeletal muscle led to improved exercise performance.

Although previous studies in our laboratory [10, 15] and by others [9, 22, 23] have demonstrated no change in LVEF or resting wall motion abnormalities after exercise training in patients with severe LV systolic dysfunction, Jugdutt *et al.* [26] reported that exercise training in selected patients initiated 15 weeks after large Q-wave anterior myocardial infarctions led to a decrease in global ejection fraction and infarct expansion. The patients in this study did not demonstrate an increase in exercise tolerance but training consisted of calisthenics and isotonic exercise for only 11 min/day, which may not have represented a significant exercise stimulus. Subset analysis of the six patients with worsening symptoms in the training group demonstrated that these patients had a decrease in global LVEF, an increase in regional left ventricular asynergy, and an increase in wall thinning in the infarct zone when compared to non-exercising controls.

Arvan [27] examined the exercise training response in 85 patients with coronary artery disease and subdivided them into four groups based on high or low LVEF (greater than or less than 0.40) and the presence or absence of a

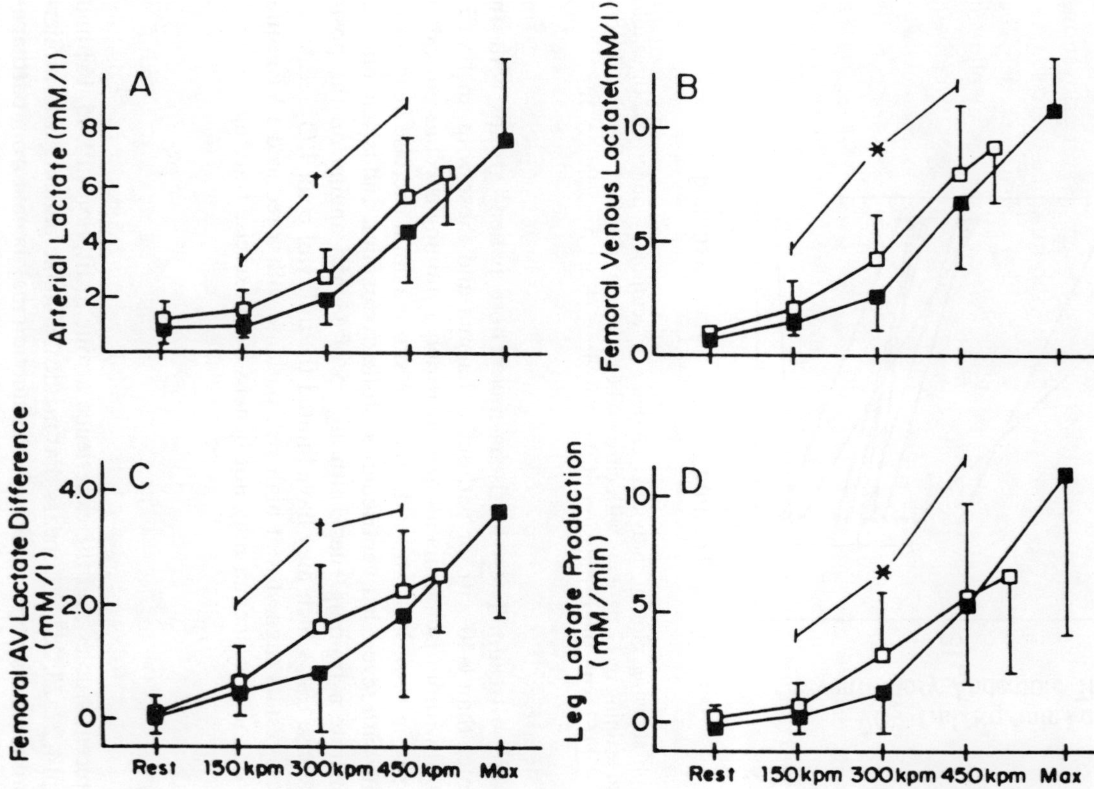

Fig. 3. Plots of resting and exercise arterial lactate, femoral venous lactate, femoral arteriovenous lactate difference and leg lactate production in patients before (□) and after (■) training. * $P < 0.05$; $^+P < 0.01$ by Wilcoxon signed-rank test. Reprinted from Sullivan *et al.* [15] with the permission of the American Heart Association, Inc.

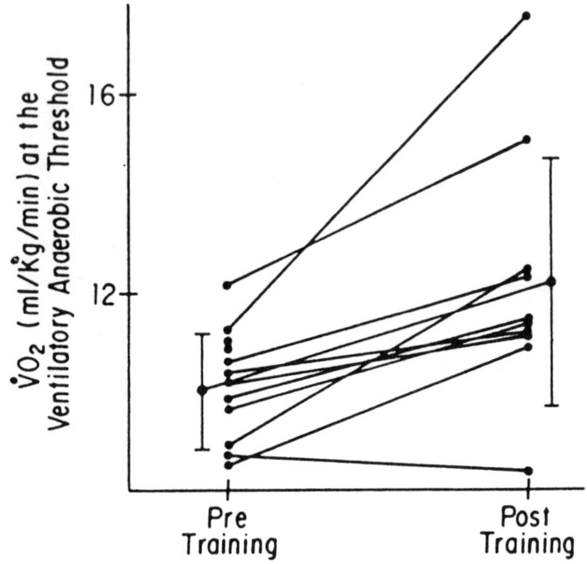

Fig. 4. Graph showing plot of individual changes in ventilatory anaerobic threshold with exercise training in 12 patients with chronic heart failure; $P = 0.01$. Reprinted from Sullivan *et al.* [16] with the permission of the American Heart Association, Inc.

positive exercise treadmill test for ischaemia. Those patient groups with an LVEF greater than 0.40 with or without ischaemia and those with an LVEF less than 0.40 without ischaemia all demonstrated a training effect as indicated by an increase in peak $\dot{V}O_2$ and a decrease in sub-maximal exercise heart rate. The patients with severe left ventricular systolic dysfunction and ischaemia did not demonstrate a training effect, although 5 of 11 had angina on the post-training exercise test, which may have limited the utility of peak $\dot{V}O_2$ measurements. These results suggest that high-risk patients with a reduced LVEF and significant ongoing ischaemia may not benefit from exercise training.

Summary

Based on recent studies and the experience at our institution [10, 15, 16] and others [11, 14, 22, 23, 28], it appears that medically stable patients with moderate heart failure and severe systolic LV dysfunction may benefit from participation in cardiac rehabilitation programmes. Patients with persistent rales and uncontrolled oedema on maximal medical therapy with digoxin, diuretics and vasodilators have not been included in previous studies and at the Duke University Center for Living generally have not participated in exercise conditioning. Patients with active ischaemia and severe LV dysfunction should probably undergo angiography and, if possible, myocardial revascularization prior to exercise training. Analogous to the coronary artery bypass grafting experience [29, 30], it is possible that patients with severe LV systolic dysfunction may achieve a benefit in terms of morbidity or mortality from exercise training precisely because they are at highest risk. However, studies examining the long-term effects of exercise training on morbidity and mortality in patients with LV dysfunction are currently unavailable. In light of recent studies [9–16, 22, 23, 25], it appears that severe LV dysfunction and stable class I–III heart failure controlled on medical therapy may benefit from participation in exercise training programmes.

Acknowledgements

This study was supported by Grant HL-17670 from the National Heart, Lung and Blood Institute, Bethesda, MD, by General Medical Research Funds from the Veterans Administration Medical Center, Durham, NC, and by Grant M01-RR-30, Division of Research Resources, General Clinical Research Centers Program, NIH. Dr Sullivan was supported by an Established Investigator Award and a Grant-in-Aid from the American Heart Association.

References

1. Thompson PD. The benefits and risks of exercise training in patients with chronic coronary artery disease. *JAMA* 1988; **259:** 1537–1540.
2. Laslett LJ, Paumer L, Amsterdam EA. Increase in myocardial oxygen consumption indexes by exercise training at onset of ischemia in patients with coronary artery disease. *Circulation* 1985; **71:** 958–962.
3. Wenger NK. Rehabilitation of the coronary patient in 1989. *Arch Intern Med* 1989; **149:** 1504–1506.
4. Clausen JP. Circulatory adjustments to dynamic exercise and effect of physical training in normal subjects and patients with coronary artery disease. *Prog Cardiovasc Dis* 1976; **18:** 459–495.
5. Varnauskas E, Bergman H, Houk P, Bjorntorp P. Hemodynamic effects of physical training in coronary patients. *Lancet* 1966; **ii:** 8–12.
6. Detry JM, Rousseau M, Vandenbroucke G, Kusumi F, Brasseur LA, Bruce RA. Increased arteriovenous oxygen difference after physical training in coronary heart disease. *Circulation* 1971; **44:** 109–118.
7. Clausen JP, Trap-Jensen J. Effects of training on the distribution of cardiac output in patients with coronary artery disease. *Circulation* 1970; **42:** 611–624.
8. O'Connor GT, Buring JE, Yusuf S, Goldhaber SZ, Olmstead EM, Paffenbarger RS, Hennekens CH. An overview of randomized trials of rehabilitation with exercise after myocardial infarction. *Circulation* 1989; **80:** 234–244.
9. Letac B, Cribier A, Desplanches JF. A study of left ventricular function in coronary patients before and after physical training. *Circulation* 1977; **56:** 375–378.
10. Cobb FR, Williams RS, McEwan P, Jones RH, Coleman RE, Wallace AG. Effects of exercise training on ventricular function in patients with recent myocardial infarction. *Circulation* 1982; **66:** 100–108.
11. Lee AP, Ice R, Blessey R, Sanmarco ME. Long-term effects of physical training on coronary patients with impaired ventricular function. *Circulation* 1979; **60:** 1519–1526.

12. Hagberg JM, Ehsani AA, Holloszy JO. Effect of 12 months of intense exercise training on stroke volume in patients with coronary artery disease. *Circulation* 1983; **67:** 1194–1199.
13. Conn EH, Williams RS, Wallace AG. Exercise responses before and after physical conditioning in patients with severely depressed left ventricular function. *Am J Cardiol* 1982; **49:** 296–300.
14. Coats AJS, Adamopoulos S, Radaelli A *et al.* Controlled trial of physical training in chronic heart failure: Exercise performance, hemodynamics, ventilation, and autonomic function. *Circulation* 1992; **85:** 2119–2131.
15. Sullivan MJ, Higginbotham MB, Cobb FR. Exercise training in patients with severe left ventricular dysfunction: Hemodynamic and metabolic effects. *Circulation* 1988; **78:** 506–515.
16. Sullivan MJ, Higginbotham MB, Cobb FR. Exercise training in patients with chronic heart failure delays ventilatory anaerobic threshold and improves submaximal exercise performance. *Circulation* 1989; **79:** 324–329.
17. Sullivan MJ, Knight JD, Higginbotham MB, Cobb FR. Relation between central and peripheral hemodynamics during exercise in patients with chronic heart failure: Muscle blood flow is reduced with maintenance of arterial perfusion pressure. *Circulation* 1989; **80:** 769–781.
18. Massie BM. Exercise tolerance in congestive heart failure: Role of cardiac function, peripheral blood flow, and muscle metabolism and effect of treatment. *Am J Med* (Suppl. 3A) 1988; **84:** 75–82.
19. Sullivan MJ, Green HJ, Cobb FR. Skeletal muscle biochemistry and histology in ambulatory patients with long-term chronic heart failure. *Circulation* 1990; **81:** 518–527.
20. Mancini DM, Coyle E, Coggan A, Beltz J, Ferraro N, Montain S, Wilson JR. Contribution of intrinsic skeletal muscle changes to ^{31}P NMR skeletal muscle metabolic abnormalities in patients with chronic heart failure. *Circulation* 1989; **80:** 1338–1346.
21. Sullivan MJ, Higginbotham MB, Cobb FR. Increased exercise ventilation in chronic heart failure: Intact ventilatory control despite hemodynamic and pulmonary abnormalities. *Circulation* 1988; **77:** 552–559.
22. Kellermann JJ, Ben-Ari E, Fisman E, Hayet M, Drory Y, Haimovitz D. Physical training in patients with ventricular impairment. *Adv Cardiol* 1986; **34:** 131–147.
23. Hoffmann A, Duba J, Lengyel M, Majer K. The effect of training on the physical working capacity of MI patients with left ventricular dysfunction. *Eur Heart J* 1987; **8:** 43–49.
24. Ferguson RJ, Taylor AW, Cote P, Charlebois J, Dinelle Y, Peronett F, De Champlain J, Bourassa MG. Skeletal muscle and cardiac changes with training in patients with angina pectoris. *Am J Physiol* 1982; **243:** H830–836.
25. Minotti JR, Johnson EC, Hudson TL, Zuroske G, Murata G, Fukushima E, Cagle TG, Chick TW, Massie BM, Icenogle MV. Skeletal muscle response to exercise training in congestive heart failure. *J Clin Invest* 1990; **86:** 751–758.
26. Jugdutt BI, Michorowski BL, Kappagoda CT. Exercise training after anterior Q wave myocardial infarction: Importance of regional left ventricular function and topography. *J Am Coll Cardiol* 1988; **12:** 362–372.
27. Arvan S. Exercise performance of the high risk acute myocardial infarction patient after cardiac rehabilitation. *Am J Cardiol* 1988; **62:** 197–201.
28. Squires RW, Gau GT, Miller TD, Allison TG, Lavie CJ. Cardiovascular rehabilitation: Status, 1990. *Mayo Clin Proc* 1990; **65:** 731–755.
29. Alderman EL, Fisher LD, Litwin P, Kaiser GC, Myers WO, Maynard C, Levine F, Schloss M. Results of coronary artery surgery in patients with poor left ventricular function (CASS). *Circulation* 1983; **68:** 785.

30. Vigilante GJ, Weintraub WS, Klein LW, Schneider RM, Seelaus PA, Parr GVS, Lemole G, Agarwal JB, Helfant RH. Improved survival with coronary bypass surgery in patients with three-vessel coronary disease and abnormal left ventricular function. Matched case-control study in patient with potentially operable disease. *Am J Med* 1987; **82:** 697.

28 The Benefit of Graded Physical Exercise in Chronic Heart Failure

Michel Koch, Jean-Paul Broustet*

Department of Clinical Cardiology A, Hôpital Cardiologique du Haut-Lévêque, Avenue de Magellan, 33604 Pessac, France

Introduction

The balance of circulatory gas exchange, as described by Wasserman [1], is upset in patients with chronic heart failure. There is therefore a disparity between cardiac output and the needs of the peripheral vessels for oxygen. The cardiogenic component of this imbalance is extremely difficult to treat. The limited number of active therapeutic treatments is witness to this. On the other hand, the peripheral component is much easier to approach. A number of cardiotonic treatments have, with use, proved to be very powerful vasodilators.

Cardiac rehabilitation is one of the active therapeutic possibilities here, as most authors emphasize [2–5]. In addition, the action it has on the weak muscle is complementary to the drug therapy used. However, this retraining poses a risk problem for those patients whose haemodynamic profile is often very impaired. It is for this reason that we have developed a "gentle" retraining method based on muscle building in graded stages. The hypothesis was that the demand put on the cardiovascular system by the training of one muscle group at a time would be such that even patients with chronic heart failure would be able to complete it.

* To whom all correspondence should be addressed.

Proceedings of the Vth World Congress on Cardiac Rehabilitation

Method

A trial was undertaken comprising 25 patients with chronic heart failure, divided at random into two groups: 13 in the control group and 12 in the group of patients to undergo rehabilitation treatment. The para-clinical explorations were carried out in simple blind fashion by independent observers. Drug treatment was continued throughout the trial and modified as necessary. This was a pragmatic trial [6]. The criteria for inclusion were: patients with heart failure at stage II or stage III of the New York Heart Association classification with an isotopic ejection fraction at rest of less than 40%, and whose condition had been stable for more than 3 months on the same drug therapy. Only patients with dilated or ischaemic cardiomyopathies not limited by angina were chosen. Patients with associated respiratory failure or a history of sustained ventricular arrhythmia were excluded from the trial. Before randomization, a detailed explanation of the programme was given to each patient, who was asked if he agreed to take part and they then drew lots.

The rehabilitation programme (Fig. 1) consisted of 40 sessions, each of 90 min duration, over a period of 90 days. The exercises were carried out on specially designed equipment (Koch bench, Genin Médical). The exercises consisted of the building up of a small number of muscle groups at a time so as to avoid too much pressure on the heart. The workloads for each patient were chosen according to the results of their exercise test and maximum muscular strength, which was measured using a dynamometer for each muscle group.

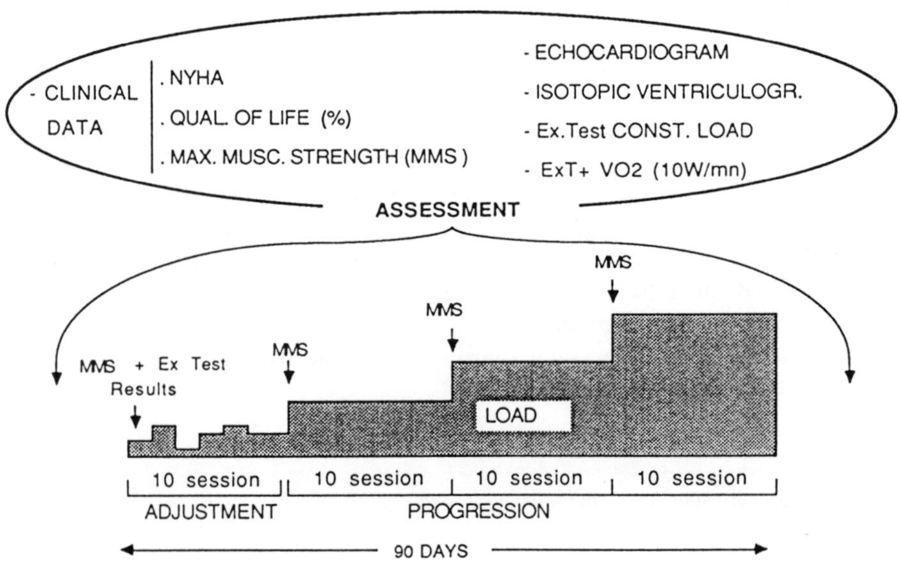

Fig. 1. Rehabilitation programme.

Using stress performance, the patients were classified at a given level and the total exercise load for that particular patient was set according to that level. Measuring maximum muscular strength enabled this load to be adapted to particular muscle groups. The sessions started on this basis, but the physiotherapist was able to adjust the loads in the first 10 sessions (Fig. 1). The programme was then divided into 3 groups of 10 sessions separated by a period in which muscular strength was measured, enabling successive loads to be adapted according to the patient's progress. The numbers of movements remained constant throughout the programme.

Assessment, which was carried out a few days before day 0 and on day 90, consisted of an echocardiogram, an exercise test with increasing load (ergometer stages: 10 W/min, symptom-limited, under treatment) and an exercise test at constant load (as in Sullivan's protocol: load at two stages under maximal stage of test with increasing load [3]), an isotopic ventriculogram and a compilation of the quality-of-life score determined as a percentage on a visual scale (percentage of overall improvement as estimated by the patient).

Results

Two patients had to be excluded from the control group: one for the onset of pulmonary neoplasia and the other had to have a cardiac transplantation. The comparability of the concomitant treatment between the two sample groups was correct, whether for clinical and echocardiographic or for ergometric variables (Table 1). Concomitant treatment was on the whole more important in the control group and these treatments were not modified for either group during the trial (Fig. 2).

Left ventricular function at rest was not significantly modified by rehabilitation (Fig. 3), whether for the end-diastolic diameter of the left ventricle, the percentage of shortening of the left ventricle or the ejection fraction at rest. During the exercise test, there were no significant bradycardic effects, either at rest (Table 2) or during exercise (heart rate for the same effort in the group undergoing rehabilitation was: day 0 = 136 $\pm$ 25, day 90 = 132 $\pm$ 24; for the control group it was: day 0 = 137 $\pm$ 24, day 90 = 138 $\pm$ 16). The systolic blood pressure at rest was not modified by the programme either. Performance during the exercise test with increasing load was improved by 34% in the group undergoing rehabilitation, while it did not improve in the control group (Fig. 4). Total muscular strength increased from 77 $\pm$ 20 to 112 $\pm$ 24 kg (Fig. 5). The improvement in the quality of life was estimated by the patients to be 63%, while the spontaneous variation in the control group was only 4% (Fig. 5).

It must be emphasized that throughout the programme, and for the patients undergoing rehabilitation, there were no side-effects: no cardiac arrhythmia and heart rate remained below 115 beats/min during exercise, with the exception of one patient who showed signs of permanent auricular fibrillation.

Table 1
Comparability of samples

Variables	Rehabilitation group ($n = 12$)	Control group ($n = 13$)	Significance
Age (years)	56 ± 11	54 ± 10	NS
Sex (no. of men)	8/12	11/13	$P < 0.01$
Weight (kg)	72 ± 16	68 ± 14	NS
NYHA (III/II)	5/7	5/8	NS
Yale scale	6.5 ± 2	7 ± 2.5	NS
EDD (mm)	65 ± 12	69 ± 8	NS
% of shortening	21 ± 6	20 ± 6	NS
LA diameter (mm)	43 ± 8	43 ± 8	NS
$\dot{V}O_2$ (ml/kg/min)	18.3 ± 5	19.5 ± 8	NS
Duration (increasing load – min)	8 ± 3	10 ± 5	NS
HR at rest (beats/min)	90 ± 16	80 ± 7	NS
SBP at rest (mmHg)	125 ± 21	118 ± 18	NS
Duration (constant load – min)	10 ± 13	13 ± 15	NS
Ejection fraction at rest (%)	26.5 ± 10	26 ± 12	NS
Ejection fraction during exercise (%)	28 ± 11	27 ± 12	NS
P/V[a]	121 ± 16	120 ± 27	NS

[a] $P/V = \frac{SBP}{ESV}$ = contractibility index.

Note: Two patients were excluded from the control group (one for neoplasia and one for cardiac transplantation). The two groups are comparable except for sex (more women in the rehabilitation group).

	REHAB PATIENTS		CONTROL	
	D 0	D 90	D 0	D 90
DIURETICS	50 %	50 %	83 %	83 %
CEI	90 %	90 %	100 %	100 %
DIGITALIS & ASSOC. DRUGS	50 %	50 %	50 %	50 %
VASODILATORS	33 %	33 %	45 %	45 %
PDI	8 %	8 %	18 %	18 %
ANTIARRYTHMIC DRUGS &/OR BETABLOCKERS	33 %	33 %	45 %	45 %

Fig. 2. Associated treatment. CEI, conversion enzyme inhibitors; PDI, phosphodiesterase inhibitors.

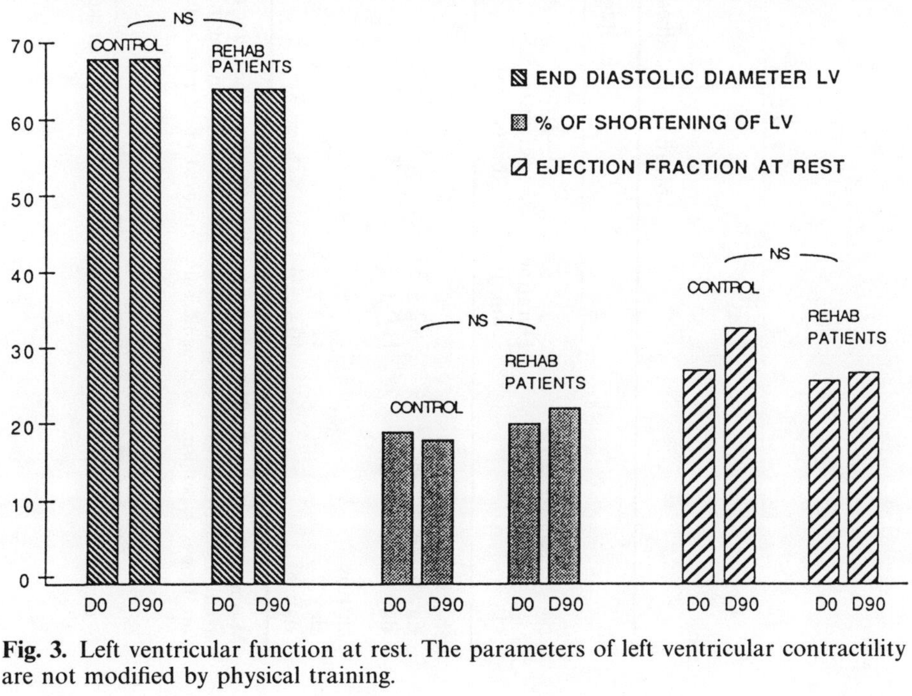

Fig. 3. Left ventricular function at rest. The parameters of left ventricular contractility are not modified by physical training.

Table 2
Mean (±SD) values of ergonometric variables

	Exercise test increasing load					
	Duration (min)	Heartrate at rest (beats/min)	HR_{max} at same perf. (beats/min)[a]	SBP at rest (mmHg)	SBP_{max} at same perf. (mmHg)[b]	Ex. test constant load (duration, min)
Rehabilitation patients						
day 0	8.2 ± 3.0	89 ± 16	136 ± 25	125 ± 21	151.7 ± 40.0	9.8 ± 13
day 90	11.0 ± 3.4	91 ± 21	132 ± 24	130 ± 12	154.6 ± 29.0	19.2 ± 14
Controls						
day 0	11.3 ± 4.8	77 ± 6	138 ± 24	121 ± 18	162.7 ± 28.7	15.3 ± 1.6
day 90	10.4 ± 4.1	85 ± 9	138 ± 16	125 ± 16	162.7 ± 31.5	18.7 ± 17

[a] Maximum heart rate for the same maximum performance (the lower of the two exercise tests). [b] Maximum systolic blood pressure (SBP) for the same maximum performance (the lower of the two exercise tests). Physical training does not significantly modify heart rate and systolic blood pressure during effort. However, performance is significantly improved whether under increasing load or endurance (constant load).

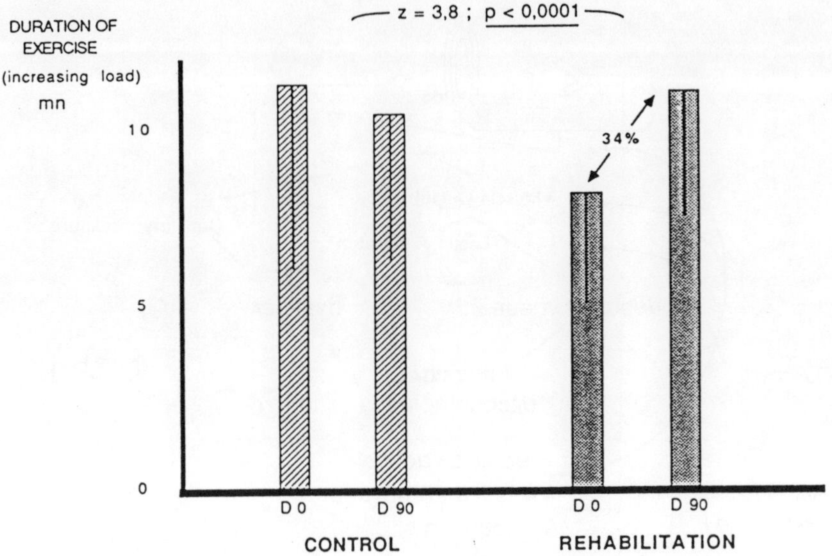

Fig. 4. Modification of performance during exercise test.

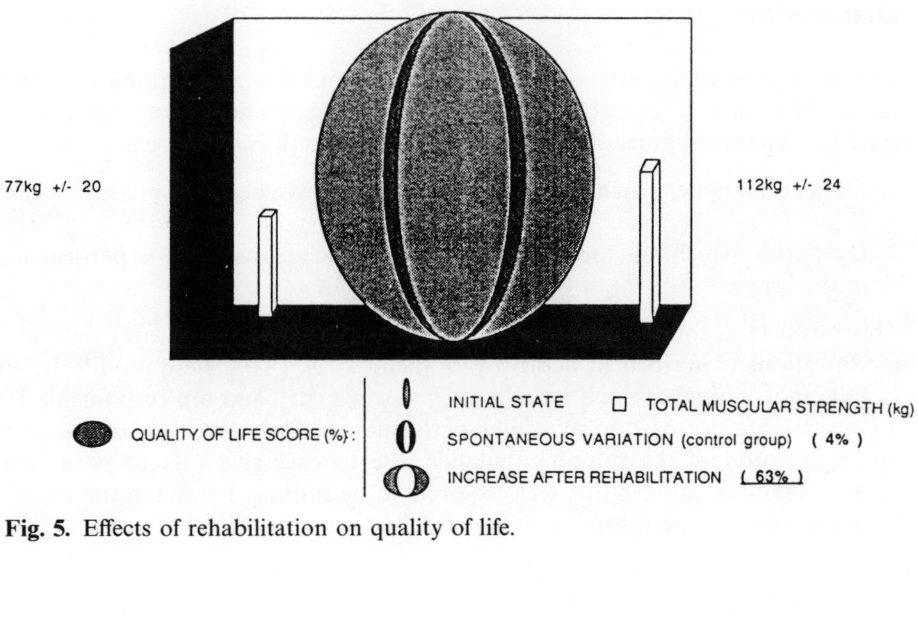

Fig. 5. Effects of rehabilitation on quality of life.

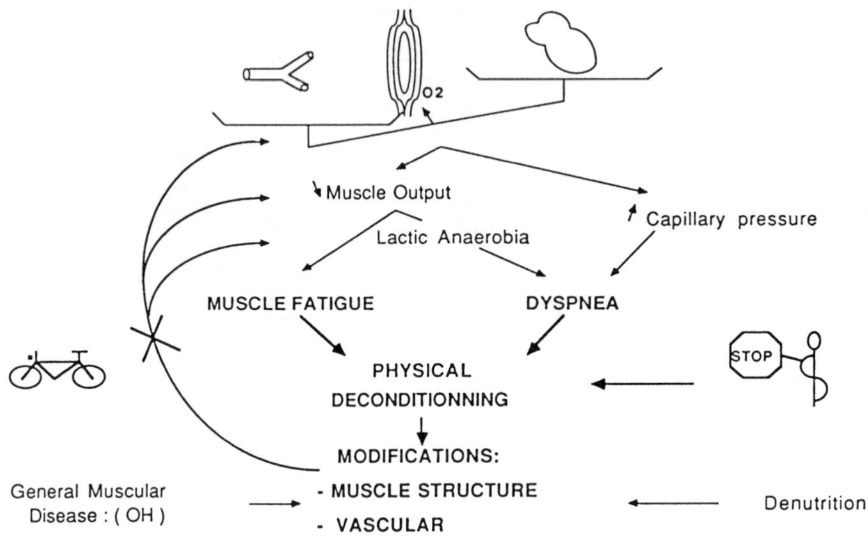

Fig. 6. Physiopathological approach to the functional handicap of the patient with chronic heart disease. It is a vicious circle, at the centre of which one finds physical deconditioning which has three causes: muscle fatigue, dyspnoea (due to the inadaptation of the heart to peripheral needs) and sedentariness (often due to advice given by doctors). This deconditioning causes modifications to the muscle structure which helps in the general deterioration of muscle performance and leads to an increase in the imbalance heart muscle/muscle requirement for oxygen.

Discussion

The imbalance which exists between the heart and the surrounding vessels is sustained by a vicious circle syndrome (Fig. 6), at the centre of which lies a state of physical unfitness. Two essential causes for this are known:

1. Muscular fatigue, which seems to be initially due to a decrease in local output [7].
2. Dyspnoea, which has multiple causes, e.g. lactic acidosis and hyperpressure in the lungs.

This physical deconditioning is itself responsible for real structural muscular modifications (described in depth by Mancini *et al.* [8]). These modifications include morphology as well as cellular histochemistry and are responsible for a considerable decrease in muscular performance. They are also the cause of an aggravation of the initial imbalance due to excessive loss of peripheral energy. Training enables this vicious circle to be broken, by giving the muscle back its ability to perform.

Graded rehabilitation does not cause any bradycardic effects at rest or during effort, since it is done in stages and is not a question of stamina. The improvement in performance (34%) in this study is one of the best to be found in the literature [2–5, 9]. It is probably due to the effect of training on the peripheral vessels [8, 10], since the function of the left ventricle is not improved. Training had no adverse effect on left ventricular systolic function at rest.

Classic rehabilitation programmes do not seem to have caused any accidents in the trials published to date [2–5]. However, these series only concern very small numbers and, given the overall character of the exercises and the very poor cardiac condition of the patients, we have been reluctant to set up such programmes.

Graded training in stages means less pressure on the heart. In addition, the patient's training is harmonious and enables considerable improvement in muscular strength at all levels. This enables patients to gain in autonomy and in quality of life. The proof is that 80% of the patients asked for training to be continued.

Conclusion

Physical training for patients with chronic heart failure means an increase in muscular strength and better adaptation to effort through a purely peripheral action. The risks appear to be very slight if the exercises are adapted to patients who have been carefully selected and who are carefully monitored. The results of the functional improvement of patients with chronic heart failure greatly outstrip those of any drug therapy.

References

1. Wasserman K, Beaver W, Whipp B. Gas exchange theory and the lactic acidosis (anaerobic) threshold. *Circulation* 1990; **81** (Suppl. II): II-14 to II-30.
2. Coats AJ, Adamopoulos S, Meyer TE, Conway J, Sleight P. Effects of physical training in chronic heart failure. *Lancet* 1990; **335:** 63–66.
3. Sullivan MJ, Higginbotham MB, Cobb FR. Exercise training in patients with severe left ventricular dysfunction: Hemodynamic and metabolic effects. *Circulation* 1988; **78:** 506–515.
4. Sullivan MJ, Higginbotham MB, Cobb FR. Exercise training in patients with chronic heart failure delays ventilatory anaerobic threshold and improves submaximal exercise performance. *Circulation* 1989; **79:** 324–329.
5. Samek L, Hauf GF, Roskamm H. Exercise training in patients with impaired left ventricular function. Symposium on Exercise Testing in Congestive Heart Failure. European Society of Cardiology, Brussels, April 1990.
6. Schwartz D, Flamant R, Lellouch J. *L'essai thérapeutique chez l'homme*. Flammarion, Paris, 1985.
7. Wilson JR, Martin JL, Schwartz D, Ferraro N. Exercise intolerance in patients with chronic heart failure: Role of impaired flow to skeletal muscle. *Circulation* 1984; **69:** 1079–1087.

8. Mancini DM, Coyle E, Coggan A, Beltz J, Ferraro N, Mountain S *et al.* Contribution of intrinsic skeletal muscle changes to ^{31}PNMR skeletal muscle metabolic abnormalities in patients with chronic heart failure. *Circulation* 1989; **80:** 1338–1346.
9. Conn EH, Williams RS, Wallace AG. Exercise responses before and after physical conditioning in patients with severely depressed left ventricular function. *Am J Cardiol* 1982; **49:** 296–300.
10. Cohen-Solal A. For the $\dot{V}O_2$ French Study Group: Improving exercise tolerance in patients with chronic heart failure: Should we treat the heart or the periphery? (Editorial). *Eur Heart J* 1989; **10:** 866–871.

29 Exercise Therapy in Coronary Patients with Severely Impaired Ventricular Function

Jan J. Kellermann

Chaim Sheba Medical Centre, Tel Hashomer,
Israel Sackler School of Medicine, Tel Aviv University,
Tel Aviv, Israel

Introduction

It is less than two decades since exercise training was first experimentally applied in selected groups of patients suffering from coronary artery disease (CAD) and a significant impaired left ventricular function. Up until now, most of our experience in this field has been based on rather short training periods and a relatively modest number of patients. In recent years, attention has focused increasingly on the management of chronic heart failure and cardiac patients with severely impaired ventricular function.

The main aim of various therapeutic modalities applied to these groups of patients has been the enhancement of the quality of survival. Increasing life expectancy, especially in the developed countries, and improved therapeutic management of chronic heart disease, are probably the factors responsible for the steadily increasing morbidity and mortality rates from heart failure. The estimated morbidity in the USA, for example, is between 1 and 2 million and the 15-year total mortality rate in the age group over 55 years is 39.1% in women and 71.1% in men [1]. These alarming figures, which have also been observed in Europe and elsewhere, underline the need for an effective therapeutic approach, and the need to prevent the clinical outburst of heart failure in those many asymptomatic patients who have an impaired ventricular function.

To date, it is still impossible to present clear scientific evidence to prove that

Proceedings of the Vth World Congress on Cardiac Rehabilitation

exercise therapy, applied in the framework of a comprehensive cardiac care programme, has an influence on prognosis and longevity.

Overview of the literature

Letac *et al.* [2] examined 15 patients who suffered from angina pectoris after myocardial infarction, both before and after a physical training programme. A maximal exercise test showed that, after training, physical capacity increased by 17% ($P < 0.02$), heart rate decreased by 13% and blood pressure decreased by 7% ($P < 0.01$). Left ventricular end-diastolic pressure, ventricular volume and ejection fraction in the total group, as well as segmental contractility in those whose contractility was considerably impaired, or in those with large dyskinetic areas or widespread akinesia, were unchanged. The authors concluded that selected patients with severely impaired left ventricular function can participate safely in conditioning programmes and also achieve a training effect.

Verani *et al.* [3] determined the effect of exercise training on left ventricular performance in 16 patients with CAD. After a 12-week training period, 15 of the 16 patients had improved exercise tolerance. Total treadmill exercise duration increased, as did the estimated maximal oxygen consumption per kg body weight. It was further observed that the left ventricular ejection fraction (LVEF) increased from $52 \pm 4\%$ to $57 \pm 4\%$ ($P < 0.02$) after training. Jensen *et al.* [4] also studied a group of 16 patients with CAD by means of radionuclide ventriculography performed before and after 6 months of exercise training. After training, no change was observed in the mean ejection fraction at rest, or during maximal exercise, but a higher maximal mean systolic blood pressure, heart rate and workload were achieved.

Lee *et al.* [5] examined 18 patients with CAD and an ejection fraction of 40% or less. Maximal-limited exercise testing and cardiac catheterization were initially performed after 12–24 months (mean, 8.5 months) of exercise training. During the follow-up period, mean functional aerobic capacity improved significantly ($P > 0.01$ and <0.05). No change was noted in left ventricular end-diastolic volume, or ejection fraction. Deniss *et al.* [6] examined 32 patients (mean age 53 years) with a mean resting LVEF of 18%, as assessed by radionuclide ventriculography. These researchers found that patients with a low ejection fraction after myocardial infarction can be as active as the symptoms permit. They further observed a significant training effect with activity levels corresponding to New York Heart Association (NYHA) class I and they concluded that ejection fraction alone may not be a good indicator of mortality in the first month after myocardial infarction.

Williams *et al.* [7] examined the effect of physical conditioning on LVEF in 53 patients with CAD who underwent exercise training for 6–12 months. This group found that although resting and peak LVEF were not significantly altered, mean LVEF at the pre-training maximal workload was increased ($P < 0.002$) after training. In addition, a significant correlation was found between training bradycardia and the increment of LVEF. The authors concluded that the relative bradycardia produced by exercise conditioning is associated with the improvement of left ventricular performance, as determined by LVEF. Nagle *et al.* [8] found that physical activity appears to enhance left ventricular function at lower exercise levels by its effect on peripheral circulation, as was evident in patients with abnormal left ventricular function. At higher exercise levels, left ventricular function was maintained, despite increased metabolic demands.

Sullivan *et al.* [9] studied the haemodynamic and metabolic effects of exercise training in patients with severe left ventricular function. They came to the conclusion that ambulatory patients with congestive heart failure (CHF) can achieve a significant training effect from long-term exercise programmes. They concluded that peripheral adaptation plays an important role in improving exercise tolerance. This group of investigators found that blood lactate levels at sub-maximal exercise were reduced without improvement in cardiac output, which would suggest that in patients with CHF peripheral metabolic or vascular factors are important in determining the onset of lactate production. This may influence exercise tolerance independent of central haemodynamics. In another paper by the same group [10], it was suggested that in patients with chronic CHF, reduced aerobic activity in the skeletal muscles plays an important role in mediating the early onset of anerobic metabolism exercise. These and other observations may further explain why there is a poor correlation between exercise performance and severity of haemodynamic changes, particularly during exercise in patients with impaired ventricular function and chronic heart failure.

Drexler *et al.* [11, 12] examined the ultra-structure of skeletal muscle. Their results demonstrated that patients with CHF developed significant ultra-structure abnormalities of skeletal muscle, reflecting a depressed oxidative capacity of working muscle. The authors concluded that these alterations to skeletal muscle contribute to a decreased exercise capacity in these patients, but are in principle reversible. Mancini *et al.* [13] addressed the problem of the contribution of skeletal muscle to general fatigue in CHF. Physical training in CHF has been shown to improve skeletal muscle function. It seems, therefore, appropriate to speculate that alterations to skeletal muscle could eventually be prevented by the timely initiation of properly adapted physical training.

Tavazzi *et al.* [14] observed that of 21 patients with LVEF, less than 30% had normal haemodynamics, whereas this feature was observed in 67% of those whose LVEF was greater than 45%. Franciosa [15] found that none of the haemodynamic variables we usually measure in patients with left heart failure, including left ventricular filling pressure, systemic arterial blood pressure, cardiac output, stroke volume or systemic vascular resistance, correlate with exercise capacity. Similarly, Litchfield *et al.* [16] found that about one-third of patients with severe left ventricular impairment achieved nearly normal levels of exercise. Adaptation, including tolerance to high pulmonary wedge pressure, increased heart rate and stroke volume during exercise, as well as ventricular enlargement and increased peripheral vascular resistance, are closely linked to the neuro-hormonal and central nervous regulation mechanism. It has to be understood that there exists an impaired exercise tolerance in patients with severe left ventricular impairment, and the work capacity as found initially in this group is significantly lower when compared to a control group with normal function.

Minotti *et al.* [17] examined the skeletal muscle metabolic response to peripheral training in heart failure. Their results indicated that training can improve muscle metabolism and endurance in CHF and that this effect is localized to the trained muscle group. Coats *et al.* [18] found that carefully selected patients with moderate to severe CHF can achieve significant improvements concerning minute ventilation and cardiac output, alterations to sympathovagal balance and a reduction in systematic vascular resistance.

Ehsani *et al.* [19] studied 25 patients during a 12-month endurance exercise programme, and an additional 14 non-exercisers who were comparable in their maximal exercise capacity and ejection fraction. In the non-exercisers, the ejection fraction remained unchanged after 12 months. Exercise-induced regional wall motion disorders worsened in the training group. It was found that intense exercise training can bring about an improvement in left ventricular function independent of cardiac loading conditions. It should, however, be noted that the exercise ejection fraction of these patients was >15%. In the trained group, the ejection fraction increased after training.

Exercise training in phase II: Rehabilitation in patients with impaired ventricular function

Arvan [20] examined post-myocardial infarction patients with significant left ventricular dysfunction and myocardial ischaemia. He discovered that a group of these patients ($n = 65$) did not benefit from an adequate training response. Jette *et al.* [21] initiated a 4-week exercise training programme for patients with large anterior infarction less than 10 weeks after the acute onset. The ejection fraction was initially measured as <30% in the control and intervention groups. The authors found that exercise training had little or no effect on haemodynamic measurements, and that training effects achieved in patients with left ventricular dysfunction are most likely due to corrected impaired vasodilatation and not necessarily to cardiac function.

Jugdutt *et al.* [22] aimed to determine the effect of a standard low-level exercise programme on left ventricular function and topography in patients who survived an acute Q-wave myocardial infarction of moderate size, referred for cardiac rehabilitation 15 weeks after the acute event. The outcome of their study brought them to the conclusion that exercise training may be injurious to patients with an extensive transmural infarct. In a letter to the editor, Fisman and Kellermann [23] questioned some of the methodological points of this study. In most of the studies, medication was not taken into account.

Gianuzzi *et al.* [24] implemented a 6-month training programme and examined left ventricular function and remodelling, before and after training, by means of two-dimensional echocardiography. They employed 25 patients in the training group and 24 in the control group. The outcome after 6-months follow-up, which only included patients with $\leq 40\%$ ejection fraction at entry, showed that there was a further global and regional left ventricular deterioration in both groups; thus physical training does not seem to be responsible for spontaneous deterioration.

Five-year follow-up study at our laboratory

Our observations, which include a 5-year follow-up of a group of patients with a low ejection fraction ($< 35\%$) and experience of other long-term exercise training interventions, indicate that impaired ventricular function in selected patients with CAD does not cause further deterioration of ventricular function.

In an uncontrolled anecdotal trial involving 22 patients (mean age 55.9 years) followed up over 60 months, 15 were post-anteroseptal myocardial infarction, 3 were post-anteroseptal and inferior infarction, and 4 were post-CABG [25]. The initial LVEF, as established by means of exercise radionuclide ventriculograph and two-dimensional echocardiography, was $30.1 \pm 9.5\%$. After 24 months follow-up, LVEF had increased to $36.2 \pm 10.2\%$, after 48 months it was $30.1 \pm 6.5\%$ and after 60 months it was $28.2 \pm 9.5\%$. In addition, we examined exercise performance expressed as workload, peak heart rate and peak rate pressure product, both using upper and lower extremity ergometry. After 3 years of training, we found significant increases in workload ($P < 0.01$), peak heart rate ($P < 0.01$) and peak rate pressure product ($P < 0.001$). After 48 and 60 months, no further changes were observed. LVEF was not statistically significant when comparing initial LVEF (pre-training) values with those after 4 and 5 years of follow-up (post-training). When considering our results, the lack of a control group should be noted. It would be inappropriate to emphasize that, in this group of patients, "contaminated" by various therapeutic interventions and with a nonunified pre-intervention baseline state, randomization becomes a most difficult undertaking, especially when long-term follow-up of more than 3 years is desired.

It is understandable that randomized studies initiated in post-myocardial infarction patients with impaired ventricular function have relatively short follow-up. In part, these studies involve patients who have unhealed scars and the results are equivocal. It is known that short-term physical training programme for groups of patients with impaired ventricular function cause a beneficial training effect; in particular, an increase in total work performance, a reduction in heart rate and systolic blood pressure for a given work task. It must be underlined, however, that the patient out to be in a stable clinical condition without signs of functional and haemodynamic deterioration.

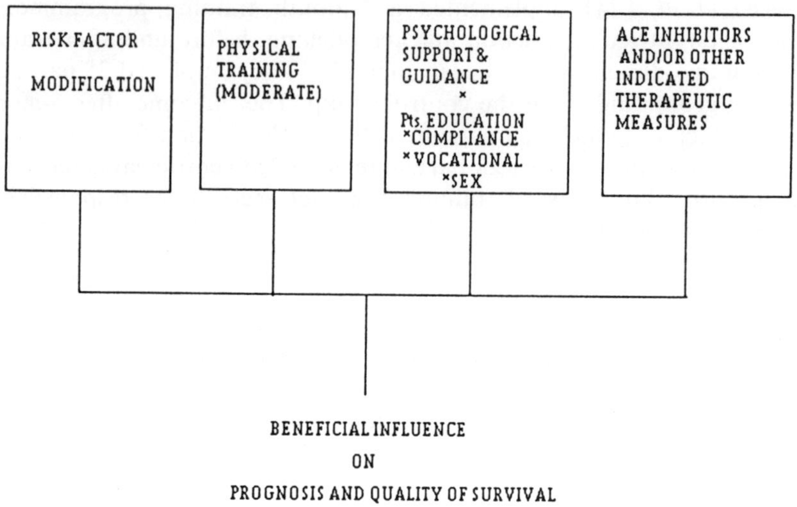

Fig. 1. Long-term comprehensive cardiac care programme consisting of risk factor modification, physical activity, psychological guidance and patient's education. ACE inhibitors are recommended in CAD patients with left ventricular impairment.

Conclusions

The results of our study indicate that it is not only possible to enhance functional capacity in patients with impaired ventricular function, but more than 80% are capable of continuing work for many years. Left ventricular dimensions remained unchanged during 5 years follow-up. Two patients died from cardiac causes, whereas the others are still continuing the long-term programme. The need for a large randomized long-term trial is not a matter for debate. The use of angiotensin-converting enzyme (ACE) inhibitors has been shown to have a beneficial effect in these patients. Therefore, it would seem reasonable that in order to maintain a good quality of life in these patients, a comprehensive cardiac care programme and the use of ACE inhibitors in asymptomatic patients with severe ventricular impairment should be implemented (see Fig. 1).

References

1. Schocken DD, Arrieta MI, Leaverton PE, Ross EA. Prevelance and mortality rate of congestive heart failure in the United States. *J Am Coll Cardiol* 1992; **20:** 301–306.
2. Letac B, Cribier A, Desplanches JF. A study of left ventricular function in coronary patients before and after physical training. *Circulation* 1977; **56:** 375–378.

3. Verani MS, Hratung CH, Hoepfel-Harris J *et al.* Improvement of exercise training on left ventricular performance and myocardial perfusion in patients with coronary artery disease. *Am J. Cardiol* 1980; **47:** 797.
4. Jensen D, Atwood JE, Froelicher V *et al.* Improvement of ventricular function during exercise studies with radionuclide ventriculography after cardiac rehabilitation. *Am J Cardiol* 1980; **46:** 770–777.
5. Lee AP, Ice R, Blessy R, Sanmarco ME. Long term effects of physical training on coronary patients with impaired ventricular function. *Circulation* 1979; **60:** 1519–1526.
6. Denniss AR, Ross DA, Russel PA *et al.* Early exercise testing, physical training and mortality in patients with severe left ventricular dysfunction. *J Am Coll. Cardiol* (Suppl.) 1983; **1:** 718.
7. Williams RS, Conn EH, Wallace AG. Enhanced exercise performance following physical training in coronary patients stratified by left ventricular ejection fraction. *Circulation* (Suppl.) 1981; **64:** IV-186.
8. Nagle RE, Murray RG, Robertson DAS. The effect of physical training on left ventricular function after acute myocardial infarction. *Circulation* (Suppl.) 1983; **68:** III-377.
9. Sullivan MJ, Higginbotham MB, Cobb FR. Exercise training in patients with severe left ventricular dysfunction. Hemodynamic and metabolic effects. *Circulation* 1988; **78:** 506-515.
10. Sullivan MJ, Higginbotham MB, Cobb FR. Exercise training in patients with chronic heart failure delays ventilatory anaerobic threshold and improves submaximal exercise performance. *Circulation* 1989; **79:** 324–329.
11. Drexler H, Riede U, Munzel T, Konig H, Funke E, Just H. Alterations of skeletal muscle in chronic heart failure. *Circulation* 1992; **85:** 1751–1759.
12. Drexler H. Skeletal muscle failure in heart failure (Editorial). *Circulation* 1992; **85:** 1621–1623.
13. Mancini DM, Walter G, Reichek N, Lenkinski R, MaCully KK, Mullen L, Wilson JR. Contribution of skeletal muscle atrophy to exercise intolerance and altered muscle metabolism in heart failure. *Circulation* 1992; **85:** 1364–1373.
14. Tavazzi L, Ignone G, Giordano A, Giannuzzi P: Cardiac rehabilitation in patients with recent myocardial infarction and left ventricular dysfunction: In: Kellermann JJ, Spodick DH (eds), *Left Ventricular Dysfunction, Advances in Cardiology*, Vol. 34. Karger: Basel, 1986; **34:** 156–169.
15. Franciosa JA, Park M, Levine TB. Lack of correlation between exercise capacity and indexes of resting left ventricular performance in heart failure. *Am J Cardiol* 1981; **47:** 33–39.
16. Litchfield RL, Kerber RE, Benge WJ, Mark AL, Sopko J, Bhatnagar RK, Marcus ML. Normal exercise capacity in patients with severe left ventricular dysfunction: Compensatory mechanisms. *Circulation* 1982; **66:** 129–134.
17. Minotti JR, Johnson E, Hudson T, Zuroske G, Murata G, Fukushima E, Cagle T, Chick T, Massie B, Icenogle M. Skeletal muscle metabolic response to peripheral training in heart failure. *J Am Coll Cardiol* (Suppl.) 1990; **15:** 258A.
18. Coats AJS, Adamopoulos S, Radaeli A, MacCance A, Meyer TE, Bernardi L, Solda PL, Davey P, Ormerod O, Conway J, Sleight P. Controlled trial of physical training in chronic heart failure: Exercise performance, hemodynamic, ventilation and autonomic function. *Circulation* 1992; **85:** 2119–2131.
19. Ehsani AA, Biello DR, Schultz J, Sobel BE, Holloszy JO. Improvement of left ventricular contractile function by exercise training in patients with coronary artery disease. *Circulation* 1986; **74:** 350–358.
20. Arvan S. Exercise performance of high risk acute myocardial infarction patient after cardiac rehabilitation. *Am J Cardiol* 1988; **62:** 197–201.

21. Jette M, Heller R, Landry F, Blümchen G. Randomized 4-week exercise program in patients with impaired left ventricular function. *Circulation* 1991; **84:** 1561–1567.
22. Jugdutt BI, Michorwski BL, Kappagoda CT. Exercise training after anterior Q wave myocardial infarction: Importance of regional left ventricular function and topography. *J Am Coll Cardiol* 1988; **12:** 3662–3672.
23. Fisman EZ, Kellermann JJ. Does exercise training deteriorate ventricular function? (Letter to the Editor). *J Am Coll Cardiol* 1989; **14:** 263–264.
24. Giannuzzi P, Giubbini R, Galli M, Mazzuero G, Lanfranchi P, Sala L, Malinverni C, Schweiger, Giordano A, Tavazzi L. EAMI – Exercise training in anterior infarction: On-going multicenter study on ventricular function and topography. *Circulation* (Suppl. II) 1991; **84:** 539.
25. Kellermann JJ, Shemesh J, Fisman EZ, Steinmetz A, Ben-Ari E, Drory Y, Lapidoth C. Arm exercise training in the rehabilitation of patients with impaired ventricular function and heart failure. *Cardiology* 1990; **77:** 130–138.

VIII Rehabilitation in Cardiac Transplantation

30 Rehabilitation after Cardiac Transplantation: 10-year Follow-up – Physiological Aspects

Serge G.L.G. Degré*, Georges Niset, Cecile Coustry-Degré

Médico-Surgical and Rehabilitation Divisions, C.U.B. Hôpital Erasme, 808 Route de Lennik, B-1070 Brussels, Belgium

Introduction

The results of human heart transplantation have steadily improved over the past several years, making it an appropriate life-saving procedure in patients with end-stage myocardial insufficiency. The introduction of cyclosporine in immunosuppressive therapy will further increase the 5- and 10-year survival rates, currently 70–75%, making heart transplantation a real alternative to end-stage cardiac disease treatment. Since 1981, 260 patients have been transplanted in our hospital, the actuarial survival rates being 75% after 5 years and 70% after 10 years. In these patients, the nature of underlying cardiac disease was ischaemic cardiopathy in 51.5%, congestive dilated cardiomyopathy in 42%, valvular cardiopathy in 3.5%, toxic myocarditis (adriamycin) in 1.5% and chronic rejection in 2.5% (retransplantation). Of our 260 patients, 13% were female and 87% male. Therapy combining cyclosporine, azathioprine and corticoids was used.

In this chapter, we report the 10-year follow-up of the first 100 male patients. They were re-investigated each year in our rehabilitation centre.

* To whom all correspondence should be addressed.

Proceedings of the Vth World Congress on Cardiac Rehabilitation

Methods

One hundred male transplant recipients aged 18–54 years ($\bar{x} = 42$ years) were investigated 1 month post-operation and every year thereafter for up to 10 years. The mean observation period was 6.6 years. The yearly investigation was as follows.

The maximal exercise test consisted of a symptom-limited exercise test using a 10 W/min profile, sitting on an electromagnetically braked bicycle. Heart rate, blood pressure (cuff method), electrocardiogram (ink-jet mingograph) and respiratory variables (ERGO Pneumotest, Jaeger) were recorded every minute during exercise. Cardiac output was measured at rest and during a sub-maximal exercise test performed in the lying position using the dye dilution technique. Maximal cardiac output was calculated by multiplying maximal heart rate by the stroke volume measured during a sub-maximal exercise test at 60% maximal working capacity. Urea, creatinine, right and left ejection fraction (radionuclide technique, ^{99m}Tc) were measured at rest. The static and dynamic respiratory volumes (Jaeger pneumotest) were also measured.

The rehabilitation programme comprised four phases.

Phase 0: pre-operative period
Phase 1: period of hospitalization (mean duration 30 days)
Phase 2: convalescence at home
Phase 3: maintenance period with secondary prevention survey

The exercise training was only performed during phase 1 due to geographical difficulties. The psychosocial and preventive aspects of the study were present at all phases. We may thus consider that the evolution of the physiological parameters at exercise reflected their natural evolution from the end of the first month until 10 years post-transplantation.

Statistical analyses of the differences were calculated using Student *t*-test. The values are given as means + standard deviations. A P value <0.05 was considered significant. All of the patients gave their informed consent. No complications resulted from any procedure.

Results

Circulatory aspects

1. *Heart rate*, expressed in relation to $\dot{V}O_2$ max, was significantly higher at rest (up to 50% $\dot{V}O_2$ max) and significantly lower at maximal exercise ($P < 0.001$) compared to the controls. During the 10-year follow-up, heart rate was significantly different between 1 month and 1 year. Resting and maximal heart rates were statistically different after 1 year and more than ($P < 0.001$) after 1 month (Fig. 1).

2. *Cardiac output.* During the steady-state exercise test performed in the lying position, the rate of rise in cardiac output at rest and at lower levels of exercise

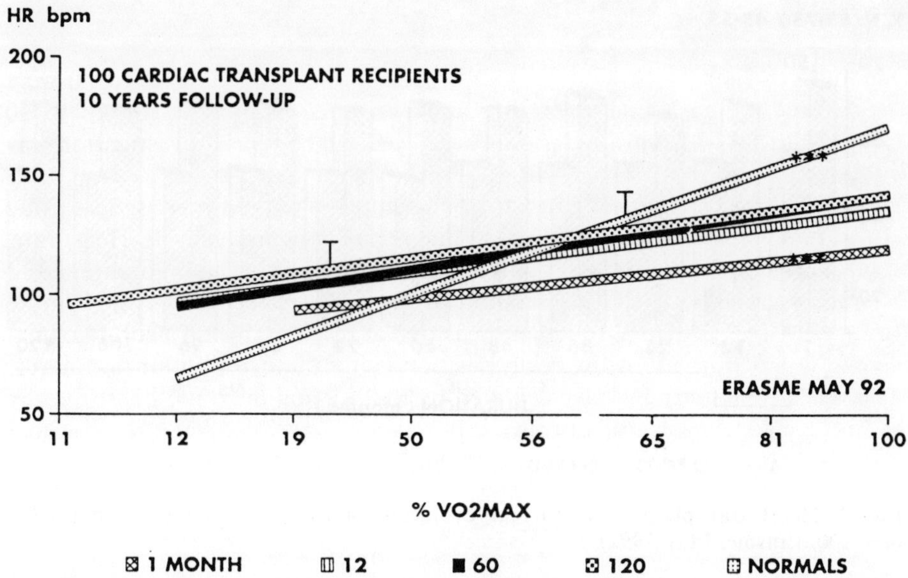

Fig. 1. Heart transplantation. Relationship between heart rate and $\% \dot{V}O_2$ max.

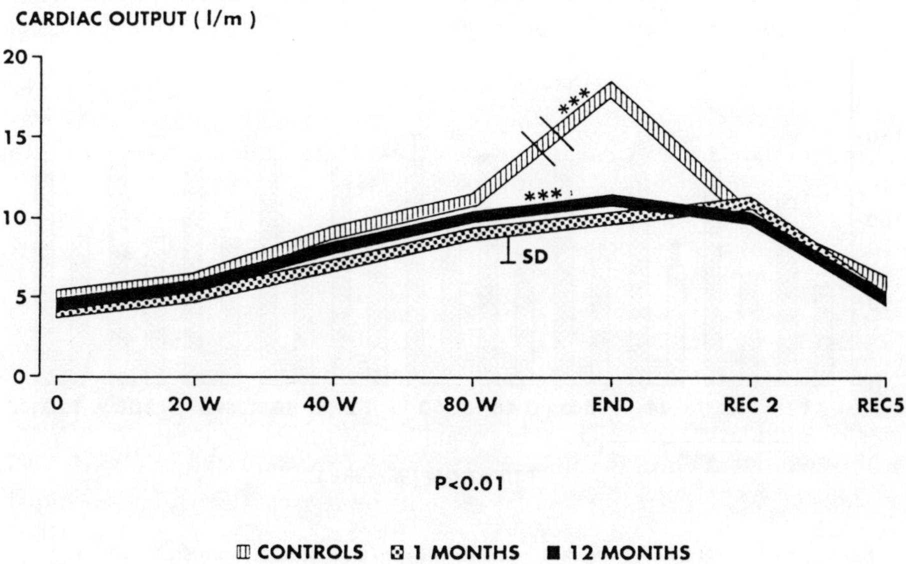

Fig. 2. Sub-maximal values. Relationship between cardiac output and energy expenditure during lying sub-maximal and maximal exercise.

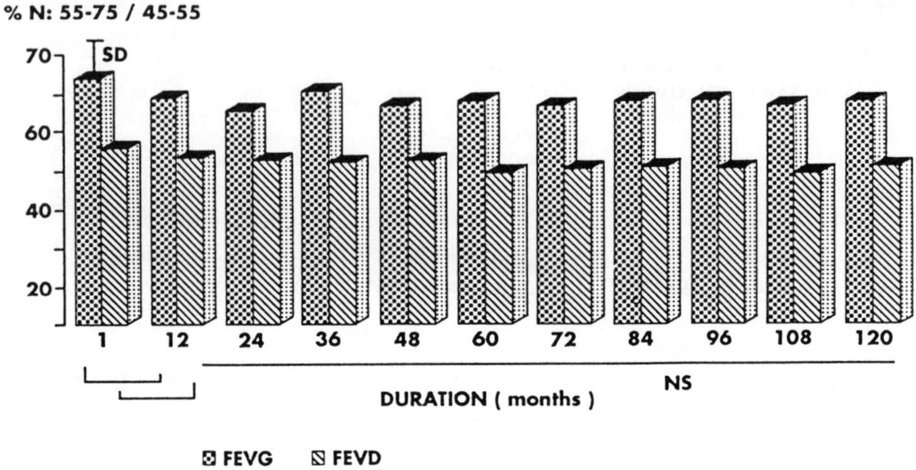

Fig. 3. Heart transplantation: 10-year evolution of right and left ejection fraction ($n = 100$, Erasme, May 1992).

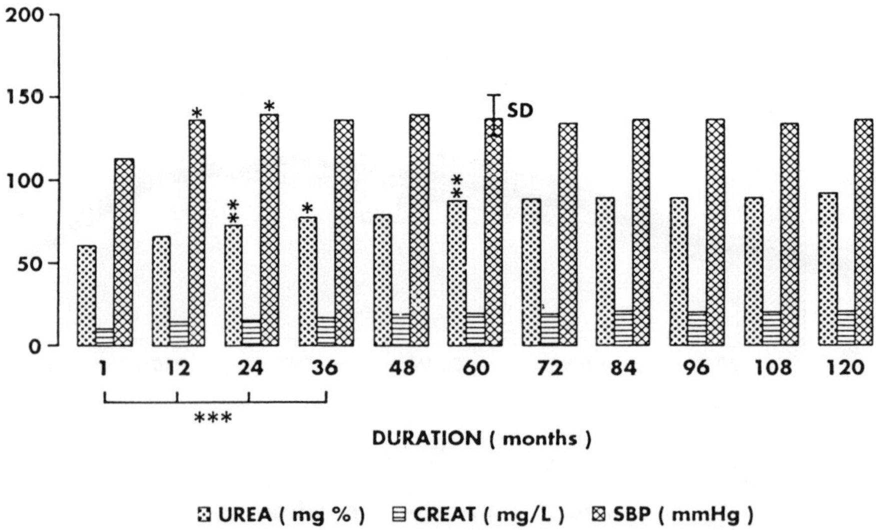

Fig. 4. Heart transplantation: 10-year evolution of resting systolic blood pressure and urea and creatinine levels (mean values; $n = 100$, Erasme, May 1992).

was normal, but calculated peak cardiac output was statistically lower in the transplant recipients compared to the controls ($P < 0.01$; Fig. 2).

3. *The right and left ejection fractions*, were significantly lower at 1 year compared to 1 month after transplantation ($P < 0.001$ and $P < 0.005$, respectively). No further modifications were observed after 1 year (Fig. 3).

4. *Blood pressure.* Resting and exercise blood pressures related to heart rate were statistically higher ($P < 0.01$) in the transplant recipients than in the controls. At rest, systolic blood pressure, despite the anti-hypertensive treatment, rose significantly between 1 and 24 months in parallel with the significant rise in levels of urea ($P < 0.018$) and creatinine ($P < 0.001$) (Fig. 4).

Metabolic aspects

According to Sue and Hansen [1], peak exercise $\dot{V}O_2$ was 42 and 58% of predicted values 1 month and 1 year post-transplantation, respectively ($P < 0.01$). No further increase in peak exercise $\dot{V}O_2$ was observed after 1 year. A mean maximal aerobic capacity close to 1.5 l/min was observed after 1 year in our patients: 43% were in class A of the Weber classification, 48% in class B, 5% in class C and 4% in class D.

Respiratory variables

Metabolic acidosis resulting from delayed circulation adaptation, persistent DLC_0 alterations (59% of predicted values according to Quanjer [2]) and

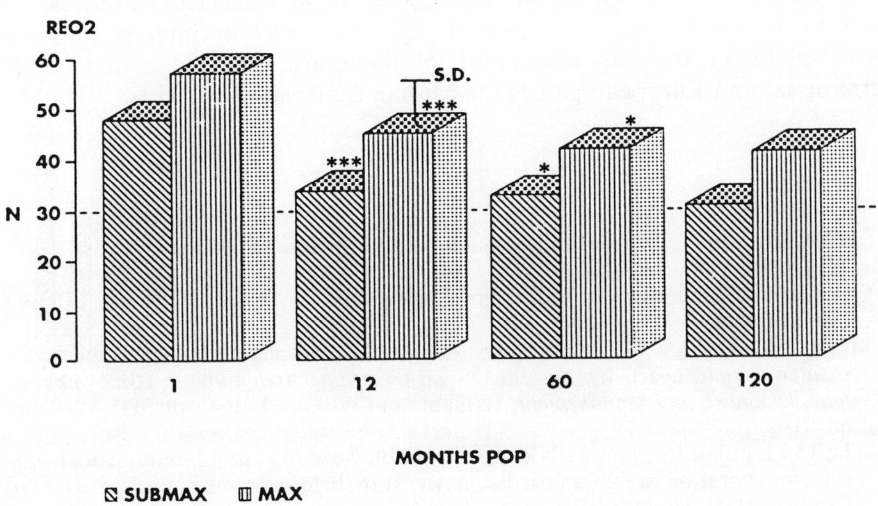

Fig. 5. Heart transplantation, exercise respiratory function: 10-year evolution of maximal and sub-maximal respiratory equivalent for oxygen (REO_2). POP, post-operative period (Erasme, May 1992).

pulmonary circulatory pressure (18 ± 5 mmHg at rest and 36 ± 5 mmHg at sub-maximal exercise) resulted in a persistent high degree of hyperventilation at exercise even after 5–10 years post-transplantation (Fig. 5).

Discussion and conclusion

The orthotopic transplant procedure cuts the nerve connections of the implanted heart. Recolonization by the nervous system does not seem to occur in humans [3, 4], and thus the heart recipient has a denervated heart which is not responsive to the actions of both the sympathetic and parasympathetic systems. This fact explains the higher resting heart rate observed in transplanted patients compared to controls, and also the longer time needed to reach steady-state during a constant sub-maximal exercise test [5]. The supply of oxygen is thus delayed in transplant recipients and responsible for acidosis and hyperventilation during exercise [6–11].

The lower maximal heart rate explains the reduced maximal oxygen consumption [7]. Exercise in cardiac transplant recipients is thus dominated by a lack of antonomic nervous system control, the presence of pre-operative respiratory (persistence of reduced lung diffusion capacity) and pulmonary circulatory dysfunction (pulmonary hypertension) and the development of systemic hypertension [12].

After transplantation, physical rehabilitation aims first to restore the ability to perform normal daily activities without dyspnoea. A mean maximal aerobic capacity close to 1.5 l/min is sufficient for most daily activities of a sedentary person. About 70% of the 1-year, 5-year and 10-year survivors are able to return to school or work and report the same level of interest in their pre-transplant leisure activities. Some of them are able to participate in international and European games for cardiac transplant recipients.

References

1. Sue DS, Hansen JE. Normal values in adults during exercise testing. *Clinics in Chest Med* 1984; **5:** 89–98.
2. Quanjer PH. Standardized lung function testing. *Bull Eur Physiopath Respir.* (Suppl.) 1983; **5:** 61–63.
3. Mason JW, Harrison DC. Electrophysiology and electropharmacology of the transplanted human heart. In: Narula OS (ed.), *Cardiac Arrhythmias: Electrophysiology, Diagnosis and Management.* Williams and Wilkins: Baltimore, MD, 1979, pp. 66–81.
4. Wharton J, Polak JM, Banner NR, Springall DR, Rose M *et al.* Immunohistochemical demonstration of human cardiac innervation before and after transplantation. *Circ Res* 1990: **66:** 900–912.
5. Stinson EB, Griepp RL, Schroeder JS, Dong E, Shumway NE. Hemodynamic observations one and two years after cardiac transplantation in man. *Circulation* 1972; **14:** 1181–1193.

6. Clark DA, Schroeder JS, Griepp RB, Stinson EB, Dong E *et al.* Cardiac transplantation in man: Review of first three years' experience. *Am J Med* 1973; **54:** 563–576.
7. Degré SGL, Niset GL, De Smet JM, Ibrahim T, Stoupel E. *et al.* Cardiorespiratory response to early exercise testing after orthotopic cardiac transplantation. *Am J Cardiol* 1987; **60:** 926–928.
8. Niset G, Coustry-Degré S. Phychosocial and physical rehabilitation after heart transplantation: 1-year follow-up. *Cardiology* 1988; **75:** 311–317.
9. Savin W, Haskell WL, Schroeder JS, Stinson EB. Cardiorespiratory responses of cardiac transplant patients to graded, symptom-limited exercise. *Circulation* 1980; **62:** 55–60.
10. Schroeder JS. Hemodynamic performance of the human transplanted heart. *Transplant Proc* 1979; **11:** 304–308.
11. Stinson EB, Caves PK, Griepp RB, Oyer PE, Rider AK *et al.* Hemodynamic observations in the early period after human heart transplantation. *J Thorac Cardiovasc Surg* 1975; **69:** 264–270.
12. Niset G, Hermans L, Depelchin P. Exercise and heart transplantation: A review. *Sports Med* 1991; **12:** 359–379.

31 On the Choice of a Cycle Ergometer Exercise Test Protocol for the Heart Transplant Patient

T. Kavanagh[1], R. J. Shephard*[1,2], D. Mertens[1], S. Qureshi[1]

[1] *Toronto Rehabilitation Centre* and [2] *School of Physical and Health Education, University of Toronto, 320 Huron Street, Toronto, Ontario M5S 1A1, Canada*

Introduction

It is common practice to infer the physical condition of both healthy individuals and cardiac patients from the heart rate observed at a given rate of working. The usual basis of such an evaluation is the supposed linear relationship that extends from 50% of maximal oxygen intake through to near peak oxygen intake [1]. The original Åstrand protocol called for 6 min of exercise at a given power output, in order to approximate a steady-state. However, such an approach makes exercise testing very time-consuming, and restricts observations to two or at most three stages of effort, thus limiting the possibility of determining the individual's ventilatory threshold. Accordingly, more recent protocols have shortened testing to 3 min, or even to 1 min per test stage, off-setting this change by making a much larger number of small increments in the intensity of exercise.

Our earlier studies [2, 3] demonstrated the acceptability of this approach in healthy normal subjects. The present research was designed to examine the situation in patients who had received cardiac transplantation, with a resultant slowing of the acceleration in heart rate during exercise. The detailed mathematical analysis of cardiac on-transients shows a distinct lag phase, a phase of rapid equilibration and a final slow increase in heart rate [4]; however, to a

* To whom all correspondence should be addressed.

Proceedings of the Vth World Congress on Cardiac Rehabilitation

first approximation, the responses of normal and cardiac transplant patients can be compared in terms of the half-time of equilibration, or the time constant of a single exponential function describing the approach to steady-state values $[1 - e^{-kt}]$.

Methods

Subjects

Twenty-seven patients with a mean age of 49 ± 6 years who had undergone orthotopic cardiac transplantation at least 6 months earlier were compared with 45 normal adults of approximately the same age (43 ± 8 years). All of the patients were in good health at the time of observation, with no clinical evidence of transplant rejection, although the majority were receiving small doses of cyclosporin and cortisol.

Exercise protocol

All of the subjects carried out a two-stage 'steady-state' exercise test on an electrically braked cycle ergometer (Elema-Schonander) operated at 60 pedal rpm. Oxygen consumption was recorded every 30 s using a Sensor-Medics Horizon II metabolic cart, and heart rate was monitored continually using a CM5 electrocardiographic lead system. Ergometer loadings were set at one-third and two-thirds of previously determined individual peak power outputs. Observations were continued at each stage until oxygen consumption had reached a plateau, the elapsed time being 6 min per stage in the majority of studies. The subjects then progressed to the second stage of the test.

A progressive cycle ergometer test was also performed by all subjects, using a standard ramp-function protocol, with 16.7-W increments of work rate every minute. Data from the progressive and the steady-state tests were compared at work rates corresponding to the two steady-state data sets.

Results and discussion

Normal subjects

The average intensities of effort for the two sub-maximal, steady-state tests were 73 and 146 W, respectively, corresponding to approximately 33 and 67% of each subject's peak aerobic power as measured on the cycle ergometer. The speed of the on-transient was of the same order as previously reported for younger individuals [4–6]. The heart rate increased on average from 72 ± 9 to 107 ± 12 beats/min over the 6 min of adaptation to the first test stage. The half-time of heart rate equilibration averaged 39 s, and after 4 min of exercise the heart rate adjustment was 89% complete. The oxygen consumption increased from its resting value of 0.31 ± 0.04 l/min to 1.12 ± 0.19 l/min during the first stage; the average half-time was 41 s, and after 4 min of exercise the oxygen consumption had attained 98% of the final value for this stage.

During the second 6-min stage, heart rate increased from an average of 107 ± 12 to 147 ± 14 beats/min Equilibration was a little slower at the higher work rate (reflecting cardiovascular drift, associated with a rise of core temperature and/or the addition of an anaerobic component to the exercise task). On average, the half-time of the second adjustment in heart rate was 108 s, and adaptation was 85% complete after 4 min of the second stage. However, the speed of adaptation of the oxygen consumption remained similar to that observed at the first stage, values rising from 1.12 ± 0.19 to 1.91 ± 0.33 l/min with an average half-time of only 35 s.

Cardiac transplant patients

The cardiac transplant patients were studied at the same relative work rates as the age-matched normal subjects, approximately one-third and two-thirds of peak aerobic effort, but because the patients had a much lower average peak aerobic power, the absolute levels of effort selected averaged only 46 and 94 W.

During the first steady-state stage, the average heart rate of the patients increased from an elevated resting value of 101 ± 9 beats/min to a 6 min value of 117 ± 10 beats/min. The half-time of adjustment was longer than in the normal subjects, averaging 73 s, and even after 4 min of exercise equilibration was only 85% complete. The oxygen consumption also increased more slowly than in the normal subjects, from a resting value of 0.29 ± 0.04 l/min to 0.89 ± 0.20 l/min at the end of the first stage of effort. The half-time of the metabolic response averaged 55 s, but after 4 min of exercise the adjustment was 100% complete.

During the second stage of submaximal exercise, there was a larger increase in heart rate, from 117 ± 10 beats/min to a final reading of 141 ± 14 beats/min. The half-time of adaptation to this stage was extended further, to an average of 118 s, and the heart rate adjustment was only 80% complete after 4 min at this intensity of effort. Oxygen consumption increased from 0.89 ± 0.20 to 1.44 ± 0.30 l/min, with a half-time averaging 42 s, and after 4 min at the second intensity of effort the oxygen consumption of the patients had attained 98% of its final value.

The slow adjustment of the heart rate in the cardiac transplant patients is readily understood from the residual mechanisms capable of inducing tachycardia. The small early increase in heart rate is probably mediated mainly via the Bainbridge reflex, and the larger, delayed reaction is dependent mainly upon the presentation of circulating catecholamines to the cardiac pacemaker. Despite some increase in the sensitivity of catecholamine receptors, a catecholamine response is still seen only with relatively vigorous effort, and even then a delay is imposed by the circulatory transit time [7].

Comparison of progressive and steady-state tests

Normal subjects

The normal subjects reached intensities of effort corresponding to the two steady-state tests after an average of 4.3 ± 0.6 and 8.6 ± 1.7 min of progressive exercise, respectively. The heart rate observed after an average of 4.3 min performance of the progressive test was 107 ± 12 beats/min, identical with the value obtained in the steady-state test, and the oxygen consumption of 1.16 ± 0.19 l/min was also only marginally and non-significantly greater than that seen in steady-state effort.

After an average of 8.6 min of progressive testing, the subjects had reached an intensity of effort that would be more likely in laboratory evaluation. The agreement between the steady-state and progressive tests was less perfect in the second stage. During the progressive test, heart rate had increased to only 139 ± 14 beats/min, substantially less than the steady-state value of 147 ± 14 beats/min ($P < 0.001$). In contrast, the oxygen consumption of 1.93 ± 0.34 l/min non-significantly exceeded the steady-state value of 1.91 ± 0.33 l/min. Thus, if progressive test data at 65–70% of peak aerobic power had been used to predict maximal oxygen intake, an average value of 3.15 l/min would have been obtained, whereas the steady-state data would have yielded an average figure of 2.85 l/min, much closer to the actually observed maximum of 2.82 ± 0.56 l/min.

Cardiac transplant patients

Because of their low levels of aerobic fitness, the cardiac transplant patients reached the required steady-state intensities of effort after average periods of 2.8 ± 0.9 min and 5.7 ± 1.5 min of progressive exercise, respectively. After 2.8 min, heart rate had increased to only 109 ± 12 beats/min, compared with the steady-state average of 117 ± 10 beats/min, a discrepancy of 8 ± 3 beats/min. The oxygen consumption of 0.8 ± 0.2 l/min was closer to the steady-state value of 0.89 ± 0.20 l/min.

These differences continued at the second intensity of effort. After 5.6 min of progressive exercise, heart rate was only 125 ± 14 rather than 141 ± 14 beats/-min, and oxygen consumption was 1.3 ± 0.3 l/min, a non-significant difference from the steady-state value of 1.44 ± 0.30 l/min. Let us again make the assumption that predictions of maximal oxygen intake were to be based on responses observed at the second work rate. In the steady-state test, the predicted maximal oxygen intake would average 2.22 l/min, somewhat in excess of the observed value of 1.91 ± 0.42 l/min, because most patients would be unlikely to attain the age-predicted maximal heart rate. However, a much greater error would arise if predictions were based on the low heart rate observed during the progressive test, the predicted maximum for this data set amounting to an unrealistic average of 2.77 l/min.

Conclusions

We may conclude that during a progressive cycle ergometer test, the consumption of oxygen approaches the steady-state value more rapidly than does the heart rate. In older normal subjects, the discrepant pattern of response is seen only at high and moderately anaerobic work rates (in our experiments, 67% of peak aerobic power). Nevertheless, this is the intensity of effort at which sub-maximal predictions of maximal oxygen intake are commonly made, and the delay in heart rate equilibration is enough to cause a 10% over-estimation of maximal oxygen intake relative to either direct measurements or steady-state predictions.

Following cardiac transplantation, heart rate equilibration occurs even more slowly. Because of slow equilibration and uncertainties regarding the attainable peak heart rate, even steady-state predictions of aerobic power over-estimate directly measured values, and the results obtained from a progressive test give a gross over-estimate of cardiorespiratory condition.

References

1. Åstrand I. Aerobic work capacity in men and women with special reference to age. *Acta Physiol Scand* (Suppl. 169) 1960; **49:** 1–92.
2. Shephard RJ. The prediction of 'maximal' oxygen consumption using a new progressive step test. *Ergonomics* 1967; **10:** 1–15.
3. Shephard RJ, Kavanagh T. On the stage duration for a progressive exercise test. In: Shephard RJ, Lavallée H (eds), *Physical Fitness Assessment: Principles, Practice and Application.* CC Thomas: Springfield, IL, 1978, pp. 335–344.
4. Shephard RJ. *Physiology and Biochemistry of Exercise.* Praeger: New York, 1982.
5. Barstow TJ, Molé PA. Linear and nonlinear characteristics of oxygen uptake kinetics during heavy exercise. *J Appl Physiol* 1991; **71**: 2099–2106.
6. Rotstein A, Sagiv M, Yaniv-Tamir A, Fisher N, Dotan R. Smoking effect on exercise response kinetics of oxygen uptake and related variables. *Int J Sports Med* 1991; **12:** 281–284.
7. Shephard RJ. Responses of the cardiac transplant patient to exercise and training. *Exercise Sport Sci Rev* 1992; **20:** 297–320.

32 Ratings of Perceived Exertion After Cardiac Transplantation: The Effect of Endurance Training

R. J. Shephard*[1,2], T. Kavanagh[2], M. H. Yacoub[3]

[1] School of Physical and Health Education, University of Toronto, 320 Huron Street, Toronto, Ontario M5S 1A1, [2] Toronto Rehabilitation Centre, Toronto, Ontario, Canada and *[3] Department of Cardiothoracic Surgery, National Heart and Lung Institute, Harefield Hospital, Harefield, Middlesex, UK*

Introduction

Cardiac transplant patients show a very slow increase in heart rate in response to a step increase in work rate [1]. Accordingly, the Borg [2] rating of perceived exertion (RPE) is commonly used in place of heart rate as a simple prescriptive guide to the intensity of exercise. The overall sensation perceived by the patient represents a mixture of central and peripheral sensations, including feelings of fatigue, pain and weakness from the skeletal muscles. Given the wasting of the skeletal muscles that is commonly induced by immunosuppressant agents in the first few months following cardiac transplantation [3], there is some danger that the peripheral component of effort ratings may increase, leading to the adoption of an intensity of exercise that is insufficient to induce gains of cardiorespiratory function. Accordingly, we thought it of interest to evaluate ratings of perceived exertion (RPE) in a group of 36 patients when they were first admitted to our cardiac rehabilitation programme, an average of some 6 months following orthotopic cardiac transplantation, repeating the evaluation 16 months later when they had completed a progressive rehabilitation procedure that had augmented their peak oxygen transport by an average of 19.5% and their lean tissue mass by an average of 3.5%.

* To whom all correspondence should be addressed.

Proceedings of the Vth World Congress on Cardiac Rehabilitation

Methods

Patients

The 36 patients had all undergone successful orthotopic cardiac transplantation at Harefield Hospital in the UK. At the time of testing, all were in good health and free of signs of transplant rejection; however, the majority were receiving small doses of cortisol and cyclosporin. Their mean physical characteristics were: age 49 ± 6 years, height 172.3 ± 9.5 cm, body mass 74.6 ± 11.3 kg, and initial peak oxygen intake 25.8 ± 6.0 ml/kg/min.

An initial progressive cycle ergometer test was performed an average of 6 months post-surgery. The patients then engaged in a progressive exercise rehabilitation programme, details of which are given elsewhere [3], and at the end of 16 months a further progressive cycle ergometer test was completed. At this stage in their treatment, peak oxygen intake had increased by an average of 19.5% and lean tissue mass by 3.5%.

Perceptions of exertion were compared with previous observations made on healthy young adults aged 30 years [4]. Further RPE data were obtained on a group of 45 control subjects whose mean physical characteristics were: age 43 ± 8 years, height 176.7 ± 6.4 cm, and body mass 79.8 ± 11.1 kg. The older normal subjects performed an identical type of progressive exercise test on one occasion only, reaching a peak oxygen intake that averaged 35.5 ± 6.2 ml/kg/min.

Exercise testing

During the progressive cycle ergometer test, the loading of an electrically braked cycle ergometer (Elema-Schonander) was increased by 16.7 W each minute until the patient reached a plateau of oxygen transport, reported an RPE of 19–20, was unable to sustain the required pedalling cadence of 60 rpm, or asked to stop the test.

The electrocardiogram (CM5 lead system) was recorded throughout and metabolic reactions were measured at 30-s intervals using a Sensor-Medics Horizon II metabolic cart. Overall perceptions of effort were reported each minute by having the subject point to an appropriate level on Borg's original 6–20 unit scale [2].

Results and discussion

Relation of RPE to heart rate

In the normal young adults, a perception of 13 units of effort on the Borg scale had been linked to a heart rate averaging 145 beats/min [4]. In the older and more sedentary normal subjects, the same perception was linked to a heart rate that averaged no more than 118 ± 20 beats/min, and in the patients a rating of 13 RPE units initially corresponded to a heart rate averaging only 111 ± 14 beats/min. After the 16 months of rehabilitation, the relationship of RPE to heart rate in the transplant patients was shifted significantly to the right, so that 13 RPE units now corresponded to 122 ± 18 beats/min ($\Delta = 10.0 \pm 17.4$, CI 3.6–16.4 beats/min).

We hypothesized that the low initial pulse rates in both the older normal subjects and the transplant patients reflected weak skeletal muscles, and a corresponding dominance of peripheral muscular sensations over central perceptions relating to heart rate, ventilation and cardiac performance. We further hypothesized that the heart rate corresponding to a fixed RPE rating would rise as the skeletal muscles became stronger. We tested this concept empirically by relating individual changes in heart rate at an RPE of 13 units to the corresponding changes in peak oxygen intake and lean body mass. As we had anticipated, the correlation was closer for lean tissue mass ($r = 0.72$) than for maximal oxygen intake ($r = 0.58$), suggesting that the perception of effort was indeed more closely linked to muscular than to central cardiorespiratory sensations.

Relation of RPE to power output

When first seen, a rating of 13 RPE units corresponded to only 59 ± 19 W in the patients, as compared with some 134 W in the younger adults and 90 W in the older normal subjects. Moreover, the relationship between perceived effort and power output was curvilinear in the patients, successive ratings from 11 to 14 units corresponding to 32, 48, 59 and 68 W; presumably, sensations increased disproportionately to power because of the onset of anaerobic effort and peripheral muscle fatigue. After the period of rehabilitation, the power output at a rating of 13 units was more variable, but on average had increased substantially to 85 ± 30 W ($\Delta = 26.3 \pm 29.2$, CI 15.6–37.1 units), close to the figure observed in the older normal subjects.

Relation of RPE to oxygen consumption

The relationships between oxygen consumption (expressed in ml/kg/min) and RPE were similar to those observed for power output. In the young adults, 13 RPE units corresponded to an oxygen consumption of some 30 ml/kg/min, but in the older normal subjects, the same rating corresponded to an average oxygen consumption of only 16.8 ml/kg/min. In the transplant patients, 13 units initially corresponded to 14.3 ± 3.6 ml/kg/min, but after the 16 months of rehabilitation, it had increased to 17.3 ml/kg/min (Δ 2.9 ± 4.6, CI 1.2–4.6 ml/kg/min), slightly more than in the age-matched normals. It is particularly interesting that the normalization of the patients' response had occurred although their final peak oxygen intake of 30.8 ml/kg/min was still only about 90.5% of that seen in the age-matched normals; this seems a further pointer to the dominance of peripheral rather than central cardiorespiratory sensations in determining the perceptions of our patients and older normal subjects.

When the data were expressed as a percentage of the individual's peak oxygen intake, the initial perception of 13 RPE units by the transplant patients corresponded to what might be considered from the viewpoint of exercise prescription a relatively acceptable average intensity of effort (66.3% of peak oxygen intake). However, the practical value of the Borg scale in advising the individual patient was quite limited, since the standard deviation was $\pm$ 11.6% of peak oxygen intake. Assuming that the data were normally distributed, 1 patient in 40 would reach 89.5% of maximal oxygen intake when seeking an RPE of 13 units, and a further 1 in 40 would attain an intensity of only 43.1% of maximum aerobic power.

After the 16 months of rehabilitation, ratings were related to percentages of the augmented peak oxygen intake. The average response to a rating of 13 RPE units showed no significant change (68.0 $\pm$ 12.2%), but again there was a very large inter-individual difference in response.

Conclusions

The present data confirm our earlier findings on younger adults [4]; the normally suggested prescription of 13 RPE units gives an appropriate average intensity of effort between 65 and 70% of peak oxygen intake. However, there is a wide inter-individual variation, corresponding to a standard deviation of some 12%, so that an exercise prescription based solely on an RPE of 13 units is not sufficiently precise to regulate the activities of an individual patient. Plainly, other indices must also be used, and because the increase in heart rate is slow after cardiac transplantation, such patients must rely mainly upon the walking of a fixed distance in a specified time.

The present observations also show that, in older adults, the intensity of sensation for a given heart rate is higher than in younger individuals, and that this trend is further increased after cardiac transplantation. The probable reason is that the overall perception of cycle ergometry in such individuals is strongly shaped by peripheral sensations, arising in the weakened skeletal muscles. Changes in the relationship of RPE to heart rate are influenced more by increments in lean mass than by increases in peak oxygen transport. Thus, the strengthening of the skeletal muscles is an important element in the improvement of function, equally so in patients who have received a cardiac transplant and in sedentary older normal individuals who have allowed their muscle strength to deteriorate.

References

1. Shephard RJ. Responses of the cardiac transplant patient to exercise and training. *Exercise Sport Sci Rev* 1992; **20:** 297–320.

2. Borg G. The perception of physical performance. In: Shephard RJ (ed.), *Frontiers of Fitness*. C.C. Thomas: Springfield, IL, 1971, pp. 280–294.
3. Kavanagh T, Yacoub MH, Mertens DJ, Kennedy J, Campbell R. Cardio-respiratory responses to exercise training after orthotopic cardiac transplantation. *Circulation* 1988; **77:** 162–171.
4. Shephard RJ, Vandewalle H, Gil V, Bouhlel E, Monod H. Respiratory, muscular and overall perceptions of effort: The influence of hypoxia and muscle mass. *Med Sci Sports Exercise* 1992; **24:** 556–567.

33 Effects of Long-term Endurance Training After Cardiac Transplantation

T. Kavanagh*[1], M. H. Yacoub[2]

[1] Toronto Rehabilitation Centre, 345 Rumsey Road, Toronto, Ontario M4G 1R7 and Department of Medicine, University of Toronto, Toronto, Ontario, Canada and *[2] Department of Cardiothoracic Surgery, National Heart and Lung Institute, Harefield Hospital, Harefield, Middlesex, UK*

Introduction

The typical heart transplantation recipient is a 45-year-old male who, as a result of severe ischaemic heart disease or cardiomyopathy, is in New York Heart Association Class IV cardiac failure [1]. He has experienced months of pre-operative invalidism, suffers from general muscle weakness, and is depressed and fearful. The first step towards recovery is the transplantation procedure itself, with its rapid alleviation of disabling cardiac symptoms and its favourable 1- and 5-year actuarial survival rates of 81 and 69%, respectively [1]. However, to take full advantage of the new heart, the patient requires an exercise rehabilitation programme to improve physical fitness, restore self-confidence and hasten return to full-time employment.

Effects of exercise training

There are only a handful of reports in the literature on the effects of training after heart transplantation (Table 1). The earliest was from Squires and co-workers [2], who trained two orthotopic transplantation recipients for 8

* To whom all correspondence should be addressed.

Proceedings of the Vth World Congress on Cardiac Rehabilitation

Table 1
Exercise rehabilitation after orthotopic heart transplantation

Author	Patients (n)	Training (months)
Squires *et al.*	2	2
Degré *et al.*	3	5
Savin *et al.*	5	4
Niset *et al.*	62	12
Kavanagh *et al.*	36	24
Keteyian *et al.*	12 (5C)	2

weeks. Benefits included a reduction in sub-maximal systolic blood pressures and perceived exertion ratings, but no significant changes in resting, sub-maximal or peak heart rates. Metabolic measurements were not carried out.

Shortly thereafter, Savin *et al.* [3] evaluated the effects of a 16-week stationary cycling programme on five orthotopic patients. Training resulted in a 45% increase in peak work output, an 18% increase in peak oxygen uptake and a 13% reduction in sub-maximal heart rates. Niset *et al.* [4] followed 62 orthotopic transplants for 1 year. The physical benefits included a 34% increase in maximal work capacity and oxygen uptake, as well as an 11% increase in peak heart rate and an 18% increase in peak blood pressure. Sub-maximal heart rates and systolic blood pressures were unchanged, but blood lactates and ventilation were reduced. Keteyian *et al.* [5] compared the results of a 10-week training regimen in 12 male orthotopes with 5 controls, and recorded a 20% increase in peak oxygen intake, a 17% increase in peak ventilation and a 14% increase in peak heart rate in the exercisers.

Most programmes have been relatively short-term in duration, often less than 16 weeks. In the longest study published to date, we had the opportunity to train 36 orthotopic transplants for 2 years [6], using a walk/jog programme described elsewhere [7]. Compliance was very good, all patients progressing to an average distance of 24 km per week at an average pace of 8.5 min/km. Eight of the highly motivated patients achieved 32 km or more a week, at an average pace of 6.5 min/km, with one of these finishing the 42-km Boston Marathon 12 months after joining the programme and 15 months after undergoing the transplantation procedure [8]. There were few episodes of rejection or infection, and these were so minor that they had little effect on the training regimen.

After training there was a 5.5% increase in body mass, of which 3.2% was lean tissue. Resting heart rate for all patients was reduced, with the greatest reduction in those who were highly compliant. Peak heart rate was significantly increased. Nevertheless, the final resting heart rates remained higher, and the final peak heart rates lower, than in a group of age-matched normal subjects. Sub-maximal heart rates were unchanged in the 28 moderately compliant

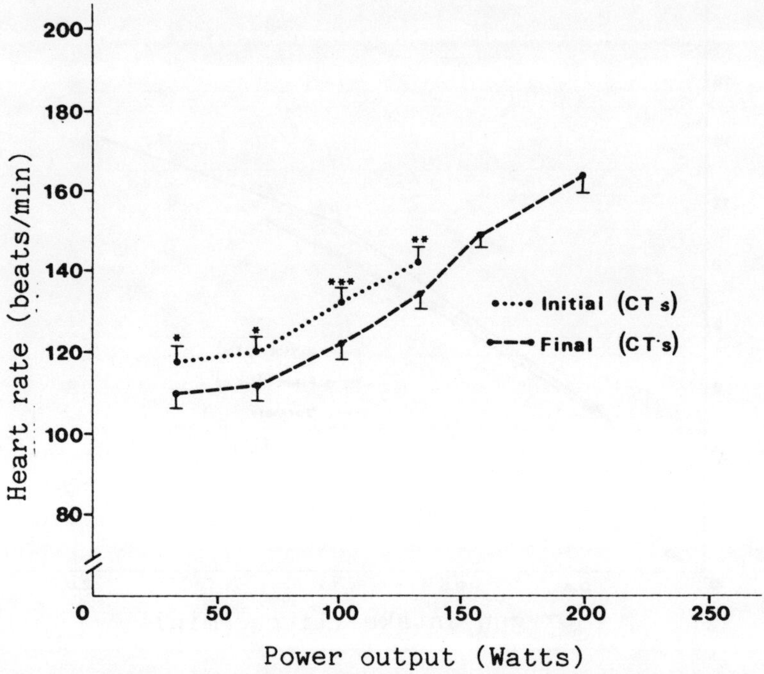

Fig. 1. Effects of long-term endurance training after cardiac transplantation.

patients, whereas in the 8 highly compliant patients the effect was quite large (Fig. 1). There was also an overall and significant marked reduction in the rating of perceived exertion, minute ventilation and diastolic blood pressure at equivalent work outputs.

The peak work output increased by 49% (65% in the 8 highly compliant subjects), peak oxygen uptake by 27% (54% in the highly compliant patients), with all patients exercising to a larger respiratory minute ventilation and a higher maximal heart rate after training. Since changes in respiratory gas exchange ratio and peak rating of perceived exertion were quite small, it is unlikely that greater voluntary effort was responsible for improved performance. Neither could any of the changes have been due to an improvement in mechanical efficiency on the ergometer, since the relationship of oxygen uptake to power output was unchanged.

The reduction in resting and sub-maximal heart rates seen in those who attained the greatest training distances was thought to be due to a drop in effort-induced levels of serum norepinephrine, and/or downregulation in the sensitivity of cardiac beta-adrenoreceptors. Both of these changes have been shown to occur in animals and humans exposed to vigorous training [9–12]. The entire group's increase in peak exercise heart rate was likely to have been due to a strengthening of the leg muscles. This peripheral adaptation would

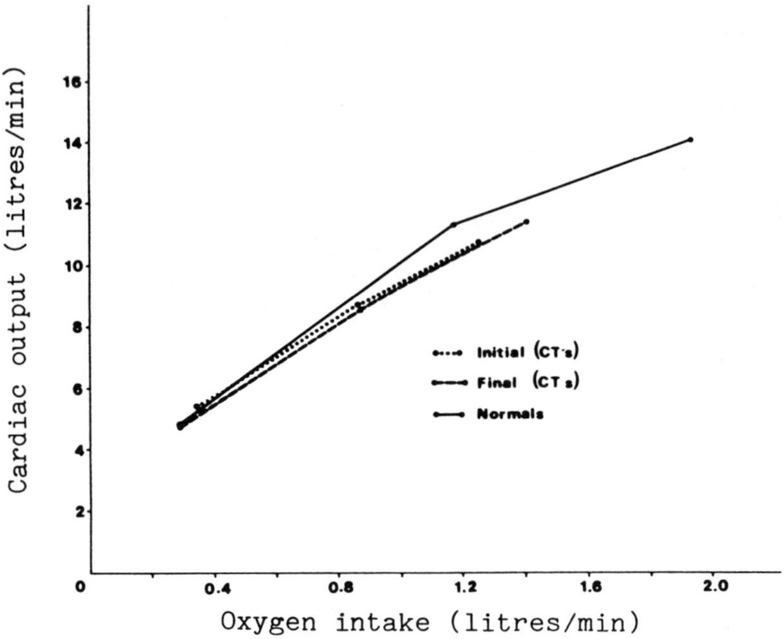

Fig. 2. Effects of exercise training.

account for the improved power output and, because of a later onset of anaerobiosis, reduced perception of effort and minute ventilation during sub-maximal exercise. Sub-maximal cardiac outputs, measured by the CO_2 rebreathing technique, did not change with training in relation to oxygen uptake (Fig. 2). This suggests peripheral rather than central improvement, although one might infer that the reduction in sub-maximal diastolic blood pressures towards normal values is an indication of improved myocardial compliance.

Currently, the heterotopic procedure comprises less than 1% of all heart transplantations, and this explains the paucity of reports on the rehabilitation of this group. Sieurat and his co-workers [13] trained eight heterotopic recipients and demonstrated an increase in peak work output and peak heart rate. Kavanagh *et al.* [14] reported on 10 male heterotopes who followed a walk/jog training programme for 18 months. After training, lean body mass increased by 4%, peak work output by 33%, peak oxygen uptake by 23% and absolute ventilatory threshold by 16%. Resting rate in the donor heart did not change significantly, but the resting rate of the recipient heart fell significantly by 14 beats/min. Sub-maximal recipient heart rates showed a training bradycardia, and demonstrated less exercise-induced ventricular ectopy than at initial testing. Donor sub-maximal heart rates were unchanged.

Accelerated coronary atherosclerosis is a serious late complication after cardiac transplantation [15]. By the third post-operative year, some 40% of patients will show angiographic evidence of this condition. Suggested causes are prolonged use of cyclosporine and/or steroids, post-operative attacks of cytomegalovirus infection, or repeated bouts of rejection [16]. The Stanford group found a high association between hypercholesterolaemia and graft atherosclerosis, and have advocated aggressive dietary and, if necessary, drug intervention [17]. The rehabilitation programme will, therefore, pay close attention to serum lipid and glucose levels, and will provide the necessary education to those who have problems in these areas.

Psychosocial aspects

Psychological changes

Information on the psychological effects of heart transplantation remains scant. Buxton *et al.* [18] have used the Nottingham Health Profile to study the quality of life in 29 patients in the UK before and after surgery. In all dimensions (physical mobility, energy, pain, emotional reaction, sleep habits and social isolation), there was a very marked improvement by 3 months; the trend was continuing, although less pronounced at the end of 1 year. Other workers have noted the high levels of anxiety and depression, the poor sense of well-being and the negative body image frequently encountered in patients awaiting a new heart. The post-transplantation months can also be highly stressful [19]. In a group of Australian heart recipients, a greater proportion (43%) were more anxious at 1 year than at discharge (19%) [20]. Causes for their concern included financial problems and being a burden on their family (50%), fear that over-exertion would harm the new heart (43%), excessive weight gain (36%) and an inability to exercise (29%).

These findings suggest that a comprehensive rehabilitation programme should have a major role to play in terms of psychosocial benefit, but to date no perspective randomized controlled trial to investigate this possibility has been carried out. Conclusions must therefore be drawn from observation reports. Niset and co-workers [4] carried out psychological assessment on 100 transplantation patients who took part in a structured exercise programme for 1 year. Acceptance of the new heart and improved quality of life was apparent in the early phases of the programme, but psychosocial items such as anxiety, coping ability, social interaction and mental alertness took longer to recover. Ultimately, however, there was a complete return to normality in all areas and in almost all patients. Kavanagh *et al.* [21] have investigated the influence of a 2-year exercise training programme upon the psychological status of 39 male patients. Although the average time elapsing between surgery and entry to the programme was 8 months, initial testing showed significant depression as well as high levels of anxiety. Training resulted in a significant reduction in depression, and this correlated well with an increase in fitness as measured by changes in peak oxygen uptake. Anxiety was also significantly lessened, although this was associated not so much with improved fitness as with the passage of time from the transplantation procedure.

Return to work

Given the high cost of the transplantation procedure and the average age of the recipients, return to work is a highly desirable goal. In those who have not been entered into a formal rehabilitation programme, the proportion obtaining work after surgery has been variously reported as being anywhere between 32 and 64% [22]. The reasons for failure to find employment are rarely medical, and include age, pre-illness employment pattern, type of work and availability of disability payments. Niset and co-workers' experience with a group attending their rehabilitation programme was that 71% of those who were working 6 months before surgery had returned to work [4]. Age seemed to be a factor in that the return rate was 82% for those under 45 years, 76% for those between 46 and 55 years and 10% for those over 55 years. The high proportion of patients returning to work (71%) suggests that a comprehensive rehabilitation programme is of value. In our own experience, 69% of patients attending our rehabilitation programme returned to work, 8% took early retirement and only 3% were finally unemployed for medical reasons [23].

Conclusions

The routine use of a comprehensive exercise rehabilitation programme following cardiac transplantation is fully justified on physiological, psychological and vocational grounds. It is a safe and effective way to maximize the benefits of surgery. There is, of course, still considerable scope for further research. Questions which remain to be answered include the precise nature of the training adaptations and the contribution made by central and peripheral factors. It is also tempting to speculate on the favourable effects of a rehabilitation programme – which includes not only exercise training but also dietary advice and weight control – on the incidence and severity of post-transplant coronary atherosclerosis, and the incidence of bouts of intercurrent infection and rejection in the immunosuppressed patient.

References

1. Kriett JM, Kaye MP. The Registry of the International Society for Heart and Lung Transplantation: Eighth Official Report – 1991. *J Heart Lung Transplant* 1991; **10:** 491–498.
2. Squires RW, Arthur PR, Gau GT, Muri A, Lambert WB. Exercise after cardiac transplantation: A report of two cases. *J Cardiac Rehab* 1983; **3:** 570–574.
3. Savin WM, Gordon E, Green S *et al.* Comparison of exercise training effects in cardiac denervated and innervated humans. *J Am Coll Cardiol* (Abstr.) 1983; **1:** 722.

4. Niset G, Coustry-Degre C, Degre S. Psychosocial and physical rehabilitation after heart transplantation: 1 year follow-up. *Cardiology* 1988; **75:** 311–317.
5. Keteyian SJ, Shepard R, Ehrman J *et al.* Cardiovascular responses of heart transplant patients to exercise training. *J Appl Physiol* 1991; **70:** 2627–2631.
6. Kavanagh T, Yacoub MH, Mertens DJ, Kennedy J, Campbell RB, Sawyer P. Cardiorespiratory responses to exercise training after orthotopic cardiac transplantation. *Circulation* 1988; **77:** 162–171.
7. Kavanagh T. The Toronto Rehabilitation Centre's Cardiac Exercise Programme. *J Cardiac Rehab* 1982; **2:** 496–502.
8. Kavanagh T, Yacoub MH, Campbell R, Mertens D. Marathon running after cardiac transplantation: A case history. *J Cardiopulmonary Rehab* 1986; **6:** 16–20.
9. Hartley LH, Mason JW, Hogan RP *et al.* Multiple hormonal responses to graded exercise in relation to physical training. *J Appl Physiol* 1972; **33:** 602–606.
10. Sylvestre-Gervais L, Nadeau A, Nguyen MH, Tancrede G, Rousseau-Migneron S. Effects of physical training on beta-adrenergic receptors in rat myocardial tissue. *Cardiovasc Res* 1982; **16:** 530–533.
11. Butler J, O'Brien M, O'Malley K, Kelly JG. Relationship of beta-adrenoreceptor density to fitness in athletes. *Nature* 1982; **298:** 60–62.
12. Butler J, Kelly JG, O'Malley K, Pidgeon F. Beta-adrenoreceptor adaptation to acute exercise. *J Physiol* 1983; **344:** 113–117.
13. Sieurat PP, Roquebrune JP, Grinneiser D *et al.* Monitoring and rehabilitation of heterotopic cardiac transplantation patients during the period of convalescence. *Arch Mal Coeur* 1986; **79:** 210–216.
14. Kavanagh T, Yacoub MH, Mertens DJ, Campbell RB, Sawyer P. Exercise rehabilitation after heterotopic cardiac transplantation. *J Cardiopulmonary Rehab* 1989; **9:** 303–310.
15. Billingham ME. Cardiac transplant atherosclerosis. *Transplant Proc* (Suppl. 5) 1987; **19:** 19–25.
16. Gao SZ, Schroeder JS, Hunt S, Stinson EB. Retransplantation for severe accelerated coronary artery disease in heart transplant recipients. *Am J Cardiol* 1988; **62:** 876–881.
17. Kuo PC, Kirshenbaum JM, Gordon J *et al.* Lovastatin therapy for hypercholesterolemia in cardiac transplant recipients. *Am J Cardiol* 1989; **64:** 631–635.
18. Buxton M, Acheson R, Caine N, Gibson S, O'Brien B. *Costs and Benefits of the Heart Transplant Programmes at Harefield and Papworth Hospitals.* HMSO: London, 1985, pp. 91–106.
19. Mai FM, McKenzie FN, Kostuk WJ. Psychiatric aspects of heart transplantation: Preoperative evaluation and postoperative sequelae. *Br Med J* 1986; **292:** 311–313.
20. Jones BM, Chang VP, Esmore D *et al.* Psychological adjustment after cardiac transplantation. *Med J Aust* 1988; **149:** 118–122.
21. Kavanagh T. The effect of exercise training on mood state following heart transplantation. In: *Proceedings of the Vth World Congress of Cardiac Rehabilitation*, Bordeaux, France, 5–8 July, 1992 (Abstract no. 1146).
22. Harvison A, Jones BM, McBride M *et al.* Rehabilitation after heart transplantation: The Australian experience. *J Heart Transplant* 1988; **7:** 337–341.
23. Kavanagh T, Yacoub M, Tuck JA. Receptiveness and compliance of cardiac transplant patients to an exercise rehabilitation program. *Circulation* (Suppl. II, abstr.) 1986; **74:** 10.

IX Home and Community-based Cardiac Rehabilitation

34 Community-Based Cardiac Rehabilitation Programmes : A View for the 1990s

Kathy Berra

Stanford Center for Research in Disease Prevention, Stanford University, 730 Welch Road, Palo Alto, CA 94304, USA

Introduction

Community-based cardiac rehabilitation programmes are designed to provide long-term exercise training and risk factor intervention specifically aimed at decreasing morbidity and mortality and enhancing the quality of life for the coronary patient. This paper will present a look into the future for cardiac rehabilitation programmes. By utilizing the community-based model, which maximizes staff-to-patient ratios, provides access to rehabilitation interventions long-term and offers cost-effective interventions, a significant impact can be made in the management of coronary disease and other chronic disease states. The programme design for the twenty-first century should be directed at diverse patient populations and at the important task of decreasing morbidity and mortality due to chronic disease.

Dr Howard Rusk [1] defined the rehabilitation continuum and the importance of our rehabilitative efforts:

> Rehabilitation is not just splints, crutch-walking, and the like. It has to meet the total needs of the individual. Those needs are physical, emotional, social and vocational, and any time you miss a cog in the link, then your morbidity goes up, and also your mortality – not the mortality of death, but the mortality of something that is sometimes more than death – the mortality of living a life of indignity, of dependence and depression.

Proceedings of the Vth World Congress on Cardiac Rehabilitation

In designing community-based programmes, it is important to ask, "Why should community organizations offer rehabilitative services?" There are three major issues which compel community organizations to commit to the rehabilitative process. These include:

1. An interest in seeking ways to impact morbidity and mortality for preventable health problems. This interest includes both primary and secondary prevention.
2. An interest in ways to impact dollars spent on rehabilitation from both acute and chronic illnesses or accidents.
3. An interest in finding ways to improve the quality of life for individuals suffering from chronic diseases or injuries.

Along with these compelling medical reasons to provide rehabilitative services, are economic and public health concerns. In 1990, health care costs in the USA included over $1 billion per day spent on health care and health-care related products. Corporate health care insurance premiums in 1959 were about $8 billion per year, and by 1980 had risen to $91 billion per year. In 1970, health care represented 7.4% of the gross national product (GNP) and in the year 2000 it is projected to represent 20%. Between 1979 and 1988 in the USA, death and death rates related to chronic obstructive lung diseases (including bronchitis, emphysema and asthma), nephritis and nephrotic syndrome rose dramatically. Death rates have improved for both cardiovascular disease (CVD) and stroke. However, since 1960, we have seen a tremendous rise in death due to chronic obstructive pulmonary disease (COPD) and chronic renal failure (CRF) [2]. In each of these categories of major disease states, CVD is often associated as the major important co-morbid disease. What we know by assessing these death rates is that in addition to the many thousands of individuals who die each year, equal numbers of individuals are chronically affected and debilitated by these diseases. The age expected death rate for men and women in the USA rose 4 and 5 years respectively between 1959 and 1986. The population living beyond 75 years in the USA rose from $7\frac{1}{2}$ million in 1970 to $12\frac{1}{2}$ million in 1986. Because we are living longer lives, we are at greater risk for the development of chronic disease. This further increases the need for rehabilitative services.

Expanding cardiac rehabilitation services

If we are to continue to offer cardiac rehabilitation services, and especially if we are to expand our services to provide longer-term, more aggressive, more cost-effective services for other chronic disease states, have we shown the model of cardiac rehabilitation to be effective? In a meta analysis of secondary prevention following myocardial infarction, May *et al.* [3] showed a 19% reduction in total mortality for patients randomized to an exercise intervention group compared to controls. No difference in non-fatal reinfarc-

Table 1
Cardiovascular complications of out-patient cardiac rehabilitation programmes

No. of patients	51,303
No. of programmes	167
No. of patient exercise hours	2,351,916
No. of cardiac arrests	21 (1 per 8.9 million hours)
No. of myocardial infarctions	8 (1 per 3.4 million hours)
No. of fatalities	3 (1 per 1.3 million hours)

Reproduced from Van Camp *et al.* [6] with permission.

tion was noted between the groups. In 1988, in a similar meta analysis, Oldridge *et al.* [4] showed a 24% reduction in total mortality and a 25% reduction in cardiovascular mortality in the intervention group compared to the control group. They also found no difference in non-fatal reinfarction. In 1989, O'Connor *et al.* [5] demonstrated similar findings. These trials indicate that morbidity and mortality are significantly impacted by rehabilitative programmes but reinfarction remains unchanged.

What about the safety of cardiac rehabilitation programmes? In 1986, Van Camp *et al.* [6] looked at the safety of patients exercising in cardiac rehabilitation programmes. They found that cardiovascular death occurred only once every 1.3 million man exercise hours. These study findings are shown in Table 1. Despite this proven efficacy and safety, cardiac rehabilitation programmes continue to face many challenges. These challenges include a shrinking reimbursement dollar, shorter hospitalization days, an ageing population with increased incidence of co-morbid diseases and a greater demand for increased revenues to the sponsoring organization. Community-based programmes can help to meet these challenges.

Community-based programmes for the high-risk coronary patient and patients with other chronically debilitating diseases

Dr Nanette Wenger [7] recently described the patient of the 1990s in cardiac rehabilitation programmes. She defined them as patients considered to be moderately complicated, plus patients previously not referred to rehabilitation programmes such as those with: cardiac enlargement; compensated heart failure; implanted pacemakers and cardiovascular/defibrillators; residual myocardial ischaemia and significant arrhythmias; medical complications including the elderly cardiac patient; and patients with multiple complex medical therapies.

Have there been any studies to support the safety and efficacy of cardiac rehabilitation interventions for the more complex coronary patient? The

Table 2
Variables predictive of excess mortality following acute myocardial infarction

1. Ejection fraction less than 0.40 at 1 week following myocardial infarction
2. Ventricular depolarizations of 10 or more per hour.
3. Advanced New York Heart Association Functional Classification (III–IV) prior to infarction
4. Rales in the upper two-thirds of the lung fields at 24–48 h post-infarction

Reproduced from the Multicenter Post-infarction Research Group [8] with permission.

Multicenter Post-Infarction Research Group (MPIP) reported in the *New England Journal of Medicine* certain prognostic indicators which would place a patient at higher risk for a recurrent coronary event [8]. These prognostic indicators are listed on Table 2. Each of these features alone increases the significance of cardiovascular risk. As these indicators occur in combination, the significance of risk multiplies. The MPIP study also found that ejection fraction alone was predictive of significant mortality following myocardial infarction. Van Camp and Peterson [9] reported similar prognostic indicators for the identification of high-risk patients in cardiac rehabilitation programmes (Table 3). Knowing that the more complex cardiovascular patient is at higher risk, do exercise training and cardiac rehabilitation programmes place them at further increased risk? Numerous studies evaluating the safety of exercise for patients with a poor left ventricular ejection fraction (LVEF) have found no increased risk of death in properly evaluated and supervised patients (10–13). As can be seen from Table 4, there was significant improvement in functional capacity by measuring MET equivalents in all patients with poor LVEF. What is important to note is the lack of measureable change in LVEF after training. It appears that a variety of physiological measures, other than changes in LVEF, should be used when evaluating the success of exercise training in the more complex coronary patients. For other disease states, more research is needed in the areas of safety and efficacy.

Table 3
Identification of the high-risk cardiac rehabilitation patient

1. Historical features of importance
   (a) History of CHF, prior cardiac arrest, ventricular tachycardia
2. Clinical features of importance
   (a) Poor exercise capacity (<4,5 min Bruce Protocol)
   (b) ST depression at a heart rate <120 beats/min
   (c) Peak systolic blood pressure <120 mmHg
   (d) Exertional hypotension (>10 mmHg drop in SBP)
   (e) Ventricular tachycardia
3. Cardiac catheterization findings of importance
   (a) LVEF <40%
   (b) Left main and/or triple vessel coronary artery disease

Reproduced from Van Camp and Peterson [9] with permission.

Table 4
Exercise training and safety in high risk coronary patients

Author	No. of patients	Age	Mean resting LVEF (%)	Length of training	No. of deaths in exercise programmes	Changes in functional capacity (METs)	% Change in LVEF after training
Cody *et al.* [10]	32	53 ± 13	18 (10–22)	12 months	0	3.7 ± 1.3 to 7.0 ± 1.8	0
Sullivan *et al.* [11]	12	54 ± 10	24 ± 10	16–24 weeks	0	4.7 ± 1.0 to 5.8 ± 1.6	0
Squires *et al.* [12]	20	53 ± 8.7	20.9 ± 3.1	8 weeks	0	6.5 ± 2.5 to 8.9 ± 2.5	0
Conn *et al.* [13]	10	57.5 ± 13.5	<27 (13–26)	2–12.7 months	0	7.0 ± 1.9 to 8.5 ± 2.9	0

Applying the model to complex coronary patients and other patient populations

The components of the cardiac rehabilitation model which can be applied to both complex coronary patients and other patient populations include:

—lifestyle evaluation,
—health education,
—individualized programme design,
—knowledge and skill in dealing with issues of chronic illness,
—a programme design that readily allows for a systematic approach to health care management, and
—a programme design dedicated to the improved quality of life as well as improved physical health status of the participant.

Other benefits include the monitoring of cardiovascular signs and symptoms and the regular evaluation of left ventricular dysfunction, myocardial ischaemia, arrhythmias and functional capacity. The frequent assessment of co-existing metabolic and orthopaedic abnormalities in addition to the evaluation of medication for side-effects can positively influence the lives of these patients. Programmes can also provide assessment of compliance to interventions and measures of quality of life. Through the provision of a group environment for support and motivation, patients are more likely to make those important lifestyle changes necessary for improved health. In rehabilitation programmes, patients can be provided the necessary encouragement to return to appropriate employment and social activities. The patient populations most likely to derive benefit are those described earlier with pulmonary diseases and chronic renal failure. In addition, patients with diabetes, peripheral vascular disease and severe neurological disease states may also benefit from the community based rehabilitation model. Children and young adults with functionally limiting diseases should also be considered as potential participants.

If this is our challenge, how are we meeting it in cardiovascular rehabilitation programmes? A survey was recently made of programmes registered with the American Association of Cardiovascular and Pulmonary Rehabilitation. The survey was designed to help determine the kinds of patient populations being served and the types of services being offered. The results of the survey showed that 96% of those responding did not incorporate support or group counselling for either patient or spouse. Also, 71% did not offer pulmonary rehabilitation, 98% did not offer rehabilitation for peripheral vascular disease, and patients with end-stage renal disease were not included as a patient population at all. There is obviously a lot of work to do in order to further develop rehabilitative efforts in the long-term care of chronic diseases.

Guidelines in the management of diverse patient populations

Guidelines and techniques for patients who are considered to be at higher risk should include slower, more progressive and more frequent bouts of exercise. In the coronary patient, prophylactic use of nitrates prior to the exercise session might be considered. The timing of the exercise session should be designed to co-ordinate with medications in order to positively influence responses to exercise. Supportive exercise such as bicycle ergometers and water-based exercises should be considered for these patients. Frequent positive physiological feedback and the setting of small achievable goals will help to ensure a greater sense of accomplishment.

Evaluation of the efficacy of rehabilitation in more complex patients

Recurrent myocardial infarction, and changes in anginal patterns, may not be the most important outcome measures for these more complex patient populations. Measures of quality of life may be as important in this patient population as hard medical outcomes are for less complex patients. The assessment of the quality of life must be incorporated into all rehabilitative efforts. Quality of life and the measurement of treatment success from the medical perspective often includes questions such as: Have we cured or regressed the disease? Have our interventions caused any serious physiological side-effects? From the patient's perspective, questions related to treatment success are more likely to be: Do I feel better? Can I return to work? Can I resume my usual lifestyle? Am I having unpleasant side-effects from the treatments? Outcome measures in clinical trials as well as in rehabilitative programmes must address quality of life as well as morbidity and mortality issues. The assessment of physical functioning, activities of daily living, stress and behavioural variables such as social support, anxiety, anger and hostility, depression, social functioning and physical functioning should have equal importance in the measurement of the "true value" of the rehabilitation programme.

Prospective studies need to further define the impact of cardiopulmonary rehabilitation programmes on the quality of life, return to work, cost of health care delivery and disability. We must look into cooperative ventures in maximizing the efficiency of our programmes and reaching out to other chronic disease states. We must look into the provision of lower-cost, longer-term management and supervision of participants in rehabilitation programmes. We must assume a more aggressive stance in the management of risk factors for all chronic diseases.

References

1. White PD, Rusk, HA, Lee PR, Williams B. *Rehabilitation of the Cardiovascular Patient.* Blakiston Division: New York, 1958.
2. US Public Health Service, National Center for Health Statistics. United States Health Department 1990; **91:** 1232.
3. May GS, Eberlein KA, Furberg CD, Passamani ER, DeMets DL. Secondary prevention after myocardial infarction: A view of long term trials. *Prog Cardiovasc Dis* 1982; **24:** 331–352.
4. Oldridge N, Guyatt G, Fisher M, Rimm A. Cardiac rehabilitation after myocardial infarction: Combined experience of randomized clinical trials. *JAMA* 1988: **260:** 945–950.
5. O'Connor GT, Buring JE, Yusuf S, Goldhaber SZ, Olmstead EM, Paffenbarger RS, Hennekens CH. An overview of randomized trials of rehabilitation with exercise after myocardial infarction. *Circulation* 1989; **80:** 234–244.
6. Van Camp SP, Peterson RA. Cardiovascular complications of outpatient cardiac rehabilitation programmes. *JAMA* 1986; **256:** 1160–1163.
7. Wenger NK. Rehabilitation of the coronary patient: A preview of tomorrow. *J Cardiopulmonary Rehab* 1991; **11:** 93–98.
8. Multicenter Post-infarction Research Group. Risk stratification and survival after myocardial infarction. *N Engl J Med* 1983; **309:** 331–336.
9. Van Camp SP, Peterson RA. Identification of the high risk cardiac rehabilitation patient. *J Cardiopulmonary Rehab* 1989; **9:** 103–107.
10. Cody DV, Denniss AR, Ross DA. Early exercise testing, physical training and mortality in patients with severe left ventricular dysfunction. *J Am Coll Cardiol (Suppl. 1.)* 1983; **2:** 178.
11. Sullivan MJ, Higginbothom MB, Cobb FR. Exercise training in patients with severe left ventricular dysfunction: Hemodynamic and metabolic effects. *Circulation* 1988; **78:** 506–515.
12. Squires RW, Lavie CJ, Brandt TR, Gau GT, Bailey KR. Cardiac rehabilitation in patients with severe ischemic left ventricular dysfunction. *Mayo Clin Proc* 1987; **62:** 997–1002
13. Conn EH, Williams RS, Wallace AG. Exercise responses before and after physical conditioning in patients with severely depressed left ventricular dysfunction. *Am J Cardiol* 1982; **49:** 296–300.

35 Patient and Family Education in Advanced Cardiovascular Disease

Erika Sivarajan Froelicher

Department of Physiological Nursing, School of Nursing and Department of Epidemiology and Biostatistics, School of Medicine, University of California, San Francisco, CA 94143-0610, USA

Introduction

Patients with cardiovascular disease can learn to manage their illness and prevent further progression or even possibly reverse their atherosclerosis through techniques about lifestyle changes that health professionals teach them. How best to teach these health management techniques to patients has been the focus of numerous research studies [1–34] and reviews [4, 8, 12]. This paper summarizes and critiques the literature on this topic, looks at the implications for clinical practice, and recommends areas for research that can improve the efficacy of patient and family education.

Literature review

This review describes the studies by (1) patient population (age, gender, and type of populations studied), (2) setting in which the studies were conducted, (3) education provider and (4) study design. It examines the types of intervention techniques, outcome, follow-up and analytical approaches. It concludes by describing the flaws and limitations of the studies; it also provides implications for educational programmes in out-patient settings, discusses threats to adherence, use of group and makes recommendations for future research. Few studies addressed "advanced" cardiovascular disease; however, the principles of patient

Proceedings of the Vth World Congress on Cardiac Rehabilitation

education that apply to cardiovascular disease for purposes of secondary prevention and rehabilitation can reasonably be applied to advanced illness when they are modified to allow for more serious conditions.

Patient populations

Age

For the most part, the studies were limited to adults. The average age was the mid-50s, ranging from the 30s to the 60s. Information on patients 70 and older is limited, yet this group is the largest population in clinical practice [10, 13]. Also, advanced age may bring sensory (vision and hearing) and memory problems that require special teaching techniques, and these have not been analysed. Little information is available on very young cardiac patients, since they are a small number.

Gender

Most studies looked at men. They provide the greatest variety and detail about educational programmes. Few studies have included women [7, 21, 29]. Studies that include women only in their sample are now under way, but the results are not yet available.

Studies combining male and female subjects suffer from three problems. First, the population of male and female subjects is in the ratio 5:1, yielding an unbalanced sample size that is inadequate for statistical analysis. Secondly, most of the studies combine the results of the male and female subjects, and obscure differences in the distributions of important variables (study variables, confounders and effect modifiers) and any differences in the outcomes under study. Thirdly, the important question of whether the same approaches and techniques in patient education and counselling are effective for both men and women remains unanswered. Understandably, given the age restrictions of many studies, males have been targeted for study because more men are available for study at an earlier age than women. The available sample size is more rapidly accrued than when women also are included. However, combining both men and women may be inadequate to answer research questions for either gender. Similarly, much needs to be learned about ethnic differences.

Populations

The majority of these studies (between 80–90%) were conducted on patients after a myocardial infarction. This group is a major target of cardiac patient education because the inception of coronary care units in the 1960s created a large number of captive audiences to provide answers to research questions. Early studies were done at these units to determine the ideal content for an education programme. Patients who underwent coronary artery bypass graft

(CABG) surgery were the second most frequently studied population. A few studies look at patients who have received percutaneous transluminal coronary angiography (PTCA). In the last 10 years or so, a few studies were done on patient education in the cardiac transplant and valve surgery population. For these patients, the need for effective education is very important, especially if life-long anti-coagulation therapy is prescribed. However, many studies have mixed patient populations, and usually do not give individual sub-group results. Differences in educational needs and outcomes depend on cardiovascular disease classification, and perceived patient needs cannot be deciphered. The literature lacks definitive studies that address patient education for those with advanced heart disease, such as congestive heart failure, those awaiting cardiac transplant surgery or those ineligible for cardiac transplant surgery. Another population that has been overlooked consists of patients with risk factors, but without a major cardiac diagnosis. We have learned most about them through secondary prevention trials, such as the exercise fitness programmes and the lipid research trials. A committee of the AACVPR with Nancy Houston Miller and co-workers [12] summarized these studies. The educational strategies for these patients are important, but are often not fully delineated in the reports on the efficacy of education and counselling.

Setting

For the most part, the early patient education studies were based on in-hospital educational programmes [22]. A summary of such studies on educational programmes in hospital and on an out-patient basis was done [7, 8, 12, 17–19, 21, 26, 27, 29]. Educational programmes in the out-patient setting are fewer and not well-delineated. Rehabilitation settings, where the out-patient rehabilitation phase includes an educational programme, are another source of interest. The home is another setting where education [17, 28, 29] is delivered either via telephone or visits by public health nurses and/or physicians, a model more common in the UK. A combination of these approaches, for example, weekly out-patient clinic appointments together with telephone follow-up, are becoming more common [17, 21, 29]. The visiting nurse service educational programmes have not been used in the USA as fully as they might be, and as they are likely to in the future, especially as our population ages.

Education providers

Most education is provided by physicians, nurses and nutritionists, and less frequently by physical therapists, occupational therapists, psychologists, psychiatrists and medical social workers. For out-patient and non-diseased populations, exercise physiologists have played a greater role in providing health education pertaining to exercise principles and practices. The physician's role as educator tends towards diagnosis and prognosis. But since the physician is the health professional that patients have the longest relationship with, physicians must bear responsibility to direct their patients towards risk factor reduction. This is particularly important for stopping smoking, controlling hypercholesterolaemia, lowering blood pressure and engaging in a regular physical fitness programme. Nurses, by far, are the most common health education providers because of their knowledge in physiology, pathophysiology, medical treatment, adjustment to illness and expected outcomes. They are the most suitable professionals to provide the majority of the health education information. In most of the literature reviewed, nurses have conducted the research studies as well.

Study design

Most study designs are descriptive and cross-sectional. They do not permit a cause-and-effect relationship to be inferred. Descriptive studies were helpful in the early phases of studying this research question in order to establish acceptance, feasibility, obtain approximations for effect size measures and identify what the major issues of concern are; however, at this point, another descriptive study is unlikely to add significantly to our knowledge base. The time has come to have better designed experimental research studies to answer specific and pertinent questions about patient education and counselling.

Interventions

Interventions have been based on educational models and effectiveness of the educational messages [2, 16, 19, 24]. Some research studies have used counselling together with education as an important intervention strategy. Here, the principles of counselling [35], education and behavioural psychology are important for effective counselling. Most of the studies were unable to separate the disciplines and use elements of all three in patient education. In recent years, a new field of behavioural medicine [3] and nursing, using behavioural interventions, has flourished. Education alone does not cause behaviour changes but has been shown to reduce anxiety and alleviate depression [4, 8, 12]; and therefore, behavioural interventions with specific approaches using social learning theory are advocated [19, 32–33]. A combination of education, counselling and behavioural intervention strategies seems to be the most effective in promoting health, reducing risk and altering lifestyle [17–19].

The unit of intervention was the patient, the couple (such as the patient and spouse or partner) [5, 11, 32], and groups of patients [19, 20, 28, 29]. The intervention frequently covered issues derived from other studies: smoking cessation and relapse prevention [23, 33]; ambulation and activity progression [17, 27]; energy conservation (particularly important in individuals with advanced heart disease) [27]; exercise prescription [15, 17, 31]; resumption of sexual activity; and return to work [29]. Dietary interventions have included management of diet and medication to control hypertension and hyperlipidaemia [19, 28, 29]. Adherence to medication regimens has been extensively studied and reported in the compliance literature [3, 6, 8, 13, 14]. This literature is also important regarding compliance with exercise interventions [13].

Outcome

The outcomes most frequently studied were knowledge acquisition [22], behavioural change, psychological adaptation [22] and compliance. More recently, quality of life and well-being have been the focus of outcome [20, 21]; earlier, the emphasis was on longevity. Economic outcomes to evaluate the cost-effectiveness of different models of patient education and counselling were studied infrequently in the past, but are likely to be included more in future research [1, 18].

Follow-up

Most studies are descriptive. They are done in a cross-sectional manner and have not included follow-up [2]. Other studies included observations spanning days [22] and weeks. They used the pre- and post-test design: a patient is tested, given information and then re-tested to see whether learning and knowledge acquisition occurred. A few studies had 3, 6 and 12 months of follow-up. Lastly, follow-up was arbitrarily selected as occurring in a given month when, ideally, follow-up ought to be viewed as a continuous variable [26, 30].

Analytical approaches

Descriptive approaches were used most often and a few experimental studies exist. Some studies used "correlational statistics" that identified relationships between predictor variables and outcome measures. Some studies about compliance aimed to define whether factors within the individual or the setting predict compliance with a medical regimen or nursing intervention. Survival analysis methods have not been used and seem to offer important analytical advantages yet to be explored in this context.

Major flaws and limitations of the literature

First, a theory to support the educational approaches and study designs is missing. Next, inadequate review of the literature and inadequate synthesis of the literature accounts, in part, for the slow progress in educational research. Sadly enough, even with the availability of computer databases, many studies summarize the review with arbitrary cut-off dates and cite studies less than 10 years old. Important classical work that predates the search time-frame is ignored. Next, inadequate synthesis of the available literature often results in research designs that do not take advantage of previous mistakes or recommendations that were made at the completion of other studies. Problems encountered in previous studies can provide the next researcher with either solutions to the problems or new research questions. Another major flaw is inadequate sample size. Hundreds of studies have, literally, 10 and 15 heterogeneous subjects, which prevents any conclusions from being made. Another flaw, mentioned earlier, is the descriptive nature of the studies. They use limited analytical approaches [4, 8]. Measurement errors that have not been adequately accommodated to minimize bias appear as flaws in many studies [25, 30]. Biases that occur due to naive study designs could be minimized. Over-interpretation, applying the study results beyond the study design, is also a flaw. Another flaw or limitation results from the multi-disciplinary approach. It offers the expertise of a variety of specialists that can produce a more enlightened, comprehensive approach to the research question; the disadvantage is that it takes a lot of time for professionals from different disciplines to work together effectively and to use the unique aspect of their discipline to guide the study design and implementation of interventions. Very often, the synergy is not created by the time funding begins, and results in ill-conceived questions, methods and analysis.

Implications for practice

Out-patient educational programmes

Studies demonstrate that in-hospital education does not cause lasting behaviour change [4, 8, 12]. This point cannot be emphasized enough because, despite hundreds of studies that demonstrate it, major efforts continue towards in-hospital education.

In-hospital teaching should be limited to the immediate needs of the patient and family [22] such as smoking cessation and relapse prevention for patients who smoke [33]. As amply documented, patients retain little of the information delivered during the hospital stay. Risk factor reduction should be introduced after hospital discharge when patients begin to deal with the realities of lifestyle changes at home, work and leisure [19, 21, 28, 29]. Education needs to be reinforced through printed materials. Even patients who cannot participate in an on-site programme can be counselled via the telephone [13, 17, 28, 29].

Considerable effort has been made to study the use of groups as an educational modality and were shown to be therapeutic by providing emotional support [5, 21, 29, 35]. Patients recognize that others have a similar problem, which alleviates their isolation. They learn from others, which increases their knowledge and sense of kinship within the group. They teach others, which increases their self-esteem. The group provides a safe place where patients can vent concerns that they earlier considered frightening or inappropriate. Early concerns that group meetings might harm cardiac patients were dispelled by researchers [2]. For more details on groups, the reader is referred to the reference list [21, 29, 35].

Outcomes

While education and learning are necessary, they do not cause behavioural change. Behavioural interventions are also necessary to achieve lifestyle change [3, 6]. Not only mortality, but quality of life and well-being are important outcomes of patient education, whereas formerly duration of life was the key focus of medical or nursing intervention [20, 21]. Lastly, compliance needs to be an important factor in any outcome study of patient education about risk factor reduction [6]. Often, the question is raised about study designs in randomized trials that insist on an analysis according to "intention to treat". The argument is that this simply is unreasonable. The public health argument would be that if a patient does not comply with an intervention, the intervention has no value. Therefore, the intervention and the public health acceptance are issues that are evaluated jointly, and intention to treat methods of analysis continue to be the standard of scientific research. Moreover, the randomized trial design theoretically allows for control of known and unknown confounders between the control and treatment group(s).

Threats to adherence

Hundreds of studies have aimed to identify predictors of non-adherence, but none is substantiated with high reliability. Only a few clues have emerged from numerous studies. Patients with erratic or irregular schedules are less compliant. Psychological distress of patients or family and the presence of other risk factors were shown to affect compliance [6]. The patient can be overwhelmed by the number of changes needed and become discouraged even from the beginning [34]. Overweight adults who were overweight as children tend to have a greater problem with adherence. Lack of social support has shown repeatedly to be an important factor in compliance. Recurrent health problems often cause the health care team to delay the lifestyle changes. The delay becomes a negative incentive for the patient. Other factors identified include blue-collar occupation, external locus of control and lack of reinforcement. Threats to adherence from the provider include social sabotage, unmet expectations, lack of skill to manage the situation, lack of feedback and lack of follow-up [6].

Use of groups

In addition to traditional patient (and patient and spouse/partner [11, 24]) educational approaches [16], several investigators have advocated and studied patient and spouse/partner groups in education and counselling programmes [2, 5, 18, 19, 21, 28]. While promising results have been documented, one-on-one, group and patient and spouse/partner have not been compared systematically. A study would reveal the most effective strategy for each education unit and the differences among them [1, 18, 21]. Further reading on group education counselling can be found elsewhere [28, 34, 35].

Recommendations for future research

Quantitative methodology that answers key questions is mandatory. The time for small-sample descriptive studies is over. Areas that demand research include:

—Most effective education methods: individual or group, in person or via telephone.
—Differences in response to education by gender, patient population, level of formal education, socio-economic standing.
—Most effective intervention by type of modification such as smoking cessation or diet modification.
—Best follow-up timetable for evaluating compliance.
—Age as a proxy variable and its effect on learning.
—Sensory (vision and hearing) and memory problems, especially in the aged, and their effects on learning.
—Analysis of interventions: measuring the behaviour that needs changing, defining the intervention, and designing a study to measure the intervention.
—Cost–benefit analysis of feasible and effective interventions.

These are just a few topics that warrant study. The field is rich and begs our analysis so that we may better serve those who come to us for answers and cure.

References

1. Ades PA, Huang D, Weaver SO. Cardiac rehabilitation participation predicts lower rehospitalization costs. *Am Heart J* 1992; **123:** 916–920.
2. Bilodeau CB, Hackett TP. Issues raised in a group setting by patients recovering from myocardial infarction. *Am J Psych* 1971; **128:** 105–110.
3. Blumenthall JA, Cliff R, Williams RS *et al.* A new frontier for behavioral medicine. *J Cardiac Rehab* 1983; **3:** 627–656.
4. Cowan MJ. Cardiovascular nursing research. *Ann Rev Nurs Res* 1990; **8:** 3–33.
5. Dracup K. A controlled trial of couples group counseling in cardiac rehabilitation. *J Cardiopulmonary Rehab* 1985; **5**: 436–442.
6. Dunbar JM, Marshall CD, Novell MF. Behavioral strategies for improving compliance. In Haynes RB, Taylor DW, Sachett DL (eds), *Compliance in Health Care.* John Hopkins Press: Baltimore, MD, 1979.
7. Foley JL, Sivarajan ES, Woods NF. Differences between men and women in recovery from myocardial infarction. *Circulation* (Suppl. III) 1983; **68:** 124.
8. Godin G. The effectiveness of interventions in modifying behavioral risk factors of individuals with coronary heart disease. *J Cardiopulmonary Rehab* 1989; **9:** 923–930.
9. Graham LE, Taylor CB, Hovell MF, Siegel W. Five-year follow-up to a behavioral weight loss program. *J Consult Clin Psychol* 1983; **51:** 322–323.
10. Hawe P, Higgins G. Can medication education improve the drug compliance of the elderly? Evaluation of an in-hospital program. *Patient Education Counsel* 1990; **16:** 151–160.

11. Hentinen M. Need for instruction and support of wives of patients with myocardial infarction. *J Adv Nurs* 1983; **8:** 579–524.
12. Houston-Miller N, Taylor B, Davidson DM, Hill MN, Krantz DS. The efficacy of risk factor intervention and psychosocial aspects of cardiac rehabilitation. *J Cardiopulmonary Rehab* 1990; **10:** 198–209.
13. King AC, Haskell WL, Taylor CB, Draemer HC, DeBusk RF. Group- versus home-based exercise training in healthy older men and women. *JAMA* 1991; **266:** 1535–1542.
14. Kinney MR, Packa DR. Nursing research in cardiovascular risk reduction. *Cardiovasc Nurs* 1988; **24:** 31–55 (whole issue).
15. Lindskog BD, Sivarajan ES. A method of evaluation of activity and exercise in a controlled study of early cardiac rehabilitation. *Cardiac Rehab* 1982; **2:** 156–165.
16. Miller A. When is the time ripe for teaching? *Am J Nurs* 1985; **85:** 801–804.
17. Miller NH, Haskell WL, Berra K, DeBusk RF. Home versus group exercise training for increasing functional capacity after myocardial infarction. *Circulation* 1984; **70:** 645–649.
18. Newton KM, Sivarajan ES, Bruce RA, Mansfield LW. Cost of hospitalization and loss of income following myocardial infarction. *Circulation* (Suppl. IV) 1981; **64:** 187.
19. Newton KM, Sivarajan ES, Clarke JL. Patient perceptions of risk factor changes and cardiac rehabilitation outcomes after myocardial infarction. *J Cardiac Rehab* 1985; **5:** 159–168.
20. Oldridge N, Guyatt G, Jones N, Crowe J, Singer J, Feeny D, McKelvie R, Runions J, Streiner D, Torrance G. Effects on quality of life with comprehensive rehabilitation after acute myocardial infarction. *Am J Cardiol* 1991; **67:** 1084–1089.
21. Ott CR, Sivarajan ES, Newton KM, Almes MJ, Bruce RA. A randomized study of early cardiac rehabilitation: The sickness impact profile as an assessment tool. *Heart Lung* 1983; **12:** 162–170.
22. Scalzi C, Burke L, Greenland S. Evaluation of inpatient educational program for coronary patients and families. *Heart Lung* 1980; **91:** 846–853.
23. Sallis JF, Flora JA, Fortmann SP, Taylor CB, Maccoby N. Mediated smoking cessation programs in the Stanford Five-City Project. *Addictive Behav* 198l; **10:** 441–443.
24. Sikowski JM. Knowledge, concerns and questions of wives of convalescent coronary artery bypass graft surgery patients. *J Cardiac Rehab* 1985; **5:** 74–85.
25. Sivarajan Froelicher ES. Nursing research in cardiovascular risk reduction: Understanding and reducing measurement error. *Cardiovasc Nurs* 1988; **24:** 48.
26. Sivarajan Froelicher ES. Ten-year prognostic value of clinical and exercise test variables in patients after myocardial infarction. Doctoral dissertation, University of California, Los Angeles, 1989.
27. Sivarajan ES, Bruce RA, Almes MJ, Green B, Belanger L, Newton KM, Mansfield LW. In-hospital exercise after myocardial infarction did not improve treadmill performance. *N Engl J Med* 1981; **305:** 357–362.
28. Sivarajan ES, Newton KM. Symposium on cardiac rehabilitation: Exercise, education and counseling for patients with coronary artery disease. *Clin Sports Med* 1984; **3:** 349–369.
29. Sivarajan ES, Newton KM, Almes MJ, Kempf TM, Mansfield LW, Bruce RA. Limited effects of out-patient teaching and counseling after myocardial infarction: A controlled study. *Heart Lung* 1983; **12:** 65–73.
30. Sivarajan Froelicher E, Perdue ST. Clinical, epidemiological, and statistical methods used in prognostic studies of survival after myocardial infarction. *J Cardiopulmonary Rehab* 1991; **10:** 16–22.
31. Sivarajan ES, Valiqette Snydsman A, Smith B, Irving JB, Mansfield LW, Bruce RA. Low-level treadmill testing of 41 patients with acute myocardial infarction prior to discharge from hospital. *Heart Lung* 1977; **6:** 975–988.

32. Taylor CB, Bandura A, Ewart CK, Miller NH, DeBusk RF. Exercise testing to enhance wives' confidence in their husbands' cardiac capability soon after clinically uncomplicated myocardial infarction. *Am J Cardiol* 1985; **55:** 635–638.
33. Taylor CB, Houston-Miller N, Haskell WL, DeBusk RF. Smoking cessation after acute myocardial infarction: The effects of exercise training. *Addictive Behav* 1988; **13:** 1–5.
34. Underhill SL, Woods SL, Sivarajan Froelicher ES, Halpenny CJ. *Cardiac Nursing*, 2nd edn. J.B. Lippincott: Philadelphia, 1989.
35. Yalom ID. *The Theory and Practice of Group Psychotherapy*, 2nd edn. Basic Books: New York, 1975.

36 Assessment of Quality of Life in Myocardial Infarction Patients

J. A. Velasco,* M. V. del Barrio, M. V. Mestre, C. Penas, F. Ridocci

Cardiac Rehabilitation Unit, University General Hospital, GV Marqués del Turia 7, 46005 Valencia, Spain

Introduction

In the developing world, the number of patients surviving a myocardial infarction (MI) has increased, as has the number of chronic cardiac patients. The American Heart Association has reported that many MI survivors and chronic patients have significant physical, psychological and social disabilities. Some recent medical interventions, such as thrombolysis, the use of beta-blockers and Aspirine, have increased the chances of survival of post-acute MI patients [1–3]. On the other hand, increasing numbers of patients with chronic heart disease, in particular congestive heart failure, now survive longer than they did a few years ago. Angiotensin-converting enzyme (ACE) inhibitors and other vasodilator drugs have been found to reduce mortality and prolong survival.

Our main task should be to prolong and improve the quality of life (QL) of patients surviving MI. Prolonging survival when there are increased occurrences of severe cardiac events (acute heart failure, reinfarction, unstable angina) and hospitalizations may not be worthwhile. As these patients become older and more isolated, and as their condition deteriorates, they become more depressed and may even contemplate suicide. However, there are

* To whom all correspondence should be addressed.

Proceedings of the Vth World Congress on Cardiac Rehabilitation

circumstances which can improve the quality of life for these patients: a reduced number of cardiac events and hospitalizations, the support of one's family, increased physical activity, etc. All of these improve the psychological stability of the patients, and increase their self-esteem and self-confidence. Measuring quality of life after interventions such as cardiac rehabilitation is therefore important.

In clinical trials, cardiovascular diseases are graded according to the severity of the symptoms, whereas quality of life is not systematically evaluated. Aspects of well-being, such as one's physical, emotional and social status, are important for assessing one's quality of life. Quality of life has been defined as "the sum of satisfactions that make life worthwhile" and as "The individual's ability to function and derive satisfaction from a variety of roles on his/her daily life".

The use of comprehensive questionnaires, having developed in the social and behavioral sciences, has now spilled over into medicine and more recently cardiology. A wide variety of instruments is available: the Sickness Impact Profile (SIP [4]), the McMaster Health Index Questionnaire [5], the Nottingham Health Profile [6] and the Quality of Well-being Scale [7]. Some of these have been administered to cardiac patients, usually after myocardial infarction. However, questionnaires specifically developed for cardiac and MI patients are lacking. Such a questionnaire would have to take into account the type of cardiovascular disease under consideration. The first such questionnaire was recently developed and validated by Oldridge and co-workers [8]; we have also developed and validated a quality of life questionnaire (QLQ) for MI patients in Spain.

Measurement of quality of life

Quality of life has three major components: functional capacity, perceptions and symptoms. Under these three headings we can list the following:

1. *Functional capacity:* activities of daily life, job satisfaction, family interactions, sexual activity, social function, intellectual function, emotional function, economic status, mobility, independence, self-care, sleep and rest, occupational and recreational activities, etc.
2. *Perceptions of:* health status, well-being, satisfaction, communication, mood changes, anxiety, anger, depression, helplessness, concerns for the future, etc.
3. *Symptoms:* dyspnoea, fatigue, pain, recurrent cardiac events, recurrent hospitalizations, amount and types of medication, side-effects of medication, etc.

Of the questionnaires previously cited, we find the SIP, as developed by Bergner and co-workers [4] at the University of Washington in Seattle in 1976, to be the most useful. This questionnaire measures illness-related behavioural dysfunction in 12 areas of living: sleep and rest; household management; eating; work; recreation and pastimes; body care and movement; mobility; ambulation; social interaction; alertness behaviour; communication; and emotional behaviour. The three main areas of the questionnaire are (1) physical, (2) psychosocial and (3) mobility and independence. The only responses required to the questions are "yes" and "no". A score of 24 points indicates the poorest quality of life and a score of 0 the best quality of life. We therefore selected the SIP as the gold standard for validating our own questionnaire. In order to get more accurate measurements, we substituted a 5-point Likert-type scale (e.g. 1 = never, 5 = always) for the yes/no option.

In the early 1980s, Oldridge and co-workers began to develop a questionnaire regarding the quality of life of MI patients, the QLMIQ, derived from the McMaster Health Index Questionnaire. Dr Oldridge kindly informed us in 1986 of his first experiences with the questionnaire before it had been validated.

Steps to develop a questionnaire of quality of life

Oldridge and co-workers first developed an item selection questionnaire based on their own experiences of treating MI patients, which they administered to 100 patients so as to select the most appropriate items. The item selection was based on the patients' responses to their illness in three different areas: physical, emotional and social. The patients were then asked whether any of the items they had not mentioned represented a particular problem for them. Finally, they were asked to rate each item on a 5-point scale (5 = extremely important, 1 = not at all important). The authors were then able to select those items with the highest scores, based on their frequency and importance. After the selection procedure, Oldridge *et al.* chose 25 items to be grouped under two main headings: *limitations* and *emotions*. These were further subdivided as follows:

1. Limitations
   - restrictions (4 items)
   - fatigue (5 items)
2. Emotions
   - emotional functions (6 items)
   - self-esteem (6 items)
   - confidence (4 items)

Development of a new Spanish QLQ (Velasco and Del Barrio)

We selected 75 items from the SIP, the QLMIQ [8] and the Index of Well-being [9] and added 10 of our own, selected after our own experience treating MI patients in Spain. We administered the item selection questionnaire to 105 patients who had previously suffered MI. We then selected 44 items with the highest scores. These can be broken down into the following nine categories:

1. *Health* (8 items), e.g. chest pain, fatigue, tiredness, missing smoking, etc.
2. *Sleep and rest* (3 items), e.g. "I can't sleep", "I lie down often", etc.
3. *Emotional behaviour* (3 items), e.g. "I am excited", "I cry without cause", etc.
4. *Concerns for the future* (3 items), e.g. "I think I am going to die soon", "I feel helpless", etc.
5. *Mobility* (5 items), e.g. "I don't like leaving home", "I only walk short distances", etc.
6. *Social interaction* (7 items), e.g. "I go out less now to visit friends", "I like to be alone", "My sex life is not as good as it was", etc.
7. *Alertness behaviour* (3 items), e.g. "My short-term memory is impaired", "I react very slowly", etc.
8. *Communication* (3 items), e.g. "I have to make an effort to maintain conversation", "I do not like using the telephone", etc.
9. *Work and leisure time* (5 items), e.g. "I work less now than I did before", "I do not like my job", etc.

As regards "concerns for the future", we believe that this area may not have been as closely related to that which we wished to measure.

We selected the following 5-point Likert-type scale where 1 = all of the time, 2 = most of the time, 3 = some of the time, 4 = a little of the time and 5 = none of the time. The highest score of 220 would indicate the poorest quality of life; a low score would indicate a good quality of life. Before administering our questionnaire, we modified the response options of the SIP and the QLMIQ so as to facilitate the work of our patients and to unify the results. For each questionnaire, we used a 5-point scale. To validate our questionnaire, we administered it, together with the SIP and the QLMIQ, to a group of 105 post-MI patients following a cardiac rehabilitation programme. We also carried out a re-test of our questionnaire 2 weeks later so as to check its reproducibility.

The validity of our questionnaire was quite good ($r = 0.85$) as was its reproducibility ($r = 0.75$). The reliability of the items was high ($r = 0.90$) as was the relation between the items ($r = 0.81$). An independent study of the reliability of each item showed that eight items were less reliable and, consequently, less related to cardiac disease.

In addition, we studied the quality of life of three groups of MI patients and a control group of normal subjects:

1. *Cardiac rehabilitation (CR) group*: 105 post-MI patients following a cardiac rehabilitation programme of 3 months to 2 years duration.
2. *Coronary Club (CC) group*: 26 post-MI patients following a year-long cardiac rehabilitation programme of 3–8 years duration. (This study was performed by MVdelB at the Coronary Club of Casa de Salud Hospital.)
3. *MI patients (MI) group*: 59 post-MI patients following conventional care by a cardiologist.
4. *Control Group*: 41 healthy subjects.

In order to validate our questionnaire and to compare the results with other questionnaires, we administered it together with the SIP and the QLMIQ to all of our subjects. The questionnaires were administered by a trained interviewer. Using this methodology, we tried to reduce the differences between the patients with a high and low cultural index. The interview lasted approximately 45 min and the interviewer was able to evaluate the reaction of the patients during the administration of the questionnaires.

Results of the Velasco–Del Barrio questionnaire

As shown in Table 1, the MI group following conventional care showed the worst quality of life (113.1) and the control group the best (72.2). Differences between the groups were assessed by ANOVA:

1. MI patients had a significantly poorer quality of life than the other groups (cardiac rehabilitation improved quality of life more than conventional care).
2. There were no differences between the control group and CC group (72.2 *vs* 77.2). That means that a year-long cardiac rehabilitation programme improves quality of life to the level of normal subjects; however, the CC group was a selected group which was able to follow a very long programme.
3. There were no differences in quality of life between the two groups following a rehabilitation programme (CR and CC).

Results of the QLMIQ

As shown in Table 1, the control group had the best quality of life (23.4), followed by the CC and CR groups; the MI patients fared worst (43.9). The results of this questionnaire were almost identical to the Spanish questionnaire. As with our questionnaire, the quality of life of the CC group and the controls was very similar.

Table 1
Results of administration of QLQs to the four groups

Questionnaire	MIG	CR	CC	CG
Velasco and Del Barrio	113.1[a]	88.1	77.2	72.2
QLMIQ	43.9[a]	31.5	25.6	23.4
SIP	68.0[a]	50.7	42.7	37.0

Abbreviations: MIG, post-MI patients receiving conventional care; CR, cardiac rehabilitation group; CC, coronary club group; CG, control group.
[a] $P < 0.05$ *vs* others. A lower score indicates a better quality of life.

Results of the SIP Questionnaire (Table 1)

As with the QLMIQ, the best quality of life was recorded by the control group (37.0) and the worst by the MI group (68.0). There were no significant differences between the CG and CC groups, whereas the quality of life of the MI patients was significantly worse compared to all of the other groups – as we found with the other two questionnaires.

Differences between MI patients and control subjects

We studied these differences using all three questionnaires. We lumped together all three groups of patients under the universal heading MI (MI, CR and CC groups). The results are shown in Table 2. The results of each questionnaire were similar. MI significantly impairs the quality of life compared with control subjects.

Influence of age on quality of life

We studied the influence of age on quality of life by splitting the patients and the controls into two groups: 50 years or younger (group 1) and older than 50 years (group 2). Table 3 shows the results of these analyses performed separately for all patients (MI patients and controls) and for MI patients alone. As Table 3 shows, the quality of life of the subjects age 51 years or more was worse than their younger counterparts. When the controls were excluded (n = 190), the same results were found.

Influence of social class on quality of life

In order to study the influence of social class on quality of life, we divided our subjects into the following social class groupings: high, medium-high, medium, medium-low and low. Table 4 shows the number of subjects in each group; eight subjects were difficult to classify and therefore they were excluded from the analysis. The classification into the five social groupings was carried out according to a code representing jobs and professions [10]. Table 4 shows the

Table 2
Differences in quality of life between MI patients and control subjects

	Spanish Q	SIP	QLMIQ
MI patients[a]	94.6	55.2	34.8
Controls	72.2	37.0	23.4
P	0.0001	0.0001	0.0001

[a] MI, all post-MI patients (MI, CR and CC).
A lower score indicates a better quality of life.

Table 3
Influence of age on measures of quality of life

	Spanish Q	SIP	QLMIQ
MI patients and healthy subjects combined ($n = 231$)			
Group 1	82.0	44.7	28.7
Group 2	96.6	56.8	35.6
P	0.0001	0.0004	0.002
MI patients only ($n = 190$)			
Group 1	86.0	48.0	30.5
Group 2	99.3	59.0	36.8
P	0.001	0.001	0.01

Group 1, ≤50 years old; group 2, >50 years old.

quality of life with respect to social class grouping. A significant difference ($P = 0.001$) was found between high and low social class for all three questionnaires. A significant difference was also found between the high and medium-low classes ($P = 0.05$) with the SIP and the Spanish questionnaire; the same was found between the medium and low social classes. Finally, quality of life is closely related to social position, especially if the subject belongs to a high or low social class. This was independent of whether or not the patient was from any of the MI groups. A high social position denotes a better education, a higher income and improved job possibilities, some of the variables that may explain differences in quality of life.

Conclusions

1. Each of the QLQs used on this study were valid measures of the quality of life of MI patients.

Table 4
Differences in quality of life in relation to social position

Social position	*n*	Spanish Q	SIP	QLMIQ
1. High	33	75.6	40.5	27.3
2. Medium-high	9	92.9	45.9	31.6
3. Medium	34	82.6	46.3	30.0
4. Medium-low	46	91.8	50.1	30.1
5. Low	103	97.2	58.0	36.4
$P = 0.001$		1 *vs* 5	1 *vs* 5	1 *vs* 5
$P = 0.05$		1 *vs* 5, 4	1 *vs* 4	NS
$P = 0.05$		3 *vs* 5	3 *vs* 5	NS

2. The quality of life of MI patients not following a cardiac rehabilitation programme is impaired when compared with patients following such a programme.
3. The selected group of patients who were able to follow the cardiac rehabilitation programme for 3–8 years registered a quality of life that was as good as that of the control subjects.
4. Nevertheless, the quality of life of patients following cardiac rehabilitation programmes was similar, independent of its duration.
5. Social position and age both influence the quality of life of MI patients.

References

1. ISSIS (Second International Study of Infarct Survival) Collaborative Group. Randomized trial of intravenous streptokinase, oral aspirin, both or neither among 17,187 cases of suspected acute myocardial infarction: ISSIS-2. *Lancet* 1988; **2:** 349–360.
2. Yusuf S, Peto R, Lewis J, Collins R, Sleight P. Betablockade during and after myocardial infarction: An overview of the randomized trials. *Prog Cardiovasc Dis* 1985; **27:** 335–371.
3. Acheson J, Archibald D, Barnet H *et al.* Secondary prevention of vascular disease by prolonged antiplatelet treatment: Antiplatelet trialists' collaboration. *Br Med J* 1988; **296:** 320–331.
4. Bergner M, Bobbit RA, Carter WB, Gilson BS. The Sickness Impact Profile: Development and final revision of a health status measure. *Med Care* 1981, **19:** 787–805.
5. Chambers LW, MacDonald LA, Tugwell P, Buchanan WW, Kraag G. The MacMaster Health Index Questionnaire as a measure of the quality of life for patients with rheumatoid disease. *J Rheumatol* 1982, **9:** 780–784.
6. Hunt SM, McKenna SP, McEwen J, Backett EM, Williams J, Papp E. A quantitative approach to perceived health status: A validation study. *J Epidemiol Commun Health* 1980; **34:** 281–286.
7. Bruschte WR, Bush JW, Kaplan RM. Successive intervals analysis of preference measures in a health status index. *Health Services Res* 1975; **10:** 181–198.
8. Oldridge N, Guyatt G, Jones N *et al.* Effects on quality of life with comprehensive rehabilitation after acute myocardial infarction. *Am J Cardiol* 1991; **67:** 1084–1089.
9. Kaplan RM, Bush JW. Health-related quality of life measurement for evaluation research and policy analysis. *Health Psychol* 1982; **1:** 61–80.
10. Hollingshead AB. Two Factors Index of Social Position. Yale Station, New York, Connecticut, 1985.

37 Physical Activity Measurement Through a Semi-structured Interview

H.W.H. Weeda, H. van der Sluys

Department of Cardiology, Building 1/C5-P, University Hospital, PO Box 9600, 2300 RC Leiden, The Netherlands

Introduction

Physical activity is an important element of physical fitness in health and disease. It is defined by Caspersen *et al.* [1] as "any bodily movement produced by skeletal muscles that results in caloric expenditure". In this context, exercise is a sub-category of physical activity which is planned, structured, repetitive and results in improvement or maintenance of one or more facets of physical fitness [2]. Where physical fitness in this study is mentioned, this concept is made concrete by defining it as aerobic power. In itself, physical activity is a rather broad concept, which relates to occupational and leisure time activity, energy expenditure and food consumption, physical fitness, inactivity as a risk factor in coronary heart disease, and functional capacity in cardiopulmonary medicine.

When it is the objective to measure physical activity through a questionnaire in relation to aerobic power, it is obvious that determining total physical activity over a whole workday cannot be the optimal solution. So, van der Sluys [3] measured habitual physical activity during a normal workday by means of an indirect time and motion study. The correlation between the habitual physical activity and the aerobic power [4] appeared to be rather modest ($r = 0.49$). Probably the mixing of all activities, ranging from light to heavy, into a sum total made this method somewhat insensitive to the aerobic power, which depends exclusively on intensive activities.

Proceedings of the Vth World Congress on Cardiac Rehabilitation

Taylor *et al.* [5] went one step further and made a distinction between light, moderate and heavy leisure time physical activity (LTPA) carried out during the previous year. Heavy activity was presumed to require at least 50% aerobic power. The energy expenditure of the various activities was taken from the literature, and the subjects had to indicate on a checklist which activities they had performed during the past year. Then, the individual's activity was characterized by four scores, i.e. one for each of these three intensities and a sum total. In this manner, the heavy activity could be correlated with the workload from a sub-maximal exercise test, at which the heart rate reached 150 beats/min. However, again the correlation was rather modest ($r = 0.52$). This result seems lower than expected, but one has to take into account that there is a substantial inter-individual variation in intensity in performing the standard activities and, furthermore, the rather long time span of 1 year might be another complicating factor.

Morrison *et al.* [6] were especially interested in the more strenuous activities when asking subjects about LTPA during a normal week. Their subjects were assigned to eight activity groups. The subjects in groups 5–8 performed strenuous exercise: group 5 once, group 6 twice, group 7 three times and group 8 four times a week. There appeared to be a significant though rather moderate correlation ($r = 0.61$, $P < 0.001$) between the intensity and frequency of LTPA on the one hand and aerobic power on the other, which was indirectly determined by means of an Åstrand-Rhyming procedure [7].

Bearing in mind the results of the above studies, we developed a LTPA questionnaire, which was based on aerobic training experience and was specifically meant to be more closely related to the aerobic power. The key element of it was the performance of vigorous exercise for at least 20 min, the weekly frequency of this exercise, and the regular performance of it during the last 3 months. Indirect validation of this questionnaire was achieved by comparing the LTPA with the aerobic power of the individual [8].

Subjects and methods

The subjects comprised 327 apparently healthy male industrial employees ranging in age from 17 to 62 years. The maximal oxygen uptake ($\dot{V}O_2$ max) was measured during a graded exercise test on a bicycle ergometer by means of an Oxycon-4 apparatus. Immediately after the exercise test, LTPA was determined through a semi-structured interview. The LTPA activity was for practical purposes defined as any activity outside working hours. Five LTPA classes were constructed. Class 1 consisted of sedentary men. Class 2 included those men who, for example, were carrying out household chores, who were active gardeners, who participated in recreational sports, and who performed vigorous exercise only once a week. We reasoned that vigorous exercise once a week would not be enough to maintain a high aerobic power and classified these subjects as class 2 LTPA, i.e. more than sedentary. Classes 3, 4 and 5

Table 1
LTPA classification

Class	*n*
1	76
2	119
3	64
4	52
5	16

comprised men who performed vigorous exercise for at least 20 min. two, three and four times a week. These groups included soccer players, for example, who played one competitive match and performed aerobic training sessions each week, and men who ran and cycled in a vigorous manner.

Results

The LTPA classification of the 327 men is shown in Table 1. The relation between aerobic power and the LTPA classes is presented in Fig. 1. The correlation between $\dot{V}O_2$ max and LTPA was $r = 0.59$ ($P < 0.001$), and that between $\dot{V}O_2$ max/kg and LTPA was $r = 0.62$ ($P < 0.001$). The relationship between $\dot{V}O_2$ max and the different LTPA classes appeared to be significantly linear [$F(1,322) = 180$, $P < 0.001$]. This is not to say that, as regards the $\dot{V}O_2$ max, there was not a large overlap between the different LTPA classes.

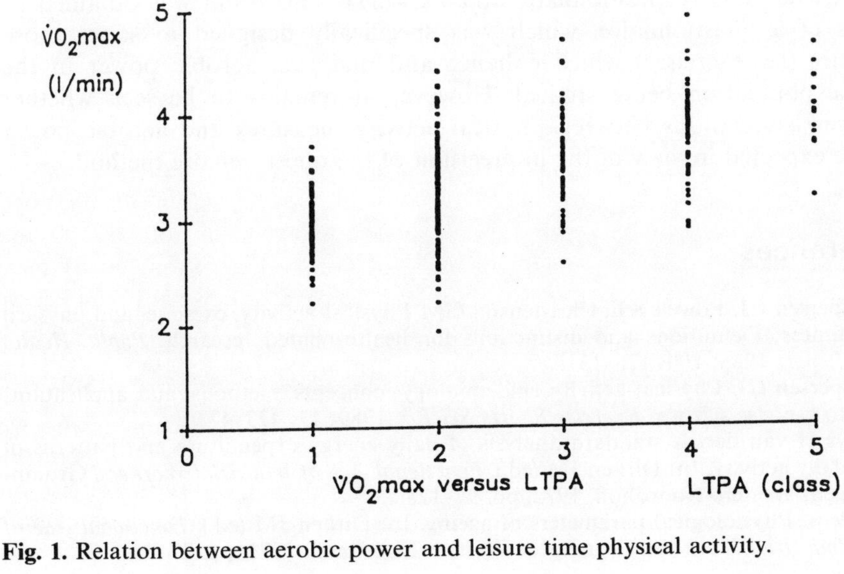

Fig. 1. Relation between aerobic power and leisure time physical activity.

Discussion

These results show that with our LTPA classification, 38% of the variance in $\dot{V}O_2$ max can be explained. This result is better than the 25% reported by van der Sluys [3] and by Taylor *et al.* [5], but not better than that reported by Morrison *et al.* [6]. Furthermore, we made the implicit assumption, as Morrison *et al.* [6] did, that the frequency of vigorous exercise was closely associated with aerobic power. This indeed appeared to be the case, because we found a linear relationship between the different LTPA classes, i.e. the frequency of vigorous exercise and aerobic power. In addition, by selecting both men who participated in competitive sports and men who ran and cycled against the clock, we introduced a certain element of competition in the classification. It might be expected that this element of competition would lead to exercising more closely to the maximum than is the case in less well motivated subjects.

The inherent weakness of the rather imprecise interview method was the estimation of the relative intensity of the physical activity. An expedient could be to inquire after indicator symptoms of intensive exertion. Examples include perceived quality of breathing (i.e. panting and breathlessness) and the ability to finish sentences without any interruption due to breathing ('talk speed'). Furthermore, sweating has been used as an indicator of exercise intensity, although seasonal influences may affect this particular indicator. However, we did not incorporate these indicators in our study.

Conclusion

We obtained a significant though moderate correlation ($r = 0.60$, $P < 0.001$) between our LTPA questionnaire and $\dot{V}O_2$ max. This result was obtained by means of a questionnaire, which was specifically designed to select those activities (i.e. exercises) which enhance and maintain aerobic power in the specific population being studied. However, it remains to be seen whether stronger associations between physical activity measures and aerobic power can be expected in view of the imprecision of the questionnaire method.

References

1. Caspersen CJ, Powell KE, Christenson GM Physical activity, exercise, and physical fitness: Definitions and distinctions for health-related research. *Public Health Report* 1985; **100:** 126–131.
2. Caspersen CJ. Physical activity epidemiology: concepts, methods, and applications to exercise science. *Exercise Sports Sci Rev* 1989; **17:** 423–473.
3. Sluys H van der. A standard analysis of daily energy expenditure and patterns of daily activity. In: Dirken JM (ed.), *Functional Age of Industrial Workers.* Groningen: Wolters-Noordhoff, 1972, pp. 97–128.
4. Bink B. Physiological parameters of ageing. In: Dirken JM (ed.), *Functional Age of Industrial Workers.* Groningen: Wolters-Noordhoff, 1972, pp. 47–65.

5. Taylor HL, Jacobs DR, Schucker B, Knudsen J, Leon AS, DeBacker G. A questionnaire for the assessment of leisure time physical activity. *J Chronic Dis* 1978; **31:** 741–755.
6. Morrison JF, Malsen S van, Noakes TD. Leisure-time physical activity levels, cardiovascular fitness, and coronary risk factors in 1015 white Zimbabweans. *S Afr Med J* 1984; **65:** 250–256.
7. Åstrand PO, Ryhming I. A nomogram for calculation of aeobic capacity (physical fitness) from pulse rate during submaximal work. *J Appl Physiol* 1954; **7:** 971–976.
8. Weeda HWH. Maximal Exercise Tests in 331 Male Employees: Relations to Age and Physical Activity. Leiden: Rijksuniversiteit Leiden, 1989, 151 pp. Dissertation.

38 Computer-assisted Program Management for Cardiac Rehabilitation

Fredric J. Pashkow

Department of Cardiology, Cleveland Clinic Foundation, 9500 Euclid Avenue, Cleveland, OH 44195-5064, USA

Introduction

Up to the present time, most cardiologists have generally encountered microprocessors as an integrated element in some piece of high-technology imaging equipment such as an imaging processor, in bedside monitoring or stress testing systems, as a means of managing fiscal information primarily for insurance and/or billing purposes, in laboratory data-retrieval systems or more rarely, in the context of a teaching system such as an algorithm-driven differential diagnostic system.

As cardiology becomes overloaded with information, the need for clinically derived programmes capable of tracking and organizing large volumes of data has become increasingly important [1, 2]. These information management or database programs start out in the minds of the clinic providers as an electronic but otherwise relatively traditional medical record, but hopefully evolve to provide highly organized, relational, information-management systems. Once available, the programs can interface with the type of software mentioned above, providing a totally different approach to the concept of systems development. Such programs while uncommon are becoming increasingly available [1, 3].

The motivating factor in the development of these programs for cardiac rehabilitation was the large volume of data requiring manipulation and storage, and the frustration and time required to process this information periodically

Proceedings of the Vth World Congress on Cardiac Rehabilitation

for the generation of reports. Cardiac rehabilitation has large informational management requirements. For example, a patient exercising in a rehabilitation program has multiple field data entries at the time of check-in and check-out (blood pressure, weight, pulse, etc.). The patient typically then participates in half a dozen exercises where the time, distance, resistance, pulse rate as well several other pieces of data may be recorded for each exercise activity. Patients usually exercise 12–15 times per month, so the dimensions of the data-tracking problem can be appreciated.

Related directly to the issues of cost containment and efficiency of program operation are patient records' management and staff-to-patient and staff-to-physician communications [4, 5]. The issue is not one of just increased record-keeping efficiency *per se*, but the design and utilization of systems that provide an administrative framework consistent with the highest professional standards and for maximizing the opportunity for positive staff and patient reinforcement, and ideally, encouraging compliance and long-term modification of lifestyle and behaviour. The technical capability to provide such systems at reasonable cost is now at hand [1, 3].

Computerized information ("database") management systems have become more of a reality for cardiac rehabilitation with the development of relatively small, powerful personal computers often referred to as PCs [3]. These computers can be coupled to relatively large (20 Mbyte and up) storage drives to provide systems eminently capable of handling patient records management for even the largest cardiac rehabilitation programs.

The ability to organize, categorize and rapidly retrieve medical and exercise information is the first and most obvious advantage of computerized information management systems. It also provides an opportunity to improve administrative efficiency and increase staff time available for direct patient care by eliminating time-consuming and tedious manual data transfer by staff. Such systems, however, when thoughtfully designed, are able to integrate with other aspects of good patient management, and provide an opportunity for reiterative education, enhanced patient communications, positive reinforcement on incremental progress, leading to improved patient compliance and better long-term outcome [6]. For example, software can be designed to provide feedback to the patient about specific information such as blood pressure, rate-response to exercise, cholesterol levels, etc. and follow progress over time and relate this to the patient's individualized goals.

Designing a computer system for cardiac rehabilitation management

When designing or buying such an information management system, the database software must accommodate all of the essential information, but allow for easy data input. Ideally, the database portion of the program should be accessible even while the computer is "busy" with another task, especially if access to certain patient information at particular times may be medically necessary. The program should operate simply enough so that staff may learn to use it without extensive training and be useable by patients to post at least a portion of their own data. This can provide an opportunity for instant feedback and the enhanced patient communication and positive reinforcement alluded to above.

Conceptually, information management programs for cardiac rehabilitation should consist of three parts. The first part is the actual database portion itself. These files must include baseline specifications, e.g. file listings of the patient demographic information, patient diagnoses, different exercises available, just to name a few. The second part handles individual patient records where information is accumulated, organized, calculated and stored on a continuing basis. The third part is the report function. What program developers have realized is that this third part of the information management system has power beyond mere summary, storage and listing. It allows for a higher level of information utilization, one that can be relational or even discriminatory. This provides the means by which the program can raise program quality, efficiency and productivity, motivate patients and staff, facilitate communication and encourage compliance.

The system should be designed to facilitate the generation of reports, particularly to patients *and* physicians, in such a way that it economizes staff time. Finally, the system should be designed so that records can be periodically archived to provide a coherent audit trail that would satisfy third-party and government quality assurance and utilization reviewers. In short, the software most suitable to fulfil the rehabilitation program's needs is the prime requisite, and the hardware necessary to run it is secondary.

Experience with a database management system

System development

Lesser [2] has pointed out that while the acquisition and maintenance of patient medical records lend themselves extremely well to computerization, there are few, if any, descriptions of successful implementations of computerized medical records in a non-institutional setting.

Since the summer of 1985, we have had experience with such a patient record/data-management system in a community-based rehabilitation setting [4, 5]. The software has evolved extensively over the last 7 years. Two versions of the program were developed, one for Apple Macintosh and another for IBM and IBM-compatible PCs, though the latter is no longer available. The Macintosh version was designed specifically to be patient-interactive and written in compiled Basic. The patient interactive aspect of the program was carefully thought-out, and the appropriate hardware configuration considered in great detail. The desired system specifications included significant "user friendliness", since the patients themselves would interact with the device at each exercise session. O'Leary *et al.* [7] have pointed out that activity that involves a personal computer can be a valuable modality in the rehabilitation of older adults, but access is a key issue. Portability, the type and availability of additional software programs, and cost were also prerequisites. This system configuration using off-the-shelf equipment costs less than $3000 is sufficiently powerful to allow for real-time access by staff to the computer during the time patients are actually exercising, and can provide staff immediate entry to such information as diagnoses, medication allergies and current medications. Whoever enters the data, whether patient or staff, has the option of logging the information as the individual exercise activities are completed, or all at once at the conclusion or after the exercise session.

Macintosh *vs* IBM and IBM-compatible PCs

While each of these PC computers has relative strengths and weaknesses, over the last few years each has become more like the other. The Macintosh high-contrast display screen accommodated the use of oversized type-fonts with black characters on a light background. A "mouse" facilitated the rapid input of data and the integration of the video screen with the central processor allowed it to be mounted on a mobile cart so that it could be moved to wherever the exercise activities took place. The same computer software program could be adapted to accommodate Phase II and Phase IV exercise programs. Patient acceptance of the Macintosh system has been excellent [4].

While the IBM system until recently lacked the patient-interactive qualities of the Macintosh version, it has had certain traditional advantages. Many hospitals and information management people have been committed to IBM-compatible systems. With large numbers of standard business analysis and statistical programs available, the IBM was more suitable for a large institution with programs for highly specialized patient populations such as renal or pulmonary patients, or for those interested in research. The MS-DOS operating software of the IBM systems, however, require much more training than the Macintosh user-interface. The current generation of IBM PCs offers some of the "user-friendly" features of the Macintosh, including pull-down menus, large fonts, etc. However, the IBM-compatible systems still do not provide the low-cost audio and graphics integration capability of the Macintosh.

Experience with the information management system

The software provides an extensive patient database and can produce instantly facsimiles of the patients' demographic data, medications, drug allergies, referring physicians, exercise prescriptions, a daily log listing staff in attendance at each session, and the display of generic group or individual messages at the time of sign-in and sign-out. All relevant medical and exercise data can be collected, collated and summarized for analysis and reporting. When heart rates are out of target range for a prescribed activity, this information is stored in a report that is assembled for the supervising staff member at the end of the session. A hard-copy summary of that session, i.e. who attended, what happened during the session, what messages were communicated to the patients during the sign-in and sign-out process, can all be produced for legal record. The patient population can be relationally summarized or an up-to-date medical/ exercise profile can be generated at any time including during the exercise session itself. Multiple end-of-period reports with graphic displays can be produced providing documentation of performance, compliance and achievement [3].

A review of 5 years' experience indicates that this can be accomplished at about half the cost of manual processing of the data over the same period of time with much less detailed reporting of the information [5]. In addition, manual processing of the information eliminates the opportunity for patient interaction, reinforcement of educational concepts and the fail-safe documentation of occurrences during the exercise sessions. We compared the computer-based management system to the manual method of records maintenance and production of reports over 5 years. The amount of time required to collate data and prepare reports was compared and net financial gain or loss was calculated. The cost of the computer and peripheral hardware was amortized over the 5 years and added to the annual cost of supplies and maintenance (= $600/year) (see Table 1).

Table 1

Financial impact of computerized program management: five years' experience

Year	No. of patients/ month	No. of reports/ year	Hours/year (manual)	Hours/year (computer)	Hours/diff.	Cost diff. ($15/h)	Net ($)
1986	44	528	176	55	121	1815	1215
1987	40	480	160	50	110	1650	1050
1988	41	492	164	51	113	1691	1091
1989	36	432	144	45	99	1485	885
1990	38	456	152	48	105	1568	968

The use of the computer resulted in a net financial gain of $5208.75 over the 5 years. This saving can be significant in a community-based rehabilitation program where lower costs can be passed through to lower patient participation fees. The computer also provides a means of quality assurance, legal documentation, automated calculation of exercise prescriptions, and monitoring of physiological parameters.

Areas of concern related to the use of computers for rehabilitation records

As with any other technology utilized in the rehabilitation or wellness environment, the application of computers will have ethical and legal ramifications [8, 9].

Reliability

This encompasses both the hardware and software aspects as well as the operational routine utilized in the application of the computerized system. The system must be maintainable in an adequate and reasonable time-frame. If vital patient information cannot be accessed on demand due to technical failure, patient safety may be jeopardized.

Privacy and access

With increasing computerization of potentially sensitive personal records, privacy has become a growing issue in recent years. A proper balance must be achieved between confidentiality of patient information and shared access to records by health care personnel [8]. Each individual having access to the computer should be assigned a unique code [10]. Ideally, the computer should be able to recall who has "signed-on" during a given time period. Certain files should be protected from entry by non-professional staff. Programs designed to upload data to mainframe systems for storage or further processing, such as billing or administrative analysis, should not transfer information that may be sensitive.

Archival and back-up

The system should be designed so that data may be appropriately archived and backed-up. Archival copies differ from routine back-ups in that, once generated, the archival copy provides a permanent record and is thereafter not altered. In addition to the obvious reason of records integrity, good archives and back-up can provide excellent documentation for legal and quality assurance purposes [9]. This also can provide a coherent audit trail and should satisfy third-party and government quality assurance and utilization reviewers.

Adequate hardware and a reasonable routine are required for this important task. While streaming-tape back-up is quite popular in industry, back-up with removable large (45–50 Mbyte) disks is less expensive and the devices can see dual service as a hard drive. Floppy disks may actually work well for a rehabilitation program archival in that data from one period, say a month, is easily stored on one diskette. Experts suggest that a different back-up copy be made on two or three successive days and that these back-ups be stored in geographically different locations. Should the previous day's data be lost or proven faulty, no more than one or two days' worth of data entry will need to be reconstructed [1].

"Interactive" and "expert" systems

Up to this point we have discussed mainly computer systems that provide automation and organization of information that essentially improve the traditional written record [2]. The ability of these systems to incorporate formulae for the calculation of exercise prescriptions is included, but even if automated, remains under the direct control of the user [3]. Software now exists that provides medical direction or alters exercise prescriptions on an algorithmic basis. These programs are referred to as "expert systems" and have been achieving increasing attention in many different areas of our society. The identification of who should review the clinical appropriateness of the algorithm and the reliability of the system, similar to issues of efficacy and safety that apply to pharmaceuticals and other medical devices, is quite controversial [8].

Education and motivation

A related future high-technology application that will have an important impact on cardiac rehabilitation programs is in the realm of patient education [11]. Sophisticated audio-visual devices using CD ROM (Compact Disc, Read-Only Memory) optical data discs or laser discs can now be easily integrated with microcomputers at reasonable cost. This technology provides the opportunity for highly dynamic, interactive learning experiences for patients and the expansion of the learning process to include goal-setting with continuous tracking of achievement. It may also provide the individualized reinforcement and motivation needed to accomplish and maintain the desired lifestyle modifications. Again, as with the computerized database systems, it is important to focus on overall program quality and content and not be seduced by the glitter of the hardware. These devices, improperly selected, can squander increasingly scarce funds for rehabilitation and risk-factor education programs [6].

Acknowledgement

I wish to thank Bryce Foens and Peg Pashkow for their tireless efforts that led to the development of the computer software discussed in this paper.

References

1. Shepard RB, Blum RI. Cardiology office computer use: Primer, pointers, pitfalls. *J Am Coll Cardiol* 1986; **8:** 933–940.

2. Lesser MF. Computerized records in clinical cardiology. *J Am Coll Cardiol* 1986; **8:** 941–948.
3. Pashkow FJ. Specialized database systems for cardiology. *Physicians and Computers* 1987; **5:** 32–35.
4. Pashkow F, Schafer M, Pashkow P. HeartWatchers - low cost, community-based cardiac rehabilitation in Loveland, Colorado. *J Cardiopulmonary Rehab* 1986; **6:** 469–473.
5. Pashkow FJ, Pashkow PS, Foens B, Winkelhake K. Computer-assisted program management for cardiac rehabilitation: Five years' experience. In: *Proceedings of the Vth World Congress on Cardiac Rehabilitation.* Bordeaux, 7 July 1992.
6. Wenger NK. Future directions in cardiovascular rehabilitation. *J Cardiopulmonary Rehab* 1987; **7:** 168–174.
7. O'Leary S, Mann C, Perkash I. Access to computers for older adults: Problems and solutions. *Am J Occ Ther* 1991; **45:** 636–642.
8. Miller RA, Schaffner KF, Meisel A. Ethical and legal issues related to the use of computer programs in clinical medicine. *Ann Int Med* 1985; **102:** 529–537.
9. Pashkow FJ. Legal aspects of computer applications in cardiac rehabilitation. *Exer Standards and Malpractice Rep* 1989; **3:** 41–43.
10. White R. Computer security: An introduction for the medical practitioner. *Urol Clin N America* 1986; **13:** 119–128.
11. Ronan J, Weisberg M, Perloff J *et al.* Cardiovascular teaching techniques: Planning and presenting effective instruction – alternative technologies of teaching in cardiovascular medicine. *J Am Coll Cardiol* 1986; **8:** 465–484.

X Psychological Aspects of Cardiac Rehabilitation

39 Social Factors Affecting Compliance and Behavioural Change

Alan J. Goble

National Heart Foundation Centre for Social and Preventive Research, Suite 1a, 333 Drummond Street, Carlton, Melbourne, Victoria 3053, Australia

Introduction

In patients with ischaemic heart disease, behaviours and compliance with behavioural change have been demonstrated to affect risk factors, resumption of work, recurrent events, admissions to hospital and deaths from subsequent episodes of coronary heart disease. The behaviours adopted by an individual following an acute myocardial infarction or following coronary bypass surgery are determined by physical, psychological and social characteristics. Those with recognized physical disability following the event are more likely to comply with advice to maintain appropriate behaviours. Those who are psychologically disturbed either because of or independently of the event, due to personality disorders and overt depression or denial, are less likely to conform to medical advice. The social factors to be discussed in this paper include level of education, occupational class, past smoking habit to the time of the cardiac event, associated or independent life events, social isolation, family structure and place of domicile. The evidence linking these social factors with outcomes comes from the recognized socio-demographic characteristics of patients, from follow-up studies of patients and from population studies. To understand the importance of epidemiological studies, relating social factors and outcomes in populations, one should recognize that "before one dies from an illness it is necessary to have that illness". Further, it should also be recognized that the vast majority of deaths from cardiovascular disease are in known patients with known

Proceedings of the Vth World Congress on Cardiac Rehabilitation

cardiovascular disease [1]. Also, cardiovascular disease death rates in populations parallel closely the death rates amongst patients [2].

Non-compliance

The risks of smoking after myocardial infarction [3–5] are well known to all health professionals and have been communicated to almost all patients with coronary heart disease. Despite this, many patients continue to smoke after myocardial infarction or coronary bypass surgery. As an example, in the Coronary Artery Surgery Study, at the time of randomization (after cardiac catheterization) approximately 40% of patients were smoking [6]. After 1 year, irrespective of randomization to medical or surgical treatment, over 30% were smoking. At 10-year follow-up, 24% of the surgical patients were smoking and 21% of medical patients were smoking. This fall in the percentage of patients smoking could have been due largely to deaths among those who continued to smoke.

In our study of the efficacy of high- and low-intensity exercise training after myocardial infarction [7], 2.5% of patients enrolled in an 8-week rehabilitation programme and reviewed at the end of that programme were smoking, at 4 months 7.5% were smoking and at 12 months 19% were smoking. Thus, although initial compliance was good, progressive recidivism occurred. It is recognized that such return to smoking is not limited to the first year.

Among subjects enrolled in the Ontario exercise training trial, comparing the outcomes of high- and low-intensity exercise over a 3-year period, approximately 40% dropped out of the programme [8]. This was independent of whether they were enrolled in high- or low-intensity exercise programmes. In this study, it was demonstrated that prior smokers were twice as likely to drop out from the exercise programmes as were non-smokers. Blue-collar workers were also significantly more likely to drop out than white-collar workers.

In the Coronary Drug Project, it was noted that there was a 15% mortality over 5 years in patients receiving either clofibrate or placebo, provided they adhered to their treatment [9]. Non-adherence to medication resulted in 24.6% deaths in the clofibrate group and 28% in the placebo group, giving relative risk ratios of 1.6 and 1.9 respectively compared with those who adhered well to their treatment. Thus, while clofibrate was not demonstrated to reduce mortality, adherence to medication, irrespective of what it was, resulted in significant and marked reduction of risk of death. From the Beta Blocker Heart Attack Trial, comparing propranolol and placebo, Horwitz *et al.* [10] reported that poor adherence to medication (propranolol) was associated with a 4.2% death rate in 12 months, compared with good adherence at 1.4%, giving a relative risk of 3.0. It was equally notable that good adherence to placebo produced a 3% mortality rate, while poor adherence resulted in a 7% mortality rate, a relative risk of 2.3%. These results were little affected by the severity of infarction, race, marital status, education, smoking, life stress, social isolation and other recognized factors associated with high mortality. Thus, it is quite clear that good adherence to medication, irrespective of what that medication may be, results in a reduction in cardiovascular deaths. Good compliance in one area is likely to be associated with good compliance in other areas.

Social markers of risk

From the Beta-Blocker Heart Attack Trial, Ruberman and colleagues [11] clearly showed that cumulative probability of death was markedly reduced among those with more education. Death was also markedly reduced among those whose life circumstances were less stressful and among those who did not have a high level of social isolation. While these patients had had myocardial infarction, similar findings were made long before by Hinkle and his colleagues [12], working from Cornell University in cooperation with the Bell System Operating Companies. They followed up approximately 270,000 men for a total of 586,294 man-years of risk. During this period (1963–65), 1020 first overt cardiac events occurred. This study showed that, for both first events and deaths, a marked benefit in the annual event rate was found among those who had received a college education. It was also shown that there was a gradient of annual event rates from workmen, to foremen, through supervisors, to managers and executives, with the highest event rates among the workmen.

In the Whitehall Study, a similar finding was noted among British male civil servants aged 40–60 years at entry, for death from coronary heart disease during 10 years of follow-up. Both all-cause mortality and coronary heart disease mortality were inversely related to the seniority of the civil servants, the least deaths occurring among the administrative class [13].

In our Family Atherosclerosis Risk Intervention Study (unpublished data) of 625 patients following myocardial infarction, bypass surgery or coronary angioplasty, white-collar workers had lower total cholesterol levels, lower systolic blood pressure and a lower body mass index than did blue-collar workers. While body mass was not significantly different, blue-collar workers were 3 cm shorter than white-collar workers. Less than average height has been demonstrated to be a risk factor for coronary heart disease, possibly related to earlier social deprivation and impaired nutrition [14].

In their study in Gothenburg between 1973 and 1982, Welin and his colleagues [15] demonstrated that among men born in 1913 and 1923, there was a clear inverse relationship between mortality and the number of activities undertaken outside the home. It appears, therefore, that a series of readily recognizable social characteristics is able to define those subjects who are at high risk of recurrent events and deaths following myocardial infarction.

Demographic markers of risk

There is evidence from the Alameida County Study to demonstrate that, for those people who live in an area of recognized poverty, the estimated survival probability is markedly reduced compared with those who live in a non-poverty area [16]. This observation held despite adjusting for multiple co-variates including age, sex, race, income, smoking, alcohol, physical activity, sleep, body mass index, symptoms, disability and other illnesses. This suggests that living in a poor area is a risk factor in itself, probably dependent upon the lack of medical and other support services.

Large epidemiological studies in the developed countries have shown that the lowest age-standardized coronary mortality rates are among the more urbanized areas and the highest coronary mortality rates in the least urbanized [17, 18].

Risk assessment

With little effort, it should be possible to construct, for each patient, a risk profile based upon socio-demographic characteristics. This would involve no testing, the use of no technology and it would be of miniscule cost, compared with the less sensitive risk stratification commonly undertaken following myocardial infarction. Technologically based risk stratification is used in the main to predict outcomes within the first year of the acute event and has some application to exercise training. Social risk stratification applies to recurrent events and deaths in the longer term. These social risks are set out in Table 1. From the hospital admission record, one knows the marital status of the patient (single, widowed or divorced), whether the patient comes from an area of poverty (dependent upon the postcode or a rural address) and whether the patient is a blue-collar worker.

The medical record should record other chronic disabilities. Self-neglect should be apparent from the patient's appearance and it should be obvious whether he or she is a smoker or not. The use of medications or excessive alcohol consumption should also be recorded. If a patient's height and weight are not measured, it should at least be noted whether they are short or overweight.

In the assessment of a patient with a view to future management, it is usual to take a social history. This will reveal the occurrence of life events (loss or threat), level of education and whether that person is socially isolated. When a patient is admitted to hospital, the level of perceived life stress prevailing at that time should be obtained by enquiring about the patient's financial concerns and whether they have any problems as regards family, social life, sexual function and work. The patient may volunteer other perceived stresses. This information, together with a simple assessment of psychological depression, denial or displacement, can be used to indicate a high, moderate or low risk of recurrent events and death. This risk is based upon anticipation of compliance *vs* non-compliance and maintenance *vs* non-maintenance of behaviours. This prediction would be more powerful than any physical or technological testing for long-term outcomes. Those at the highest risk require the greatest

Table 1
Risk of non-compliance, adverse behaviours, recurrence and death

Admission record
Blue-collar occupation
Unmarried male
Poor area of domicile
Rural dweller
Medical record
Other disability
Self-neglect
Smoker
Poor compliance to medication
Alcohol excess
Short in stature
Overweight
Social history
Life-events (loss or threat)
Years of education
Social isolation
Perceived stress
• Financial
• Family
• Sexual
• Occupational
• Other
Physical inactivity

attention and support throughout their illness and afterwards. Sadly, they are the least likely to get it. Efforts should be made to rectify this serious socio-medical problem.

References

1. Kuller L, Cooper M, Perper J. Epidemiology of sudden death. *Arch Int Med* 1972; **129:** 714–719.
2. Perth MONICA Data Book 1984–1990. University of Western Australia, Department of Public Health, 1992.
3. Sparrow D, Dawber TR, Colson T. The influence of cigarette smoking on prognosis after a first myocardial infarction. *J Chron Dis* 1978; **31:** 425–432.
4. Salonen JT. Stopping smoking and long-term mortality after myocardial infarction. *Br Heart J* 1980; **43:** 463–469.
5. Mulcahy R. Influence of cigarette smoking on morbidity and mortality after myocardial infarction. *Br Heart J* 1983; **49:** 410–415.
6. Rogers WJ, Coggin CJ, Gersh BJ *et al.*, and the CASS Investigators. Ten year follow-up of quality of life in patients randomized to receive medical therapy or coronary artery bypass graft surgery: The Coronary Artery Surgery Study (CASS). *Circulation* 1990; **82:** 1647–1658.

7. Goble A, Hare DL, Macdonald PS, Oliver RG, Reid MA, Worcester MC. Effect of early programmes of high and low intensity exercise on physical performance after transmural acute myocardial infarction. *Br Heart J* 1991; **65:** 126–131.
8. Oldridge NB, Donner AP, Buck CW *et al.* Predictors of dropout from cardiac exercise rehabilitation: Ontario Exercise-Heart Collaborative Study. *Am J Cardiol* 1983; **51:** 70–74.
9. Coronary Drug Project Research Group. Influence of adherence to treatment and response of cholesterol on mortality in the Coronary Drug Project. *N Engl J Med* 1980; **303:** 1038–1041.
10. Horwitz RI, Viscoli CM, Berkman L *et al.* Treatment adherence and risk of death after a myocardial infarction. *Lancet* 1990; **336:** 542–545.
11. Ruberman W, Weinblatt E, Goldberg JD, Chandhary BS. Psychosocial influences on mortality after myocardial infarction. *N Engl J Med* 1984; **311:** 522–559.
12. Hinkle LE, Whitney LH, Lehman EW *et al.* Occupation, education and coronary heart disease. *Science* 1968; **161:** 238–246.
13. Marmot MG, Shipley MJ, Rose G. Inequalities in death – specific explanations of a general pattern? *Lancet* 1984; **1:** 1003–1006.
14. La Vecchia C, Decarli A, Negri E, Ferraroni M, Pagano R. Height and the prevalence of chronic disease. *Rev Epidem et de Sante Publ* 1992; **40:** 6–14.
15. Welin L, Tibblin G, Svardsudd K *et al.* Prospective study of social influences on mortality: The study of men born in 1913 and 1923. *Lancet* 1985; **i:** 915–919.
16. Haan MN, Kaplan GA, Camacho T. Poverty and health: Prospective evidence from the Alameda County Study. *Am J Epidemiol* 1987; **125:** 989–998.
17. Fulton M, Adams W, Lutz W, Oliver MF. Regional variations in mortality from ischaemic heart and cerebrovascular disease in Britain. *Br Heart J* 1978; **40:** 563–568.
18. Salonen JT, Puska P, Kottke TE, Tuomilehto J, Nissinen A. Decline in mortality from coronary heart disease in Finland from 1969 to 1979. *Br Med J* 1983; **286:** 1857–1860.

40 Psychological Factors in Behavioural Change and Compliance

Marian C. Worcester

National Heart Foundation Centre for Social and Preventive Research, Suite 1a, 333 Drummond Street, Carlton, Melbourne, Victoria 3053, Australia

Secondary prevention of coronary heart disease involves the modification of risk factors. Patients are usually advised to change their lifestyles following an acute cardiac event and medication may be prescribed for the control of blood pressure and lipids. The main behavioural changes targeted for secondary prevention of coronary heart disease are smoking cessation, reduced saturated fat intake, reduced weight and increased physical activity.

A number of studies have demonstrated benefits in terms of secondary prevention from achieving these behavioural changes. For example, the benefits from reduced smoking have been reported in studies by Wilhelmsson, Mulcahy, Galan and their colleagues [1–3]. Positive effects of dietary change upon secondary prevention of coronary heart disease have been shown [4], although they are less easily demonstrated. The important role of physical activity in the secondary prevention of coronary heart disease is now accepted [5,6].

Despite these potential benefits to the secondary prevention of cardiovascular disease, however, many cardiac patients fail to comply with advice regarding smoking, diet and physical activity. Studies show that above one-third of cardiac patients continue or resume smoking after an acute event [7,8]. High drop-out rates from exercise rehabilitation programmes [9] or a return to a sedentary lifestyle upon completion of a formal exercise programme [10] have also been reported. Non-compliance with dietary advice among cardiac patients is known to be high but it is difficult to measure.

Proceedings of the Vth World Congress on Cardiac Rehabilitation

There have been few long-term studies of compliance in cardiac patients, but those conducted with different populations indicate non-compliance with advice is more likely if patients are given long-term and complex regimens [11]. Because of the chronicity of coronary artery disease, long-term regimens are often prescribed. Moreover, cardiac patients are usually required to modify simultaneously multiple lifestyle habits which are difficult to change.

It is becoming increasingly recognized that psychological factors – both intrapersonal and interpersonal – play a crucial role in determining whether or not patients adopt and maintain improved health behaviours. A number of theories have been developed to explain psychological factors in behaviour change. A key component of such theories is motivation to change, which is strongly influenced by both cognitive and affective responses of the patient.

One model of compliance which addresses cognitive influences upon behaviour change is the well-known Health Belief Model developed by Rosenstock and colleagues [12]. According to this model, behavioural change after an acute event is strongly influenced by the patient's beliefs, perceptions and expectations. For example, the belief that smoking was a major cause of the heart attack might increase the patient's motivation to quit smoking. A number of studies have examined this proposition. For example, in a study of 256 post-myocardial infarction (MI) patients in hospital, Newton and colleagues [13] found a significantly greater percentage of patients who thought smoking was important decreased or quit smoking at 3 months and 6 months after MI. Moreover, patients who perceived being overweight as important reported more weight loss. Other investigators, however, have not found any correlation between the patient's rating of smoking as important and subsequent behaviour change [14]. In the Austin Hospital Rehabilitation Trial [15] in Melbourne, a high proportion of post-MI patients claimed that smoking was a cause of their heart attack but there was no association between such perceptions and resumption of smoking after hospital discharge.

Furthermore, the Health Belief Model suggests that perception of the heart attack as severe, with future cardiac events being likely and possibly with a fatal outcome, might reinforce the patient's desire to stop smoking or lose weight. The patient's perception that the required behaviour change is feasible is one of the most important ingredients of this model of behaviour change. Patients may appreciate the benefits of stopping smoking or changing their diet, but may feel the barriers and costs of attempting to adopt new lifestyles are too great.

The failure of cardiac patients to comply with regimens is likely to be a result of inadequate motivation. Motivation is recognized as a key ingredient of the behaviour change process, which involves three fundamental stages: decision and commitment to change, initial change and maintenance of change. Prochaska and DiClemente [16] have expanded these stages to include pre-contemplation and contemplation as well as a phase for relapse to former behaviours. An important conceptual advance of their model is the emphasis upon a circular rather than a linear model of change. Linear models have changes which occur in a specific sequence, with relapse occurring at the last stage, whereas a circular model shows relapse leading back to an earlier stage from which a further attempt to change can be made.

Another important theoretical contribution to our understanding of behaviour change is the theory of self-efficacy, initially developed by Bandura [17]. Self-efficacy is a person's belief that he or she can respond effectively to a situation by using available skills. Thus, the cardiac patient needs to know not only which behaviours to change, and how, but also to feel confidence in his or her ability to achieve and maintain the desired behaviour changes. Several studies, such as that by Condiotte and Lichtenstein [18], have found measures of self-efficacy associated with positive outcomes.

As well as cognitive factors such as self-efficacy, perceptions and beliefs regarding the illness, compliance with advice and behavioural change in cardiac patients are significantly affected by affective responses to the illness, especially anxiety and depression, and by coping strategies employed to handle these emotions, particularly denial. There have been relatively few long-term studies of psychosocial outcome and lifestyle change following myocardial infarction, but those which have been undertaken confirm that emotional responses have a significant impact upon behavioural change [19–21].

Of the 224 patients studied in the Austin Hospital Rehabilitation Trial [15], 108 (48%) were smokers on admission to hospital. Of these, 15 were smoking at 4 months and 39 at 1 year. Non-compliers were not identified by any socio-demographic or medical characteristics but had significantly higher anxiety and depression scores than non-smokers on the Spielberger State Trait Anxiety Inventory and the IPAT Depression Questionnaire in hospital and at 4 months. These associations were not found at 12 months. However, patients who resumed smoking later in the year commonly reported feeling depressed, even though their depressed mood was not reflected in the scores on psychological inventories. Analysis of levels of physical activity during leisure in these patients also revealed that inactive patients had higher anxiety and depression than active patients at entry and at 4 and 12 months. These findings highlight the relevance of affective responses to adherence to advice regarding lifestyle change and suggest that anxious and depressed patients may need extra support from the rehabilitation team to help them to adopt and maintain healthier behaviours.

While an individual's motivation for behaviour change is determined in part by his or her cognitive and affective responses, interpersonal factors play an essential part in reinforcing motivation. There are a number of potentially powerful influences upon the cardiac patient, including spouse, doctor and others in the rehabilitation team, as well as other cardiac patients.

The spouse and family can assist the patient's adherence to advice through providing emotional support and acting as a buffer against stresses in the patient's life, such as those experienced on first resuming work. They can also help the patient comply by offering encouragement and reinforcement. For example, they may explicitly discourage or disallow inappropriate behaviour (such as smoking in the house) or give practical assistance (such as cooking the prescribed meals). Finally, the spouse and family can provide essential supervision of the patient's behaviour over a long period, reinforcing lifestyle advice and assisting the patient to avoid relapses. Studies have shown that family support and encouragement are associated with greater success in quitting smoking [22], losing weight [23] and adhering to an exercise programme [24].

In his comprehensive review of the literature on behavioural approaches to secondary prevention of coronary artery disease, Godin [25] emphasizes the importance of family involvement in rehabilitation, asserting that more attention should be paid to the influence of social support at initiation of health behaviour change among cardiac patients. Thus, actively involving the patient's spouse in the cardiac rehabilitation programme is clearly desirable. Counselling sessions regarding dietary and other lifestyle changes should include both patient and spouse. Where possible, active participation of the spouse in the exercise programme should be encouraged. In a Melbourne study of 43 men after a first heart attack, non-attendance of wives at the rehabilitation programme was strongly associated with overall non-compliance of the patients [26]. The wives of non-compliers rarely attended.

Studies show that doctors can exert a powerful influence upon patients to cease smoking [21]. Behaviourally oriented programmes are now being developed in Australia and elsewhere to strengthen the doctor's role in promoting behavioural change for the primary and secondary prevention of cardiovascular disease. The doctor can readily apply behavioural modification principles during consultations. For example, the doctor can praise the patient for reducing the amount of smoking and encourage further reduction. This approach is likely to be more effective than reproaching the patient's failure to quit totally. The doctor can provide continuing support, reinforcing the patient's motivation and coping skills for avoiding relapse, and can encourage the patient to monitor his or her behaviour and to become more aware of situations where lapses occur (such as time, place, social setting, mood) and suggest how such situations might be avoided in the future. However, the doctor should also recognize when to refer a patient to another health professional for further help in modifying his or her lifestyle.

Because of its subtle presentation, depression in cardiac patients is often overlooked. The doctor has a critical role to play in its detection and management because, as previously noted, a depressed mood often leads to poor compliance. Depression is common during convalescence at a time when the patient is often attempting to adopt new patterns of behaviour [27]. Participation in a group cardiac rehabilitation programme during convalescence may provide the necessary emotional and social support to minimize such depression. Compared with the very large number of studies investigating the physical benefits of exercise programmes, relatively few studies have examined their effectiveness in promoting psychological recovery after a cardiac illness. Nor has their potential in facilitating behaviour change been fully explored.

Group exercise programmes can promote behavioural change in a number of ways. They offer patients regular access to expert advice and provide explicit guidelines for physical activity. Furthermore, others in the group provide a yardstick for the patient to measure his or her level of fitness or weight loss. They may also act as models for successful behavioural change. For example, patients in the group may encourage each other to stop smoking and offer assistance if lapses occur. In a study by Taylor *et al.* [28], patients in the group exercise training programme were more successful than others in decreasing their cigarette smoking.

The potential of group exercise programmes to improve the psychological functioning of patients during convalescence is considerable. In particular, participating in a supervised exercise programme demonstrates to patients that they are physically capable, increasing their self-confidence and reassuring them that it is safe to exercise and to undertake other activities outside the sessions. The exercise group also provides camaraderie and opportunities for social interactions which enhance well-being.

In summary, a patient's ability and willingness to comply with advice regarding behavioural changes are closely linked to his or her health attitudes and psychological well-being. The support of "significant others", including spouse, family, doctor, other health professionals and fellow patients can promote early psychological recovery which, in turn, should facilitate the adoption of a healthier lifestyle. The availability of a group exercise programme during convalescence provides an ideal and supportive environment for such interaction and lifestyle change to take place.

References

1. Wilhelmsson C, Vedin JA, Elmfeldt D, Tibblin G, Wilhelmsen L. Smoking and myocardial infarction. *Lancet* 1975; **1:** 415–420.
2. Mulcahy R. Influence of cigarette smoking on morbidity and mortality after myocardial infarction. *Br Heart J* 1983; **49:** 410–415.
3. Galan KM, Deligonul U, Kern MJ, *et al.* Increased frequency of restenosis in patients continuing to smoke cigarettes after percutaneous transluminal coronary angioplasty. *Am J Cardiol* 1988; **61:** 260–263.
4. Campeau L, Enjalbert M, Lesperance J, *et al.* The relation of risk factors to the development of atherosclerosis in saphenous-vein bypass grafts and the progression of disease in the native circulation: A study 10 years after aortocoronary bypass surgery. *New Engl J Med* 1984; **311:** 1329–1332.
5. Fletcher GF, Blair SN, Blumenthal J *et al.* Statement on Exercise. Benefits and recommendations for physical activity programs for all Americans: A Statement for health professionals by the Committee on Exercise and Cardiac Rehabilitation of the Council on Clinical Cardiology, American Heart Association. *Circulation* 1992; **86:** 340–344.
6. Oldridge NB, Guyatt GH, Fischer ME, Rimm AA. Cardiac rehabilitation after myocardial infarction: Combined experience of randomized clinical trials. *JAMA* 1988; **260:** 945–950.
7. Baile WF, Bigelow GE, Gottlieb SH *et al.* Rapid resumption of cigarette smoking following myocardial infarction: Inverse relation to myocardial infarction severity. *Addictive Behav* 1982; **7:** 373–380.

8. Burt A, Illingworth D, Shaw TRD *et al.* Stopping smoking after myocardial infarction. *Lancet* 1974; **i:** 304–306.
9. Oldridge NB *et al.* Compliance and dropout in cardiac exercise rehabilitation. *J Cardiac Rehab* 1984; **4:** 166–177.
10. Carmody TP, Sennerm JW, Malinow MR, Matarazzo JD: Physical exercise rehabilitation: Long-term dropout rate in cardiac patients. *J Behav Med* 1980; **3:** 163–168.
11. Becker MH, Naiman L. Sociobehavioural determinants of compliance with health and medical care recommendations. *Med Care* 1975; **13:** 10–24.
12. Rosenstock IM. The health belief model and preventive health behaviour. *Health Education Monographs* 1974; **2:** 354–386.
13. Newton KM, Sivarajan ES. Patient perceptions of risk factor changes and cardiac rehabilitation outcomes after myocardial infarction. *J Cardiac Rehab* 1985; **5:** 159–168.
14. Croog SH, Richards NP. Health beliefs and smoking patterns in heart patients and their wives: A longitudinal study. *Am J Public Health* 1977; **67:** 921–930.
15. Goble AJ, Hare DL, Macdonald PS *et al.* Effect of early programmes of high and low intensity exercise on physical performance after transmural acute myocardial infarction. *Br Heart J* 1991; **65:** 126–131.
16. Prochaska JO, DiClemente CC. Stages and processes of self-change of smoking: Toward an integrative model of change. *J Consult Clin Psychol* 1983; **51:** 390–395.
17. Bandura A. Self-efficacy: Toward a unifying theory of behavioural change. *Psychol Rev* 1977; **84:** 191–215.
18. Condiotte MM, Lichtenstein E. Self-efficacy and relapse in smoking cessation programs. *J Consult Psychol* 1981; **49:** 648–658.
19. Finlayson A, McEwen J. Coronary Heart Disease and Patterns of Living, Croom Helm: London, 1977.
20. Wiklund I, Sanne H, Vedin A, Wilhemsson C. Psychosocial outcome one year after a first myocardial infarction. *J Psychosom Res* 1984; **28:** 309–321.
21. Croog SH, Levine S. The Heart Patient Recovers: Social and Psychological Factors. Human Sciences Press: New York, 1977.
22. Mermelstein RJ, Lichtenstein E, McIntyre KO. Partner support and relapse in smoking cessation programs. *J Consult Clin Psychol* 1982; **51:** 465–466.
23. Brownell KD, Heckerman CL, Westerland RJ, Hayes SC, Monti PM. The effect of couples training and partner cooperativeness in the behavioural treatment of obesity. *Behav Res Ther* 1978; **16:** 323–333.
24. Wankel LM. Decision-making and social support strategies for increasing exercise involvement. *J Cardiac Rehab* 1984; **4:** 124–135.
25. Godin G. The effectiveness of interventions in modifying behavioural risk factors of individuals with coronary heart disease. *J Cardiopulmonary Rehab* 1989; **9:** 223–236.
26. Worcester MC. Processes and patterns of recovery following acute myocardial infarction. PhD thesis, Melbourne, 1979.
27. Hackett TP, Cassem NH. Adjusting to coronary artery disease: Coping with the problems of convalescence following myocardial infarction. In Mathes P, Halhuber MJ (eds). *Controversies in Cardiac Rehabilitation.* Springer-Verlag: Berlin, 1982.
28. Taylor CB, Houston-Miller N, Haskell WL, DeBusk RF. Smoking cessation after acute myocardial infarction: The effects of exercise training. *Addictive Behav* 1988; **13:** 331–335.

41 Maintenance of Behaviour Change After a Coronary Event

Brian Oldenburg*, Andrew Martin

Department of Public Health, University of Sydney, Sydney, New South Wales 2006, Australia

Introduction

Various reviews and meta-analyses published in recent years [1–4] indicate that a variety of physical, psychosocial and rehabilitative interventions conducted with cardiac patients have been effective in modifying coronary heart disease (CHD) risk factors and reducing mortality. The most recent meta-analysis, conducted by Mullen *et al.* [4], examined 28 controlled studies of cardiac patient education interventions and noted the following effects: a significant improvement in blood pressure, a significant improvement in dietary and exercise outcomes, and an almost 20% improvement in mortality.

Other research (reviewed by May *et al.* [1]) indicates that the direct control of risk factors in those individuals at high-risk of CHD can also lead to substantial reductions in mortality. Increased exercise has been shown to lower mortality by 15–25% [5], hypertension control can positively affect mortality by 20% [6], cession of smoking can reduce mortality by 20–50%, and lipid-lowering programmes have resulted in a wide range of mortality improvements.

In summary, these results suggest that the promotion of healthy lifestyle behaviours is an important goal in the management of the cardiac patient. Clearly, there are a variety of means of achieving this end, and the challenge remains to identify those approaches and strategies which are most likely to

*To whom all correspondence should be addressed

Proceedings of the Vth World Congress on Cardiac Rehabilitation

be associated with high levels of compliance and long-term maintenance. There is a considerable amount of evidence to indicate that unhealthy behaviours, such as smoking, are resistant to long-term change. In fact, most reviews of the field have found that at least one-third of all cardiac patients fail to comply with any recommended regimen. This is particularly disturbing, as secondary preventive research indicates that healthy behaviours must be sustained for many years in order to achieve substantial cardiac benefit.

There are three different types of intervention strategies which have been used in clinical settings as an adjunct to routine medical and nursing care [5]. First, the instructional or educational approaches generally provide information about the disease process, CHD risk factors, and simple advice regarding lifestyle changes or CHD treatment. Secondly, the motivational approaches attempt to motivate individuals to modify their lifestyle by encouraging attitudinal change. Finally, the behavioural approaches aim to directly modify particular behaviours which increase an individual's risk of heart disease.

Obviously these different strategies are not mutually exclusive, and many cardiac rehabilitation programmes attempt to incorporate them all. The next section will examine the comparative outcomes associated with the use of these different approaches. In the final section, we will make some recommendations regarding the more effective use of such approaches in the secondary prevention of cardiovascular disease.

Over the past 10 years, we have conducted three randomized controlled trials of educational and behavioural interventions with cardiac patients. The first two of these were conducted with patients who had suffered a myocardial infarction (MI) [6, 7], while the most recent trial was conducted with coronary artery bypass (CABG) patients [8].

A controlled trial of psychological and educational intervention during the hospitalization phase of MI patients

In this study [6], we compared the effectiveness of three intervention conditions which varied by type and also intensity. These conditions were: routine care with regular follow-up; an educational programme which provided information on MI, CHD risk factors and lifestyle change; and a behavioural counselling intervention which explored patient anxiety in counselling sessions, detailed behavioural strategies for lifestyle change, and also included the aforementioned educational component.

The individuals who received the counselling intervention changed their lifestyles (e.g. smoking, dietary and exercise habits) to a significantly greater extent than the other two groups. This difference increased at the 12-month follow-up, and was probably attributable to the degree of relapse occurring in the control and educational conditions. In terms of quality-of-life outcomes, however, there were no differences between the counselling and educational interventions; although at 12 months these groups, on average, reported significantly less psychosocial distress than individuals receiving only routine care.

A controlled trial of behavioural and educational intervention during the out-patient phase of MI patients

As in the previous study, three conditions were compared [7]. The routine care group obtained standard medical care and regular follow-up assessments. The educational group received not only a variety of educational materials, but also the opportunity to attend a group education programme while in hospital and also after discharge. The behavioural counselling group was offered, in addition to the educational programme, an overall cardiac rehabilitation intervention which addressed patients' individual risk factors and included an exercise regimen. This latter intervention employed a range of behavioural strategies, including behavioural contracting, goal-setting, self-monitoring and stress management.

Over the 12-month follow-up period, the two intervention groups performed significantly better than the routine care group on a variety of quality-of-life and physical outcomes – in particular, exercise test performance and smoking relapse rates. Although there were some initial differences on the dietary outcomes, these were not maintained in the long term. Contrasting the two intervention conditions, the behavioural counselling group tended to do better than the educational group on the lifestyle-related measures of smoking and exercise test performance; however, few differences emerged between these groups on the physical and quality-of-life outcomes.

The results for this study were similar to those obtained in the earlier study. The interventions were generally more effective than standard medical care alone, and a difference between the educational and behavioural interventions was detected for some of the lifestyle or risk factor outcomes but not for the quality-of-life outcomes.

A controlled trial of educational and behavioural intervention in post-CABG patients

Our most recent study [8] has evaluated the effectiveness of a behavioural and educational programme to modify coronary risk factors and improve the quality-of-life of coronary bypass surgery individuals. In this study, however, there were two conditions: a routine care condition which involved standard medical and nursing care and regular follow-up, and a behavioural intervention condition. Individuals in the latter group received an individualized programme with goal-setting, a group-based risk factor reduction programme, printed materials and regular follow-up. The exercise component of the intervention consisted mainly of group walking and encouragement to include more walking and activity in daily life.

All of the patients were assessed at baseline (in hospital and within 3 weeks of discharge), and after 4, 8, and 12 months. The patients were assessed on cardiovascular risk factors, a variety of quality-of-life measures and self-reported lifestyle outcomes. For the quality-of-life and physical outcomes, both groups on average experienced a significant 15% reduction in psychological distress, and around a 50% improvement for symptoms over the 12-month follow-up period. The most impressive significant difference between the two groups on risk factor outcomes was on exercise testing. At 12-months, the intervention group's estimated aerobic capacity was 10% higher than that of the control group. There was also some suggestion that the behavioural intervention achieved higher HDL- cholesterol levels and lower smoking relapse rates than the routine care condition.

Discussion

Comparing the results of this most recent study with CABG patients against those of the MI patient studies raises some interesting issues concerning the management and rehabilitation of bypass and MI patients. The intervention employed in the CABG trial appears to have been relatively less effective in achieving change beyond the effects of standard medical care than the comparable interventions used in the earlier studies with MI patients.

This finding may be indicative of certain differences between the treatment needs of these two groups of CHD patients. Perhaps there is a stronger motivation for MI patients to change their lifestyles as they see themselves recovering from an "illness", while bypass surgery patients might see themselves as having been "cured". It is also possible that CABG patients simply comprise a more "hard-core" group of CHD patients who are more difficult to change. Prior to the intervention, for example, 55% of the CABG patients had previously experienced a MI, 52% had undergone blood pressure treatment, 16% had participated in other intervention programmes, and 15% had already undergone coronary artery surgery. Future trials in CHD secondary prevention would do well to explore the differences between the needs of MI and CABG patients so that future interventions can be tailored accordingly. Furthermore, it is clear that long-term maintenance of lifestyle change remains a major challenge with both MI and CABG patients. From the research that we and others have conducted with MI patients, it seems clear that the more behaviourally focused and intensive lifestyle change interventions tend to yield not only more initial change, but change which is also more resilient to relapse in the longer term.

These findings are supported further by the programme ingredients Mullen *et al.* [4] identified in their meta-analysis as being predictors of programme success. They suggest that intervention programmes should employ reinforcement, give feedback on patient progress, offer individualized programmes, facilitate behaviour change and be relevant to patients' needs and abilities.

Furthermore, recent research by Prochaska and DiClemente [9], summarized by Oldenburg *et al.* [10], indicate that individuals move through a number of stages in the lifestyle change process, namely:

1. The preparation stage, during which the individual is contemplating change.
2. The action stage, in which the individual is actually making attempts at change.
3. The maintenance stage, in which the individual strives to maintain change.

Identifying which stage an individual is in, and using strategies appropriate to that stage, is also likely to enhance the maintenance of significant lifestyle change.

References

1. May GS, Eberlein KA, Furberg CD, Passamani ER, DeMets DL. Secondary prevention after myocardial infarction: A review of long- term trials. *Prog Cardiovasc Dis* 1982; **24:** 331–352.
2. Oldridge NB, Guyatt GH, Fischer M, Rimm A. Cardiac rehabilitation after myocardial infarction: Combining data from randomized clinical trials. *JAMA* 1988; **260:** 945–980.
3. O'Connor GT, Buring JE, Yusuf S, Goldhaber SZ, Olmstaed EM, Paffenbarger RS, Hennekens CH. An overview of randomized trials of rehabilitation with exercise after myocardial infarction. *Circulation* 1989; **80:** 234–244.
4. Mullen PD, Mains DA, Velez R. A meta-analysis of controlled trials of cardiac patient education. *Patient Education and Counseling* 1992; **19:** 143–162.
5. Glanz K. Patient and public education for cholesterol reduction: A review of strategies and issues. *Patient Education and Counseling* 1988; **12:** 235–257.
6. Oldenburg B, Perkins RJ, Andrews G. A controlled trial of psychological intervention in myocardial infarction. *J Consult Clin Psychol* 1985; **53:** 852–859.
7. Oldenburg B, Allan R, Fastier G. The role of behavioural and educational interventions in the secondary prevention of coronary heart disease. In: Lovibond P, Wilson P, (eds), *Clinical and Abnormal Psychology.* Elsevier Science Publishers: Amsterdam, 1989.
8. Oldenburg B, Martin A, Greenwood J, Bernstein L, Allan R. A controlled trial of behavioural and educational intervention in coronary artery bypass surgery (in prep.).
9. Prochaska JO, DiClemente CC. Towards a comprehensive model of behavioural change. In: *Treating Addictive Behaviours: Processes of Change.* Plenum Press: New York, 1986: pp. 3–27.
10. Oldenburg B, Gomel M, Graham-Clarke P. Cardiovascular risk reduction through lifestyle change in clinical settings. *Ann Acad Med Singapore* 1992; **21:** 114–120.

42 Rehabilitation after Cardiac Transplantation: 10-year Follow-up – Psychological Aspects

Cecile Coustry-Degré*, Françoise Platieau

Médico-Surgical and Rehabilitation Divisions, C.U.B. Hôpital Erasme, 808 Route de Lennik, B-1070 Brussels, Belgium

Introduction

Between March 1982 and May 1992, 260 heart transplantations were performed on patients suffering end-stage cardiac diseases (87% male, 13% female) in our hospital.

Methods and materials

In May 1992, a representative sample of 85 patients (both males and females) were given a questionnaire about their psychological reactions to the transplantation and their quality of life. Two groups of patients were considered: 21 patients who underwent transplantation more than 5 years previously and 64 patients who underwent transplantation less than 5 years previously. Their median ages were 45 and 51 years, respectively. This age difference was due to the selection criteria at the time of transplantation.

The socio-professional status of the patients was as follows: 12% independent, 29% executives, 28% clerks, 27% manual workers, 4% others. Their educational status was as follows: 23% of the patients went on to University

* To whom all correspondence should be addressed.

or other forms of higher education, 15% completed their secondary schooling, 31% left school at age 14 and 31% followed professional or technical training.

Results

1. Anxiety regarding rejection, infection and medication

Table 1

	Transplantation more than 5 years previously	Transplantation less than 5 years previously
Rejection	44%	52%
Infection	33%	42%
Medication	23%	23%

The anxiety [1] of those patients who had recently undergone transplantation was higher than that of the older transplant recipients. Attitudes regarding medication are similar for both groups, and they are particularly anxious about hypertension, renal insufficiency, decalcification and cancers.

2. Global anxiety after transplantation. Both groups remain anxious for their future, their life-expectancy and also for the potential undesirable side-effects of their treatment [1, 2, 6]. The group receiving transplantation less than 5 years previously is less anxious because transplantation is now more commonplace; the group receiving transplantation more than 5 years previously is more anxious because of the poor survival rates 10 years post-operation.

3. Return to work [3, 4]. In our sample, 16% of the patients are unable to return to work, 38% are retired, 8% are on the point of returning to work and 38% have returned to work. In comparison, a "normal" Belgian sample (Belgian Social Legislation) would show 66% at work, 24% disabled and 10% on the point of returning to work.

4. Family support. Transplant recipients require vigorous support from their families [1, 2, 5, 6]. The general experience is that the quality of family support is of prime importance for successful re-insertion into family and social life.

Table 2

	Transplantation more than 5 years previously		Transplantation less than 5 years previously	
	During illness	Now	During illness	Now
Yes	9%	66%	89%	62%
No	9%	34%	8%	31%
Undecided			3%	7%

5. Sexual life. The patients undergoing transplantation less than 5 years previously, being younger, were more sexually active than the other group of patients. Our results are in agreement with those of a control cardiac population. The concerns of the patients included: impotency, decrease of libido, fear of spouse, side-effects of medical therapies.

6. Adaptation of lifestyle after transplantation

Table 3

	Transplantation more than 5 years previously	Transplantation less than 5 years previously
Yes	57%	52%
No	43%	40%
Undecided		8%

After transplantation, patients of both groups have positive and negative reactions:

better life-events;
the most possible enjoyment from life-events;
more realistic adaptation;
more philosophical and tolerant behaviour;
"life first", more egoistic;
time is of first importance;
less projects for the future;
fear for the future;
more careful;
more nervous and impulsive (drugs);
changes in relationship with family and society [1, 6].

7. Ability to cope with medical and dietetic obligations

Table 4

	Transplantation more than 5 years previously	Transplantation less than 5 years previously
Good	70%	67%
Less good	30%	25%
Less bad	—	33%
Bad	—	5%

The most serious difficulties confronted include: poor adaptation to dietary restrictions; poor adaptation to medication (undesirable side-effects, body changes, etc.) [1, 2, 6]; and stress resulting from medical therapies and diet.

Conclusions

The majority of patients adapt to the lifestyle of a transplant recipient [7, 8] and their quality of life is good [1, 3, 4]. They enjoy their new life, are active and take advantage of work possibilities. Nevertheless, difficulties do arise for a number of patients:

tension in family life [1, 6];
sexual inactivity [1, 2];
poor adaptation to changes in body appearance;
fear of the future, and of the new heart being rejected, and the consequences of medical therapies [1, 2].

The group receiving transplantation less than 5 years previously are better adapted in general to life changes.

References

1. Beidel DC. Psychological factors in organ transplantation. *Clin Psychol Rev* 1987; **7:** 677–692
2. Lough ME, Lindsey AM, Shinn JA, Scotts NA. Life satisfaction following heart transplantation. *J Heart Transplant* 1985; **4:** 446–449.
3. Niset G, Coustry-Degré C, Degré S. Psychosocial and physical rehabilitation of the heart transplantation: 1-year follow-up. *Cardiology* 1988; **75:** 311–317.
4. Meister MD, McAleer MY, Meister YS, Riley YE, Copeland YG. Returning to work after heart transplantation. *J Heart Transplant* 1986; **5:** 154–161.
5. Suszycki LH. Social work groups on a heart transplant program. *J Heart Transplant* 1986; **5:** 166–170.
6. McAleer MJ, Copeland J, Fuller J and Copeland JG. Psychological aspects of heart transplantation. *Heart Transplant* 1985; **4:** 232–233.
7. Christopherson LK, Griepp RB, Stinsom EB. Rehabilitation after heart transplantation. *JAMA* 1976; **236:** 2082–2084.
8. Christopherson LK. Cardiac transplantation: A psychological perspective. *Circulation* 1987; **75:** 57–62.

43 Psychological Stress Following Myocardial Infarction and Long-term Prognosis: Potential for Altering Outcomes

Nancy Frasure-Smith

McGill University and Montreal Heart Institute,
5000 Belanger East, Montreal, Quebec H1T 1C8, Canada

Introduction

Over the past 10 years, there has been increasing evidence that psychosocial factors including life stress, depression and social isolation may play as important a role following a heart attack as the more traditional risk factors of smoking, obesity and lipid levels. For example, in 1984, Ruberman *et al.* [1] carried out secondary analysis of data collected on 2319 patients who took part in the Beta-blocker Heart Attack Trial. They found that patients judged to have had high stress levels prior to their myocardial infarction (MI) had about twice the risk of death over the subsequent 3 years as other patients. Judgements about stress levels were based on a *post-hoc* combination of questions about job satisfaction, social class and memories of the impact of a few selected life events. Control for standard cardiac risk variables did not alter the pattern of results. Clearly, there are problems with the measurement of stress in this study, but it remains a landmark in the literature. Since its publication, several other teams have demonstrated similar significant relationships between post-MI psychological status and post-MI prognosis.

Ahern and his colleagues [2] analysed data from the Cardiac Arrhythmia Pilot Study and found that scores on the Beck Depression Inventory (a measure of symptoms of depression) administered within 60 days after an MI, predicted 1 year cardiac death/arrest rates in a sample of 351 patients with significant arrhythmias at baseline. In another study, Follick *et al.* [3] administered the

Proceedings of the Vth World Congress on Cardiac Rehabilitation

SCL-90 in hospital to a sample of 125 post-MI patients who took part in a 1 year study of the telephone transmission of portable electrocardiographic (ECG) readings. Global SCL-90 scores, which measure psychological distress, significantly predicted the occurrence of ventricular arrhythmias on ECGs randomly collected throughout the first post-MI year. In Germany, data from 560 males involved in the Post-infarction Late Potential Study showed that high degrees of depressive symptomatology in hospital significantly predicted cardiac deaths in the first 6 months following MI [4]. The impact remained significant after controlling for previous MI, and the presence of late potentials on the in-hospital electrocardiogram. Finally, a team in Sweden reported that among 201 post-MI patients, those anxious enough to be taking minor tranquillizers 3 months after their infarct had significantly higher 1 year and 5 year death/MI recurrence rates than patients not taking these medications [5].

In summary, it appears that some aspect of post-MI psychological status, something related to life stress, depressive symptoms, distress and anxiety, perhaps negative affect in general, has important long-term prognostic significance following MI. This suggests that one way to improve the odds for MI survivors might well involve psychological, supportive and educational techniques aimed at relieving the psychological distress, depression and uncertainty accompanying myocardial infarction. In fact, over the past 15 years, our research team in Montreal has been involved in developing and evaluating just such an approach.

The ischaemic heart disease life stress monitoring programme

Although the evidence linking psychosocial factors with post-MI prognosis is much stronger now than it was 15 years ago when my colleague Dr Raymond Prince of the Department of Psychiatry at McGill University began clinical research in this area, studies examining the impact of life change events were already beginning to suggest that periods of increasing life stress were particularly dangerous for post-MI patients [6]. Prince tried to draw clinical applications from this work, and reasoned that if periods of increasing life stress do precede and predict cardiac events, then regular psychological stress monitoring coupled with timely interventions to reduce stress might prevent at least some cardiac episodes among post-MI patients. The clinical approach based on this reasoning was originally called the Ischaemic Heart Disease (IHD) Life Stress Monitoring Programme [7]. There are three key parts to this 1-year programme: first, monthly telephone monitoring of psychological symptoms of stress using a standardized measure, the General Health Questionnaire (GHQ) [8]; secondly, individually tailored home nursing visits for patients reporting high levels of stress symptoms during monthly telephone calls; and, thirdly, weekly team meetings in which a psychiatrist and other project members help project nurses develop plans of care tailored to each patient's own sources of stress.

The GHQ includes 20 cognitive-behavioural symptoms which people undergoing periods of life stress frequently report; for example, not being able to concentrate and feeling nervous or uptight. No physiological symptoms of distress (such as sweaty palms or a rapid heart beat), which might be confused with cardiac symptoms, are included. For each of the 20 symptoms on the GHQ, patients are asked to compare their current status with what is normal or usual for them. Patients are considered to have one symptom of psychological stress each time they report that a particular symptom is worse or much worse than usual. Thus, scores on the 20-item GHQ can range from 0 to 20. Scores of 5 or more reflect a high level of psychological symptoms of stress [9], and in the IHD Life Stress Monitoring Programme patients who reported this level of stress were considered to be in need of interventions to lower their stress. These interventions involved home visits from project nurses. Since the symptoms of stress measured by the GHQ are non-specific and can be triggered by a variety of problems needing a variety of solutions, the treatments for each patient were matched in terms of type, amount and timing to the specific needs of each high-stress patient. The nurses' mandate was to visit patients with high stress levels and to attempt to discover aspects in each patient's life which may have produced high stress. Later, in consultation with the project team (a psychiatrist, a psychologist and other project nurses), the nurses' task was to do whatever was relevant to help the patient deal with his problems and lower his number of stress symptoms. Each nurse had her own caseload, and in practice the nursing interventions involved an individually tailored combination of teaching, support and consultation or referral. Nursing visits continued until the patient's stress score came down to normal and the team felt that the patient's problems had been resolved.

A preliminary evaluation of this approach involving 461 males assigned randomly to the treatment programme ($n = 232$) or usual care ($n = 229$) showed that the programme lowered stress symptoms ($P = 0.03$) and reduced cardiac deaths by 50% over the programme year ($P = 0.07$), but made no difference in re-admissions [7]. Long-term follow-up based on Quebec medicare data, death certificates and hospital records showed a post-programme impact on MI recurrences beginning at about 18 months post-MI (6 months after the end of the programme), and continuing up until at least 5 years post-MI (5-year relative risk = 0.58, $P = 0.008$) [10]. After control for baseline differences between the treatment and control groups, the first year mortality impact was no longer significant ($P = 0.21$), but the long-term impact on MI recurrences remained ($P = 0.028$). These results were achieved at relatively little cost. Only about half the treated patients required nursing intervention, and the average high-stress patient received only 6 h of nursing contact. In addition, physician costs were no higher in the treatment than in the control group.

Programme impact in terms of in-hospital stress levels

Given the recent evidence linking psychological status in hospital after an infarction with long-term prognosis, we felt that it was important to consider how programme impact may have interacted with baseline levels of psychological distress [11]. We hypothesized that with usual post-hospital care, that is, in the control group, high levels of stress in hospital would have a negative long-term prognostic impact, but that with participation in the IHD Life Stress Monitoring Programme, high levels of stress in hospital would not increase long-term risk.

Stress was measured using the patients' baseline in-hospital GHQ scores obtained before randomization to the treatment or control conditions. Scores of 5 or more were considered to indicate high stress and scores of 4 or less were considered to be low. The sample was divided into four groups based on in-hospital GHQ scores and treatment and control groups. Data analysis was based on the time from the index infarct to death from cardiac causes. Kaplan-Meier survival curves were compared using the generalized Mantel-Cox test.

With usual post-hospital care, patients with high in-hospital stress scores were almost three times as likely to die of cardiac causes within 5 years as patients with low scores (relative risk = 2.81, $p = 0.0003$). Background comparisons between high- and low-stress patients in the control group showed that high-stress patients were significantly younger, more likely to be single, less likely to exercise regularly and more likely to have had non-Q-wave infarctions than low-stress patients. However, the increase in risk associated with high levels of stress in-hospital remained after statistical control for these imbalances. In contrast, within the treatment group, that is among those patients who took part in the year-long programme of telephone monitoring and nursing visits, there was no increase in risk associated with high stress (relative risk = 0.81, $P = 0.57$). Control for background variables did not alter the outcomes. Similar patterns of results occurred when the data were examined for long-term MI recurrences. In short, the marked stress-related increase in long-term risk in the control group disappeared in the treatment group.

We also examined the data from the point of view of treatment impact among high-stress patients in contrast to treatment impact among low-stress patients. Within the high-stress group treated patients had less than half the risk of cardiac mortality over 5 years as the control patients (relative risk = 0.36, $p = 0.006$), and this difference remained after control for background differences between the groups. In comparison, there was no evidence of treatment impact among the low-stress patients (relative risk = 1.25, $P = 0.41$). Similar results occurred for MI recurrences. Thus, treatment impact was mostly restricted to patients reporting high levels of psychological stress symptoms in hospital.

Limitations

In light of recent evidence linking various psychological factors with post-MI prognosis, the outcomes of the IHD Life Stress Monitoring Programme, and the results of the subsequent secondary analyses in terms of in-hospital stress level are intriguing. However, because of study limitations, it is too soon to encourage widespread programme implementation. After controlling for background variables, the 1-year treatment impact was of only marginal statistical significance for the sample as a whole, and it is possible that overall programme outcomes, as well as the results of the secondary analyses, may represent chance phenomena. In addition, methodological problems with the study may have accounted for group differences [10]. Furthermore, it is not clear that the programme really acted by reducing stress. There is evidence that the mechanisms may have been increased compliance with beta-blocking medication and/or advice to quit smoking. In addition, the study only included male patients. Finally, post-MI medical treatment has evolved considerably since the last patient was recruited to the study in 1981. It is unclear what impact the programme would have in today's era of thrombolysis, early revascularization, aspirin and beta- and calcium blockade.

Montreal Heart Attack Readjustment Trial (M-HART)

In order to obtain better information about the value of this approach, we are currently involved in a large-scale randomized controlled trial involving a target sample of 1630 post-MI patients, including 734 women. This trial, which we call the Montreal Heart Attack Readjustment Trial or M-HART, is funded by Health and Welfare Canada and the National Heart, Lung and Blood Institute in the USA. My co-investigators include Drs François Lespérance, Martin Juneau and Martial Bourassa of the Montreal Heart Institute and Dr Raymond Prince of McGill University. The M-HART study has three objectives: to assess the replicability of programme results using an expanded sample size; to obtain additional information about programme mechanisms including compliance, improved access to medical treatment and changes in negative emotions; and to compare programme impact for men and women. Extensive baseline data on cardiac variables is being collected so that we can stratify the sample in terms of post-MI risk. Costs will be studied in terms of physician contact data from Quebec Medicare records. In about 3 years, we should have better answers about the importance of psychosocial factors in post-MI prognosis, and the value of a cost-effective intervention aimed at altering these factors.

References

1. Ruberman W, Weinblatt E, Goldberg JD, Chaudhary BS. Psychosocial influences on mortality after myocardial infarction. *N Engl J Med* 1984; **311:** 552–559.
2. Ahern D, Gorkin L, Anderson J *et al.* Biobehavioral variables and mortality or cardiac arrest in the Cardiac Arrhythmia Pilot Study (CAPS). *Am J Cardiol* 1991; **66:** 59–62.
3. Follick M, Gorkin L, Capone R *et al.* Psychological distress as a predictor of ventricular arrhythmias in a post-myocardial infarction population. *Am Heart J* 1988; **116:** 32–36.

4. Ladwig K, Keiser M, Konig J *et al.* Affective disorders and survival after acute myocardial infarction: Results from the post-infarction late potential study. *Eur Heart J* 1991; **12:** 959–964.
5. Wiklund L, Oden A, Sanne H *et al.* Prognostic importance of somatic and psychological variables after a first myocardial infarction. *Am J Epidemiol* 1988; **128:** 786–795.
6. Rahe R, Romo M, Bennett L, Siltanen P. Recent life change, myocardial infarction, and abrupt coronary death. *Arch Int Med* 1974; **133:** 221–228.
7. Frasure-Smith N, Prince R. The Ischaemic Heart Disease Life Stress Monitoring Program: Impact on mortality. *Psychosom Med* 1985; **47:** 431–445.
8. Goldberg DP. *The Detection of Psychiatric Illness by Questionnaire.* Oxford University Press: Oxford, 1972.
9. Prince R, Miranda L. Monitoring life stress to prevent recurrence of coronary heart disease episodes: Report on a feasibility study. *Can Psych Assoc J* 1977; **22:** 161–169.
10. Frasure-Smith N, Prince R. Longterm follow-up of the Ischaemic Heart Disease Life Stress Monitoring Program. *Psychosom Med* 1989; **51:** 485–513.
11. Frasure-Smith N. In hospital symptoms of psychological stress as predictors of longterm outcome following acute myocardial infarction in men. *Am J Cardiol* 1991; **67:** 121–127.

44 Outcome of Psychological Intervention in Heart Disease

Elizabeth L. Cay

Astley Ainslie Hospital, Grange Loan, Edinburgh EH9 2HL, UK

Introduction

The aim of cardiac rehabilitation (CR) is to improve function and to enhance the patient's quality of life by relieving symptoms and slowing progression of the underlying disease. Secondary prevention, an integral part of CR, has the specific goal of reducing rates of reinfarction and cardiac mortality through the lowering of known risk factors for ischaemic heart disease (IHD). This may entail considerable and permanent changes in life style, which many patients find difficult to achieve on their own. As a result, rehabilitation programmes have been set up for patients after myocardial infarction (MI) and coronary artery bypass graft surgery (CABGS) and, more recently, for those with angina pectoris, cardiac failure and following cardiac transplantation.

Quality of life

When outcome is equated with quality of life, an important first step is the recognition that physician and patient do not necessarily agree on what is a good outcome; the physician is interested in improvement and cure of disease, whereas the patient wants a feeling of well-being and health and the ability to lead a normal active life. Descriptive studies of the results of comprehensive

Proceedings of the Vth World Congress on Cardiac Rehabilitation

CR have shown that there are positive gains from intervention. Traditionally, these have been divided into physical, psychological and social outcomes:

1. *Physical benefits*: increase in maximal work capacity of 20%; less angina.
2. *Psychological benefits*: increased energy, enthusiasm, well-being; decreased depression and anxiety; improved self-image; improved ability to deal with stress; improved sexual activity; fewer tranquillizers, hypnotics.
3. *Socio-economic benefits*: increased optimism, enthusiasm, creativity; less illness, absenteeism; shorter invalidism; reduced expenses, benefits.

As a result, it is possible to understand quality of life as applicable to the patient with IHD. It depends on the ability to perform the tasks of daily living with the least physical and psychological restrictions and the least threat to life and health [1].

The determining factors of quality of life have been identified: functional capacity, psychological state, personal functioning (activities of daily living) and symptoms and risks as a result of the disease process [2]. These factors are interrelated and determine outcome of cardiac rehabilitation. They are influenced by a variety of social, cultural and environmental factors [1].

Implications

There are implications when outcome is equated with quality of life:

1. Assessment becomes multifactorial.
2. The needs of the individual have to be taken into account to a greater extent than before.
3. In theory, outcome can be different in each patient. For a good outcome, what is perceived by the physician as feasible must match what the patient wants.
4. Patients lose their passive role. They have to become responsible for their own life-style changes.
5. CR must become more flexible, with programmes tailored to the needs of the individual. To do this, the components of a comprehensive programme must be examined separately to see which one gives the best results both in the short and long term.

Results of psychological intervention

Before examining the results of various different kinds of psychological intervention, it is important to remember that having a MI has a considerable psychological impact on the individual. Following their infarct, one-third of patients reported increased physical activity, improved eating habits and less stress and competition at work. Half were very glad to be alive and put greater store on enjoyment of hobbies, family life and having good health, where previously they had rated success at work as being most important [3]. Obviously, immediately after MI, patients are motivated to change and educational programmes have been developed to capitalize on this and attempt to produce long-term benefits.

On the whole, education and advice have proved somewhat disappointing. With increasing length of time after an infarct or CABGS, patients revert to previous bad habits [4, 5]. An educational programme before surgery, while of benefit in the short term, had little or no effect on areas that required long-term behavioural changes [6]. An important factor may well be that, while there has been much stress for many years on the value of educating patients about their disease, it is only recently that patients' own perceptions of the cause of their MI and their knowledge of risk factors have been studied. Psychological factors (overwork, stress, worry) were the most frequently cited causes of their MI according to the patients, with smoking, being overweight and overeating the most frequently cited risk factors [7]. This contrasts with medical opinion which emphasizes biological causes. A post-surgical group did not think that they had been at all well prepared for operation and its aftermath, particularly in areas that affected their quality of life [8]. Unless these specific areas of concern are addressed, patients feel that they get little help with the most life-threatening aspects of their disease, and the result is likely to be poor compliance and high psychological morbidity. Where these issues are taken into account, educational programmes have been more successful, with gains lasting at least a year after MI. In a controlled trial, counselling did not have any advantage over education [9].

Programmes using more formal psychological techniques have shown benefits. A daily programme of individual psychotherapy produced marked improvement in physical and emotional state 4 months after MI compared to controls with standard medical care [10]. Stress management and relaxation training resulted in improved psychological and vocational outcome 6 months post-MI [11]. Other studies have reported significant cardiological and secondary preventive effects using psychological methods of intervention: fewer deaths, lower rates of reinfarction, fewer supraventricular arrhythmias in a coronary care unit, less medication and fewer readmissions to hospital [10, 12–15]. An intensive behavioural modification programme resulted in comprehensive lifestyle changes and regression of atherosclerosis [16].

It appears that psychological intervention is effective, yet its value is largely ignored. In practice, psychological factors are not considered and many patients lead miserable unproductive lives after the diagnosis of IHD is made; they lack the confidence to resume any physical activity even after successful revascularization and unnecessarily become cardiac invalids.

Current practice

Advances in treatment of acute episodes, new investigative techniques and the advent of CABGS and balloon angioplasty have increased the workload of the cardiologist and used up often scarce resources. Patients spend less time in hospital. As a result, the cardiologist has become more specialized with less time to spare for rehabilitation issues. On the other hand, rehabilitation physicians have instituted expensive, elaborate in-patient and out-patient programmes which require a team of specialist staff. Instead of CR and secondary prevention becoming an integral part of patient care, it is seen as the province of the specialist and, as such, available only to a few patients.

There is evidence that the picture is slowly changing. Cardiologists are becoming more aware of the benefits of CR and secondary prevention; there has been increasing interest on the part of those involved in rehabilitation in developing simple rehabilitation interventions. To this has been added an increase in patient demand for CR. They are more knowledgeable about what they can expect of treatment, they are encouraged to voice their own beliefs and hopes and to become more responsible for their health, as they have been subjected to intense media coverage on the effects of a healthier life style.

Simplifying rehabilitation

An example of one way of bringing rehabilitation within the reach of almost every patient after MI is the development, by a clinical psychologist in the Rehabilitation Medicine Unit, Edinburgh, of a 6-week self-administered cardiac rehabilitation programme (The Heart Manual) which contains all the components of a comprehensive CR programme. Emphasis is laid on the correction of erroneous beliefs and that the onus is on the individual to change his or her lifestyle. The manual is introduced before the patient leaves hospital and spouses are included. A controlled trial has demonstrated that patients using the manual have greater self-confidence, less emotional distress, an improved quality of life, greater changes in dietary habits and are less dependent on medical services over the next year when compared to controls [17].

Cardiac rehabilitation: A cheaper alternative

Another approach is to demonstrate that psychological intervention may offer a cheaper alternative to other methods of treatment. Patients with continuing angina use a great many resources: readmissions to hospital, reinvestigations and revascularization procedures. The clinical psychologist at the Rehabilitation Unit, Edinburgh has used pain management techniques to develop a 7-

week course for patients with angina. They attend hospital in groups twice a week. The preliminary results of a controlled trial have included decrease in symptoms, increased physical activity and less dependence on medication. Fifty percent of patients on the waiting list for elective CABGS who attended the course have not required operation and these beneficial results are persisting over a year.

These are two examples of possible advances. More innovative approaches are needed if the goal of making cost-effective CR available to all patients is to be achieved.

References

1. Imperial ES. Approach to cardiac rehabilitation. *Clin Rehab* 1987; **1:** 203–210.
2. Wenger NK. Quality of life: Concept and approach to measurement. *Adv Cardiol* 1986; **33:** 122–130.
3. Laerum E, Johnsen N, Smith P, Larsen S. Myocardial infarction may induce positive changes in life-style and in the quality of life. *Scand J Prim Health Care* 1988; **6:** 67–71.
4. Higgins C, Schweiger MJ. Smoking termination patterns in a cardiac rehabilitation population. *J Cardiac Rehabil* 1983; **3:** 55–59.
5. CASS Principal Investigators and their Associates. Coronary Artery Surgery Study (CASS): A randomised trial of coronary artery bypass surgery. Quality of life in patients randomly assigned to treatment groups. *Circulation* 1983; **68:** 951–960.
6. Steele LE, Ruzicki D. An evaluation of the effectiveness of cardiac teaching during hospitalisation. *Heart Lung* 1987; **16:** 306–311.
7. Maeland JG, Havik OE. After the myocardial infarction: A medical and psychological study with special emphasis on perceived illness. *Scand J Rehabil Med* (Suppl. 22.) 1989.
8. Stanton BA, Jenkins CD, Savageau JA, Thurer RL. Functional benefits following coronary bypass graft surgery. *Ann Thor Surg* 1984; **37:** 286–290.
9. Oldenburg B, Perkins RJ, Andrews G. Controlled trial of psychological intervention in myocardial infarction. *J Consult Clin Psychol* 1985; **53:** 852–859.
10. Gruen W. Effects of brief psychotherapy during the hospitalisation period in the recovery process in heart attacks. *J Consult Clin Psychol* 1975; **43:** 223–232.
11. Langosch W, Seer P, Brodner G, Kallinke D, Kulick B, Heim P. Behaviour therapy with coronary heart disease patients: Results of a comparative study. *J Psychosom Res* 1982; **26:** 475–484.
12. Brenner H. Themzentierte gesprache und verhaltensubungen zur einstellungsund verhaltensanderung von hertzinfarktpatienten. In: *Psychosoziale Probleme und Psychotherapeutische Interventionsmoglichkeiten bei Herzinfarktpatienten.* Minerva Publikation: Muchen, 1980, pp. 201–226.
13. Brenner H. Heizinfarkt und selbstverantwortung. *Pravention* 1981; **4:** 13–18.
14. Fielding R. Behavioural treatment in the rehabilitation of myocardial infarction patients. In: *Research in Psychology and Medicine*, Academic Press: London, 1979, pp. 176–182.
15. Freidman M, Thorensen CE, Gill JJ, Ulmer D, Thompson D, Powell L, Prive V, Eleck SR, Rabin DD, Breall WS, Piaget G, Dixon T, Bourg E, Levy RA, Tasto DL. Feasibility of altering type A behaviour pattern after myocardial infarc tion. Recurrent coronary prevention project study: Methods, baseline results and preliminary findings. *Circulation* 1982; **66:** 83–92.

16. Ornish D, Brown SE, Scherwitz LW, Billings JH, Armstrong WT, Ports TA, McLanahan S, Kirkeeide RL, Brand RJ, Gould KL. Can life-style changes reverse coronary heart disease? The Life-Style Heart Trial. *Lancet* 1990; **336:** 129–133.
17. Lewin B, Robertson IH, Cay EL, Irving JB, Campbell M. Effects of self-help post-myocardial-infarction rehabilitation on psychological adjustment and use of health services. *Lancet* 1992; **339:** 1036–1040.

XI Regression of Atherosclerosis

45 Can Lifestyle Changes Reverse Coronary Heart Disease? The Lifestyle Heart Trial

Dean Ornish

Preventive Medicine Research Institute, 1001 Bridgeway, Suite 305, Sausalito, CA 94965, USA

Can atherosclerosis regress?

The Lifestyle Heart Trial is a randomized, controlled clinical trial to determine if ambulatory patients can be motivated to make and sustain comprehensive lifestyle changes and, if so, whether regression of coronary atherosclerosis can occur due to lifestyle changes alone. The Lifestyle Heart Trial is in two phases: phase 1 (after 1 year of intervention, completed) and phase 2 (the same patients after 4 years, still in progress) [1–7]. Two previous trials in 1977 and 1980 assessed the short-term effects of lifestyle changes on coronary heart disease using non-invasive endpoint measures. These two studies measured improvements in cardiac risk factors, functional status, myocardial perfusion [8] and left ventricular function [9, 10].

In the Lifestyle Heart Trial, patients were randomly assigned to an experimental group asked to make comprehensive lifestyle changes or to a usual care control group who followed more conventional recommendations. Average percent diameter stenosis (%D) regressed from 40.0 to 37.8% in the experimental group, yet progressed from 42.7 to 46.1% in the control group ($P = 0.001$). When only lesions greater than 50% stenosed were analysed, average %D regressed from 61.1 to 55.8% in the experimental group and progressed from 61.7 to 64.4% in the control group ($P = 0.03$). Overall, 82% of the experimental group patients had an average change which was in the direction of regression. Degree of overall adherence was strongly related to

Proceedings of the Vth World Congress on Cardiac Rehabilitation

changes in %D in a "dose-response" relationship ($r = 0.62$, $P = 0.003$). Thus, comprehensive lifestyle changes may cause significant regression of even severe coronary atherosclerosis to begin occurring after only 1 year, whereas more moderate changes resulted in significant progression of atherosclerosis.

In the Lifestyle Heart Trial, patients with angiographically documented coronary artery disease at baseline who were not taking cholesterol-lowering drugs were randomly assigned to an experimental group or to a usual care control group. All patients who were eligible and volunteered were accepted into the study. Experimental group patients were prescribed a lifestyle programme that included a low-fat vegetarian diet, moderate aerobic exercise, stress management training, smoking cessation and group support. Control group patients were not asked to make lifestyle changes, although they were free to do so. Progression or regression of coronary artery lesions was assessed in both groups by quantitative coronary angiography at baseline and after approximately 1 year. Cine-arteriograms made in San Francisco were sent to the University of Texas Medical School at Houston for quantitative analyses [11].

The patients completed a 3-day diet diary at baseline and after 1 year to assess nutrient intake and dietary adherence [12]. They were asked to complete a questionnaire describing smoking behaviour and the type, frequency and duration of exercise and of each stress management technique. Information from these adherence questionnaires was quantified using a formula determined *a priori.* To reduce the possibility that knowledge of group assignment may bias the outcome measurements, the technicians responsible for all medical tests remained unaware of patient group assignment. Different personnel provided the lifestyle intervention, performed the tests, analysed the results, and computed statistical analyses.

The patients in the experimental group were asked to consume a low-fat vegetarian diet for at least one year, which included fruits, vegetables, grains, legumes and soybean products without caloric restriction. No animal products were allowed except for egg whites and one cup per day of non-fat milk or yoghurt. The diet contained approximately 10% calories as fat (P/S ratio >1), 15–20% protein and 70–75% predominantly complex carbohydrates. Cholesterol intake was limited to 5 mg/day or less. Salt was restricted only for hypertensive patients. Caffeine was eliminated, and alcohol was limited to no more than 2 oz per day or equivalent. The stress management techniques included stretching exercises, breathing techniques, meditation, progressive relaxation and imagery [3, 13–15]. The patients were asked to practise these stress management techniques for at least 1 h/day. The patients were individually prescribed exercise levels (typically walking) according to their baseline treadmill test results. They were asked to exercise for a minimum of 3 h/week and to spend a minimum of 30 min/session exercising within their target heart rates. The twice-weekly group discussions provided social support to help patients adhere to the lifestyle-change programme [3, 16, 24–25].

Differences in the baseline characteristics of the experimental and control group patients were tested for statistical significance by use of conventional

t-tests. Comparisons of these two study groups with respect to baseline coronary artery lesion characteristics (measured by quantitative coronary angiography) and changes in lesion characteristics from pre- to post-intervention were examined via a mixed model analysis of variance with clusters of varying sizes [17]. Mean changes in other endpoint measures were analysed for statistical significance by repeated-measures analysis of variance.

At baseline, there were no significant differences between the experimental and control groups in demographic characteristics, diet and lifestyle characteristics, functional status, cardiac history, or risk factors. HDL and apolipoprotein A-I were significantly higher in the control group, but ratios of total cholesterol/HDL and LDL/HDL were not significantly different between groups at baseline. At baseline, the experimental and control groups did not significantly differ in disease severity as measured by minimum diameter (D_{min}), percent diameter reduction (%D), normal diameter (D_{norm}), or stenosis flow reserve (SFR).

In the experimental group, adherence to the diet, exercise and stress management components of the lifestyle programme was excellent. The patients in the control group made more moderate changes in lifestyle consistent with more conventional recommendations, including a diet consisting of approximately 30% fat and 200 mg dietary cholesterol. In the experimental group, total cholesterol decreased from 226.5 to 171.5 mg/dl (24.3%) and LDL cholesterol fell from 151.4 to 94.8 mg/dl (37.4%). These decreases occurred even though many patients already had made some dietary changes prior to baseline testing. HDL cholesterol did not change significantly in either group. In the experimental group, apolipoprotein B decreased from 104.0 to 78.9, but it did not change appreciably in the control group. Neither group had significant changes in apolipoprotein A-I.

Functional status improved considerably, and in many patients dramatically. The patients in the experimental group reported a 91% reduction in the frequency of angina, a 42% decrease in the duration of angina and a 28% decrease in the severity of angina. In contrast, the patients in the control group reported a 165% increase in frequency, a 95% increase in duration and a 39% increase in severity of angina. In our earlier studies, we found that similar improvements in functional status occurred in only 1 month [8–10], suggesting that improvements in angina may precede regression of coronary atherosclerosis, perhaps by altering platelet–endothelial interactions, vasomotor tone, or other dynamic characteristics of stenoses.

All detectable lesions were included for analysis. Altogether, 195 coronary artery lesions were detected and quantitatively analysed. When all the lesions were included, average %D regressed from 40.0 to 37.8% in the experimental group, yet progressed from 42.7 to 46.1% in the control group ($P = 0.001$, two-tailed). When only lesions greater than 50% stenosed were analysed, average %D regressed from 61.1 to 55.8% in the experimental group and progressed from 61.7 to 64.4% in the control group ($P = 0.03$, two-tailed).

Eighteen of the 22 patients (82%) in the experimental group had average lesion change scores ($\%D_{post} - \%D_{pre}$) in the direction of regression of coronary atherosclerosis (including the one woman in the experimental group). In contrast, 10 of the 19 control group patients (53%) had average lesion change scores in the direction of progression of coronary atherosclerosis; in contrast, all of the four women in the control group had average lesion change scores in the direction of regression of coronary atherosclerosis.

Within-group secondary analyses were performed to determine if the experimental group showed "true regression" rather than simply less progression than the control group. In this analysis, the experimental group showed 2.11 ± 0.98 units in the direction of regression ($P = 0.03$, two-tailed); the control group showed 4.23 ± 2.91 units in the direction of progression ($P = 0.15$, two-tailed).

In the experimental group and in the combined groups, overall adherence to the lifestyle changes was strongly related to changes in lesions in a "dose–response" relationship, suggesting a causal relationship between lifestyle changes and coronary atherosclerosis. These differences in overall adherence are sufficient to explain the observed differences in $\%D$. To assess whether programme adherence was related to lesion changes, patients in the experimental group and in the combined groups were divided into three equal tertiles based on overall adherence score. Degree of adherence directly correlated with changes in $\%D$.

This clinical trial demonstrated that a heterogeneous group of patients with coronary heart disease were motivated to make comprehensive changes in lifestyle for at least 1 year in an ambulatory population. These lifestyle changes substantially reduced total cholesterol, LDL cholesterol and apolipoprotein B, while HDL cholesterol and apolipoprotein A-I remained about the same. These lipid changes are comparable to those seen in studies in which cholesterol-lowering drugs are used. This intervention appears to be safe and compatible with other treatments of coronary heart disease.

After 1 year, the patients in the experimental group began to demonstrate significant overall regression of coronary atherosclerosis (decreased $\%D$) as measured by quantitative coronary arteriography. Since coronary atherosclerosis occurs over a period of decades, one would not expect to find larger changes in only 1 year. Perfusion is a fourth power function of coronary artery diameter, so even a small amount of regression in a critically stenosed artery has a disproportionate effect on myocardial perfusion and thus on functional status and clinical significance. In contrast, the patients in the usual care control group who were making less comprehensive changes in lifestyle demonstrated significant overall progression of coronary atherosclerosis. This suggests that conventional recommendations for patients with coronary heart disease (such as a 30% fat diet) may not be sufficient to cause regression to occur in many patients, and that more comprehensive lifestyle changes may be required.

The strong relationship between programme adherence and lesion changes indicated that most patients needed to follow the lifestyle programme as prescribed in order to show regression. Those who made even more changes demonstrated even greater improvement. Since degree of lifestyle change was correlated with degree of stenosis change across the entire range of adherence, even moderate changes in lifestyle may slow the progression of atherosclerosis, whereas substantial changes in lifestyle may be required in order to halt or reverse coronary atherosclerosis.

The five women in the study were the notable exceptions. One woman was randomly assigned to the experimental group and four women were randomly assigned to the control group. All five of these women made only moderate lifestyle changes, yet all showed overall regression. All five were post-menopausal, and none were taking exogenous oestrogens. The four women in the control group showed more regression than any of the men in that group, even though some men made greater changes in lifestyle. While the numbers are small, these data raise the interesting question if gender may influence progression and regression of atherosclerosis.

Five men in the control group also demonstrated very small changes in average $\%D$ in the direction of atherosclerosis regression. These patients exercised more often, for longer periods, and consumed fewer calories and less cholesterol than the control group patients who showed progression of atherosclerosis.

The more severely stenosed lesions showed the greatest improvement. Although this is opposite of what was expected, the finding is important since more severely stenotic lesions are of greatest clinical significance. More work is needed to determine to what extent the relationship between change and initial site of lesions is influenced by the statistical phenomenon known as regression to the mean.

Some important questions remain unanswered. Whether or not these comprehensive lifestyle changes can be sustained in larger populations of patients with coronary heart disease remains to be determined. What is optimal is not always easy. Further research will be necessary to determine the mechanisms of changes in coronary atherosclerosis. It would be especially interesting to examine the effects of lifestyle changes in a larger sample of post-menopausal women with coronary atherosclerosis. Also, direct comparisons of intensive lifestyle changes with pharmacological or surgical interventions are interesting questions needing study. The Lifestyle Heart Trial suggests that comprehensive lifestyle changes may begin to reverse coronary atherosclerosis in only 1 year [11, 19].

If so, what can be done to achieve regression of human atherosclerosis?

Regression of coronary atherosclerosis in humans has been reported, either in controlled clinical trials or in anecdotal reports, in response to comprehensive lifestyle changes, various cholesterol-lowering drugs, partial ileal bypass surgery, or plasmapheresis. Each of these interventions may be appropriate in some circumstances, either solely or in combination with other interventions. Given these possibilities, what criteria should determine our choice of intervention?

The following criteria may be helpful: medical effectiveness, cost-effectiveness, risk-benefit ratio and patient motivation/adherence.

1. *Medical effectiveness.* Comprehensive lifestyle changes may cause significant improvement in risk factors and regression of coronary atherosclerosis. In comparison with other interventions, the Lifestyle Heart Trial measured a greater degree of overall regression in a shorter period of time. However, one should interpret comparisons between studies with caution given the variations from one study to another in patient populations, recruitment, endpoint methodologies and statistical methods.

2. *Cost-effectiveness.* Cholesterol-lowering medications are costly. Lovastatin, for example, may cost $1500/year; these costs are considerable when multiplied by the large numbers of people with hypercholesterolaemia. As the goals for desirable plasma cholesterol levels become lower (from 260 to 200 to below 150 mg/dl), the number of people whose plasma cholesterol levels are defined as too high increases. Partial ileal bypass surgery and plasmapheresis are expensive and invasive. In principle, at least, a vegetarian diet, moderate exercise, smoking cessation and stress management may be learned at moderate cost. While no-one has tested this hypothesis, it would not be surprising if comprehensive lifestyle changes may lower utilization of medications (e.g. lipid-lowering drugs) or surgery (e.g. angioplasty or coronary artery bypass surgery), thereby lowering health care costs.

3. *Risk-benefit ratio.* All drugs, including lipid-lowering medications, have risks and side-effects, both known and unknown, as well as potential benefits. The same is true for plasmapheresis and partial ileal bypass surgery. In contrast, the only side-effects of lifestyle changes are generally desirable ones.

4. *Patient motivation/adherence.* Clearly, the major obstacle to widespread adoption of comprehensive lifestyle changes is patient adherence. It is often easier to submit to surgery or take medications than to change one's lifestyle. Paradoxically, however, it may be easier to motivate patients to make and maintain comprehensive changes in lifestyle than more moderate ones. When a patient makes only moderate changes in diet and lifestyle, there is often a feeling of deprivation but without substantial improvements in symptoms or plasma cholesterol levels. However, comprehensive lifestyle changes often cause marked reductions in frequency of angina and plasma cholesterol levels, so the choices and benefits become clearer. Patients who, for whatever reason, do not wish to make comprehensive changes in lifestyle, should be offered cholesterol-lowering drugs or other options after a clear discussion of the relative risks and benefits of each approach.

In the Lifestyle Heart Trial, we found that adherence to lifestyle changes was strongly correlated with changes in coronary atherosclerosis in a "dose–response" pattern across the entire range of adherence in both the experimental and control groups. Regression tended to occur when adherence was high, even when plasma cholesterol levels did not fall below 150 mg/dl or even 200 mg/dl. Serum cholesterol levels are important, but coronary heart disease is a multifactorial illness. Evidence suggests that dietary cholesterol and fat may contribute to coronary atherosclerosis in part independent of the effects on plasma cholesterol levels [18,19]. Algorithms for treating hypercholesterolaemia may tend to focus too much on plasma cholesterol levels; attention also should be given to dietary and lifestyle factors.

Is regression of human atherosclerosis measurable?

Using the methods of quantitative coronary arteriography (QCA) pioneered by Brown [20], Blankenhorn [21], Gould [11] and others, it is now possible to measure the degree of coronary atherosclerosis with reasonable accuracy and reproducibility. This accuracy makes feasible clinical trials with smaller cohorts and shorter durations. However, coronary arteriography, even when quantitatively analysed, has some inherent limitations:

1. Atherosclerosis exists to a considerable degree before it impinges into the arterial lumen. Glagov *et al.* [22] demonstrated that human coronary arteries undergo compensatory enlargement in the presence of coronary atherosclerosis to preserve the cross-sectional area of the lumen. Coronary arteries enlarge as the lesion area increases, and luminal stenosis may be delayed until the lesion occupies more than 40% of the internal elastic lamina, after which the lumen diminishes markedly. This phenomenon would make it more difficult to detect regression or progression in lesions that are less than 40–50% stenosed at baseline, since compensatory changes in the cross-sectional area of the lumen may occur. In contrast, there would be less compensation in more severe lesions, so progression or regression would be easier to measure. Emerging technologies such as intravascular ultrasound may give a more accurate picture of the true extent of coronary atherosclerosis.
2. It is difficult to distinguish between changes in atherosclerosis and changes in vasomotor tone. If one defines "regression" as "clinical improvement", then the question is less important, for both improvements in coronary atherosclerosis and in vasomotor tone increase myocardial perfusion. Giving nitroglycerin at the time of angiography may reduce coronary vasoconstriction; however, this may introduce another confounding variable, for nitroglycerin may not always affect vasomotor tone to the same degree each time in a given patient.
3. There is no consensus on the best endpoint measure in QCA. Traditionally, percent diameter stenosis ($\%D$) has been used, but there are limitations. $\%D$ is a function both of D_{min} and the "normal" segment adjacent to it. However, as discussed by Glagov *et al.* [22] even seemingly normal segments are likely to have disease. Also, one may have an apparent improvement in $\%D$ if the proximal or distal "normal" segments narrow and D_{min} is unchanged, since $\%D$ is a relative difference between D_{min} and $\%D$. On the other hand, up to a point, a reduction in D_{norm} may paradoxically improve perfusion if D_{min} remains constant due to a reduction in exit losses.

The use of relative percent diameter narrowing as a clinical measure of severity does not account for other important geometric characteristics of stenoses, such as length, absolute cross-sectional luminal area, multiple lesions in series, or eccentric narrowing which may be worse in one view compared to another view. The concept of stenosis flow reserve (SFR) is one way of addressing this dilemma, but it, too, has limitations. The anatomic-geometric approach utilizes all of the X-ray determined geometric dimensions of a stenosis, including percent narrowing, absolute diameter and length effects. These dimensions are integrated throughout the length of the stenosis using fluid dynamic equations to predict the pressure flow characteristics of the SFR as a single integrated measure of its severity, reflecting all of the combined effects of percent narrowing, absolute diameter and length. Determination of stenosis flow reserve by this quantitative analysis of coronary arteriograms correlates well with directly measured flow reserve in animals and with perfusion effects in man. In practice, however, SFR is a close function of $\%D$ and may not add much additional information. Also, there is little change in SFR until a lesion becomes severely stenosed.

4. Atherosclerosis is only one of several mechanisms affecting perfusion. Changes in coronary vasomotor tone, platelet adherence and aggregation, collateral circulation, free fatty acid metabolism, local endothelial factors, preload/afterload factors, and other mechanisms may affect myocardial perfusion. Since perfusion is the "bottom line" in coronary heart disease, functional measures of perfusion (e.g. cardiac PET imaging) may be a better "gold standard" than anatomical measures such as coronary arteriography. Both anatomical and functional measures provide complementary information.

5. "Not everything that counts can be counted" (Burkitt). We focus on what is measurable, but what is measurable may not necessarily be what is most interesting or important. In the FATS study by Brown *et al.* [23], for example, there was a 73% reduction in clinical events, yet only a 0.7–0.9% diameter stenosis regression in the experimental group. Thus, other mechanisms than regression of coronary atherosclerosis may play important roles. Psychosocial factors are more difficult to measure, although these, too, may play important roles in both adherence and in outcome [18].

References

1. Ornish DM, Brown SE, Scherwitz LW, *et al.* Can lifestyle changes reverse coronary atherosclerosis? The Lifestyle Heart Trial. *Lancet* 1990; **336:** 129–133; *Yearbook of Medicine* and *Yearbook of Cardiology*. C.V. Mosby: New York, 1991.
2. Gould KL, Ornish D, Kirkeeide R, *et al.* Improved stenosis geometry by quantitative coronary arteriography after vigorous risk factor modification. *Am J Cardiol* 1992; **69:** 845–853.
3. Ornish D. *Reversing Heart Disease.* Ballantine Books: New York, 1992.
4. Ornish D. Reversing heart disease through diet, exercise, and stress management. *J Am Dietetic Assoc* 1991; **91:** 162–165.

5. Ornish D. Can life-style changes reverse coronary atherosclerosis? *Hospital Practice*, May 1991.
6. Ornish D. Lessons from the Lifestyle Heart Trial. *Choices in Cardiology* 1991; **1:** 1–4.
7. Ornish D. Can you prevent – and reverse – coronary artery disease? *Patient Care* 1991; **25:** 25–41.
8. Ornish DM, Gotto AM, Miller RR, *et al.* Effects of a vegetarian diet and selected yoga techniques in the treatment of coronary heart disease. *Clin Res* 1979; **27:** 720A.
9. Ornish DM, Scherwitz LW, Doody RS, *et al.* Effects of stress management training and dietary changes in treating ischemic heart disease. *JAMA* 1983; **249:** 54–59.
10. Ornish DM. *Stress, Diet, & Your Heart.* Holt, Rinehart and Winston: New York, 1982.
11. Gould KL. Identifying and measuring severity of coronary artery stenosis: Quantitative coronary arteriography and positron emission tomography. *Circulation.* 1988; **78:** 237–245.
12. Stuff JE, Garza C, Smith EO, *et al.* A comparison of dietary methods in nutritional studies. *Am J Clin Nutr* 1983; **37:** 300–306.
13. Benson H, Rosner BA, Marzetta BR, Klemchuk HM. Decreased blood pressure in pharmacologically treated hypertensive patients who regularly elicited the relaxation response. *Lancet* 1974; **i:** 289–291.
14. Patel C, North WR. Randomised controlled trial of yoga and bio-feedback in management of hypertension. *Lancet* 1975; **ii:** 93–95.
15. Patel C, Marmot MG, Terry DJ, Carruthers M, Hunt B, Patel M. Trial of relaxation in reducing coronary risk: Four year follow up. *Br Med J* 1985; **290:** 1103–1106.
16. Orth-Gomer K, Unden AL, Edwards ME. Social isolation and mortality in ischemic heart disease. *Acta Med Scand* 1988; **224:** 205–215.
17. Dixon WS *et al.* (eds). *BMDP3V* statistical software. University of California Press: Berkeley, CA, 1983.
18. Blankenhorn DH, Johnson RL, El Zein HA, *et al.* Dietary fat influences human coronary lesion formation. *Circulation* (Suppl. II) 1988; **78:** 11.
19. Shekelle RB, Stamler J. Dietary cholesterol and ischemic heart disease. *Lancet* 1989; **i:** 1177–1179.
20. Brown BG, Bolson EL, Dodge HT. Arteriographic assessment of coronary atherosclerosis: Review of current methods, their limitations, and clinical applications. *Arteriosclerosis* 1982; **2:** 2–15.
21. Barndt R, Blankenhorn DH, Crawford DW, *et al.* Regression and progression of early femoral atherosclerosis in treated hyperlipoproteinemic patients. *Ann Intern Med* 1977; **86:** 139–146.
22. Glagov S, Weisenberg E, Zarins CK *et al.* Compensatory enlargement of human atherosclerotic coronary arteries. *N Engl J Med* 1987; **316:** 1371–1375.
23. Brown BG, Alberts JJ, Fisher LD *et al.* Regression of coronary artery disease as a result of intensive lipid-lowering therapy in men with high levels of apolipoprotein B. *N Engl J Med* 1990; **323:** 1289–1298.
24. Ruberman W, Weinblatt E, Goldberg JD, Chaudhary BS. Psychosocial influences on mortality after myocardial infarction. *N Engl J Med* 1984; **311:** 552–559.
25. House JS, Landis KR, Umberson D. Social relationships and health. *Science* 1988; **241:** 540–545.

46 Physical Activity and the Risk of Coronary Heart Disease

Henry Blackburn, David R. Jacobs

School of Public Health, University of Minnesota, 1300 South 2nd Street, Minneapolis, MN 55454, USA

Introduction

The role of physical activity in the cause and prevention of cardiovascular disease (CVD) and other diseases is a major issue for the public health. We review here the epidemiological evidence from observational and experimental studies about the relationship of habitual physical activity and fitness to coronary heart disease (CHD) risk and total mortality in healthy populations and cardiac patients living in affluent societies. This subject has been extensively studied and exhaustively reviewed so that this update will include only recent studies and statistical summaries.

Background

Mass diseases result from profound changes in cultural patterns of behaviour against an evolutionary genetic legacy. The cultural changes and accompanying epidemics are dynamic, often changing direction in less than a generation. An anthropological view finds that mass physical inactivity is a pervasive recent change in the human condition. In this view, modern humans are still hunter-gatherers metabolically and the sedentariness of civilization is regarded as a major environmental stress on an evolutionary legacy [1]. Modern industrial societies create "sick and well" populations as well as sick and well individuals

Proceedings of the Vth World Congress on Cardiac Rehabilitation

[2], while physical inactivity as a risk factor for coronary heart disease may act differently among individuals than among populations [3].

Meta-analyses

The "new-fangled business" of meta-analysis, that is, the mathematical synthesis of multiple study results, can be hazardous if used indiscriminantly. It can serve a useful purpose, however, in reviewing many similar sources of evidence. The systematic application of agreed definitions, criteria and analyses tends in itself to strengthen any process of synthesis. That logic is more important to a sound review than a given level of "statistical significance" eventually assigned to the outcome.

Trials of cardiac rehabilitation

Individual randomized clinical trials (RCT) of rehabilitation programmes involving exercise following myocardial infarction have all had samples too small to detect potentially important reductions in mortality, or to elucidate any specific role of exercise. The major statistical reviews of these trials combined will therefore be considered, among equally scholarly if less mathematically formal syntheses attempted by numerous investigators over recent years [4-7].

Table 1 presents the first statistical summary attempted of the RCT of cardiac rehabilitation [8]. Criteria for entry of studies into this analysis were not as formal then as currently used ones, but the authors concluded that exercise rehabilitation might reduce mortality as much as 20%, particularly if started within 3 months after the infarction. They appropriately pointed out, however, that the pooled results indicated randomization of 5000–10,000 patients would be required to demonstrate this difference (20%) with confidence. In the autumn of 1970, a WHO Working Group on Cardiac Rehabilitation meeting in Bordeaux made comparable estimates of 3000–5000 randomized subjects required to detect an anticipated 25% effect of rehabilitation [9]. And there we remain today.

This preliminary effort at a statistical overview [8] was followed by two broader, more thoroughgoing syntheses, one by Oldridge and colleagues in 1988 [10], which pooled only the "10 best" trials, and the other by O'Connor and colleagues in 1989 [11], based on a worldwide survey. The meta-analysis of risk by Oldridge and colleagues used rigorous clinical and analytical criteria to include, in a statistical summary, 10 of the better-designed RCT among a world wide survey of studies. Table 2 presents their results and indicates an estimated 24% reduction (risk ratio, RR = 0.76) of deaths from all causes in patients undergoing cardiac rehabilitation and a 25% reduction in CVD mortality overall, both of which estimates are clinically important and significant statistically. There was, however, a 15% greater incidence (RR = 1.15) of non-fatal myocardial infarction (not statistically significant) in treated groups

Table 1
Meta-analysis of randomized clinical trials (RCT) of exercise rehabilitation post-infarction

	Experimental	Control	Pooled odds ratio	Confidence intervals
Total mortality				
Started early	115/642 (18%)	152/652 (23%)	0.71	(0.54–0.94)
Started up to 3 years	51/702 (7%)	50/682 (7%)	0.98	(0.66–1.47)
All trials	166/1344 (12%)	202/1334 (15%)	0.79	(0.63–0.99)
Non-fatal myocardial infarction				
	134/1344 (10%)	116/1334 (9%)	1.2	(0.89–1.5)

Source: Collins *et al.* [8].

combined, and a 32% excess (approaching nominal levels of statistical significance) in treated groups among which cardiac rehabilitation was begun very early, that is, within 8 weeks after myocardial infarction. The data suggest that programme emphasis on risk factor reduction *vs* enhanced physical activity made no discernible difference in outcome, but that longer programmes result in greater reduction in mortality risk.

Table 3 presents the results of a study by O'Connor *et al.* [11], giving pooled odds ratios and confidence intervals on 22 RCT having "objective and re-

Table 2
Cardiac rehabilitation after myocardial infarction: Risk ratios from a meta-analysis of RCT

	All deaths	CVD deaths	Non-fatal myocardial infarction (MI)
All RCT	0.76*	0.75*	1.15
Intervention started			
early after MI	0.78	0.73	1.32
late after MI	0.72	0.80	0.99
Type of intervention			
risk factor emphasis	0.81	0.74	1.28
exercise emphasis	0.89	0.78	1.06
Duration of intervention			
<12 weeks	0.92	0.99	1.15
12–52 weeks	0.76	0.65	1.29
>36 months	0.62*	0.71	1.08

Source: Oldridge *et al.* [10].
* $P < 0.0125$ (adjusted).

Table 3
Summary of odds ratios by endpoints and intervention group

	All interventions			Exercise only			Exercise plus other interventions[a]		
Endpoints	OR	95% CI	Studies (*n*)	OR	95% CI	Studies (*n*)	OR	95% CI	Studies (*n*)
Total mortality (*years*)									
1	0.77	0.59, 1.01	20	0.93	0.62, 1.39	6	0.67	0.47, 0.96	14
2	0.74	0.59, 0.92	19	0.67	0.45, 0.98	5	0.77	0.59, 1.02	14
≥3	0.80	0.66, 0.96	21	0.81	0.60, 1.10	6	0.79	0.62, 1.01	15
CVD mortality (*years*)									
1	0.78	0.58, 1.04	19	0.98	0.61, 1.50	5	0.68	0.48, 0.98	14
2	0.78	0.60, 1.01	17	0.81	0.46, 1.43	3	0.77	0.57, 1.03	14
≥3	0.78	0.63, 0.96	20	0.85	0.59, 1.22	5	0.74	0.57, 0.96	15
Sudden death (*years*)									
1	0.63	0.41, 0.97	15	1.62	0.54, 4.86	2	0.54	0.34, 0.85	13
2	0.76	0.54, 1.06	16	1.12	0.45, 2.80	2	0.71	0.49, 1.02	14
≥3	0.92	0.69, 1.23	17	1.38	0.73, 2.59	3	0.83	0.60, 1.15	14
Fatal MI (*years*)									
1	0.67	0.48, 0.94	17	0.70	0.33, 1.47	3	0.67	0.46, 0.97	14
2	0.73	0.54, 0.97	16	0.77	0.34, 1.73	2	0.72	0.53, 0.98	14
≥3	0.75	0.59, 0.95	18	0.73	0.44, 1.19	4	0.75	0.57, 0.99	14
Nonfatal MI (*years*)									
1	1.09	0.76, 1.57	17	0.78	0.43, 1.44	3	1.31	0.83, 2.05	14
2	1.10	0.82, 1.47	17	0.90	0.55, 1.50	3	1.22	0.85, 1.74	14
≥3	1.09	0.88, 1.34	20	1.01	0.74, 1.37	5	1.16	0.87, 1.56	15

Source: O'Connor *et al.* [11].
Abbreviations: OR, odds ratio; CI, confidence interval; CVD, cardiovascular disease; MI, myocardial infarction.
[a] These included smoking cessation, dietary modification and stress reduction.

producible entry criteria", while it excluded 14 studies from a worldwide survey of the literature. Analysis was primarily influenced by results in 40- to 60-year-old men, involving 502 deaths (82% CVD) among 4554 subjects. The 20% reduction found in the 3-year overall mortality risk was generally similar for the "exercise only" trials (RR = 0.81) and the "exercise plus other" interventions (RR = 0.79). The results were similar for CVD deaths (up to 3 years follow-up) and for sudden deaths during the first year. There was, however, no apparent effect of rehabilitation on non-fatal myocardial infarction (RR = 1.09).

These three pooling results, analysing the same and separate trials, found approximately a 20% reduction in deaths. The authors argued that neither heterogeneity of studies nor confounding were likely contributors to the overall differences, nor were incomplete ascertainment of deaths or publication bias. We conclude from these thorough-going summaries of secondary prevention trials that such programmes probably reduce post-infarction deaths from cardiovascular disease and all causes but apparently have no effect on the risk of recurrent non-fatal myocardial infarction. When initiated very early, they may be associated with excess risk of non-fatal infarction. A positive interpretation of the overall effects of rehabilitation trials is strengthened by the similar direction of results in most of the studies, carried out at different times, with different protocols and populations, and by different investigators.

Primary prevention of CHD

The larger question is about the role of physical activity and fitness in the primary prevention of CHD and atherosclerosis and in the prevention of elevated CVD risk in the first place. This issue is not likely to be tested by rigorous experiment because of the inability to enforce compliance in activity programmes and the immense cost of intervention and testing in the large samples required. We depend, therefore, on inference from the observational evidence about activity, fitness and risk, attempting to identify and adjust for the confounding effects of lifestyle and characteristics other than physical activity.

In 1987, Powell and colleagues [12] performed the pioneering and classic statistical summary of observational studies on the relation of activity to primary risk of CHD and laid the groundwork for subsequent reviews. They made a systematic search of the literature in which 54 studies were garnered and 43 selected for analysis based on prior criteria about the availability of individual activity measurement, adherence, data collection methods, disease classification, confounding variables, population representativeness and loss to follow-up (under 20%). The overall quality of studies was assessed on three major components, the measures of physical activity, the classification of disease and the epidemiologic methods. In 1990, Berlin and Colditz [13] added another important statistical summary of the same and newer studies and contributed further to methods of analysis by developing a continuous score for study quality and isolating occupational and leisure activity for separate analysis. These two efforts were seminal, not only in performing the first statistical summaries of the relations, but for contributions about the type, amount and intensity of exercise and dose–response relations, about standardized CHD diagnoses (showing the effect of diagnostic misclassification), and understanding how relatively small differences in the definition of vigorous activity (e.g. 6 *vs* 7.5 *vs* 10 kcal/min) can account for the different reported results of mortality associations with vigorous activity [14]. They also showed how heterogeneity among studies, within types of activity or disease endpoints, reduces the risk ratios and must be accounted for in the analysis. They both dealt systematically with study quality and devised continuous scores for analyses which showed that study quality was the strongest predictor of RR, stronger in fact than all other variables (e.g. amount of activity); that is, the higher the study quality, the greater the apparent contribution of inactivity to excess risk Berlin and Colditz's regression of quality scores on CHD risk, for example, estimated a ratio of 1 (no correlation) for zero (poor) quality studies and 2.3 for a score of 6 (highest quality).

These two works were also the first to consider systematically and to conclude that rigorous epidemiological criteria for causal inference from statistical associations were fully satisfied by the relationship of inactivity to risk. They confirmed the earlier computations of Paffenbarger and colleagues [15] about the population attributable risk (PAR) or "community risk" of physical inactivity. All concluded that the RR for inactivity, applied to the high prevalence of sedentary people in the population, provides estimates that a substantial proportion of the population risk of CHD is attributable to physical inactivity. Shaper and Wannamethee's [16] study, the only major observational study to appear since these statistical reviews, also made unique contributions to methods by their continuous score for activity validated against heart rate, and by exploring relationships in older and younger men and in symptomatic and asymptomatic coronary patients as well as in the healthy.

Main results

The analysis of Powell *et al.* [12] provided its results according to standard criteria for causal inference for epidemiological associations:

1. *Consistency*: about two-thirds of studies reported a statistically significant association, a graded response, or both.
2. *Strength:* the RR of CHD associated with inactivity ranged from 1.5 to 2.4 with a median value of 1.9 (2.4 for studies with high-quality scores). These values are only a little lower than those for the major CHD risk factors.
3. *Temporality:* two-thirds of studies demonstrated the essential characteristic that the activity classification preceded the CHD event.
4. *Graded response:* 17 of the 25 studies (68%) having appropriate data on dose–response, found lower CVD risk with greater activity.
4. *Plausibility:* experimental exercise reduces levels of several risk factors for atherosclerosis and for myocardial infarction and sudden death and raises levels of "protective" factors.

The summary data of Powell *et al.*, according to an index of calories expended in exercise per week, indicated a lower RR for vigorous activity than for regular activity, and also a "plateau" of association above 3500 kcal/week [14].

Table 4 summarizes the results of the second major meta-analysis, that of Berlin and Colditz [13], giving RR and confidence intervals (CI) for CHD manifestations of incidence, death, myocardial infarction (MI) and MI plus sudden death, according to energy expended in leisure time physical activity (LTPA). The gradient of RR by LTPA class was also found for occupational activity. The authors concluded that the results are consistent with an inverse and graded association of physical activity and CHD. They also considered that if the effect of exercise were only to reduce severity rather than frequency

Table 4
Pooled relative risk for leisure time activity[a]

Physical activity levels compared	CHD	CHD death	Myocardial infarction	Myocardial infarction or sudden death
High *vs* moderate[b]		1.3 (1.0–1.7)	1.4 (1.4–1.7)	
High *vs* low[c]	1.6 (1.3–1.8)	1.9 (1.0–3.4)	1.3 (1.0–1.7)	2.3 (1.5–3.6)
High *vs* sedentary[b]		1.6 (1.2–2.2)	2.9 (1.9–4.5)	

Source: Berlin and Colditz [13].
[a] Same studies as Powell *et al.* [12].
[b] Studies that separated both moderate and sedentary comparison groups.
[c] Studies that did not separate moderate and sedentary comparison groups.

of CVD events, there should be a higher RR for CHD death than for incidence, a pattern not found. They confirmed Powell and co-workers' [12,14] findings of the importance of study quality as the strongest predictor of RR. In the few studies in their analysis where confounding variables could be accounted for, the RR was not significantly altered. They acknowledged, however, an inability to demonstrate conclusively the independence of physical activity from other and related risk factors. They considered that publication bias was unlikely because many of the studies analysed did not find statistically significant results and because positive rather than negative associations were found between study quality and CHD risk.

Figure 1, from the more recent study of these relations by Shaper and Wannamethee [16], shows the risk of "heart attack" significantly lower with a higher index of habitual activity. Moderate and moderately vigorous activity were associated with less than half the level of CHD rates seen in inactive men. The association was greatest in those without pre-existing coronary disease and increased up to classes of moderately vigorous activity. The most vigorously active men, however, had higher rates of heart attack than the men with moderate or moderately vigorous activity, which was entirely accounted for by events in younger men (40–49 years). This excess risk appeared to be related to the degree and type of sporting effort and the presence of hypertension. They found that the overall relationship between physical activity and CHD risk was independent of other risk factors. Symptomatic heart disease patients showed a lower rate of heart attack at light or moderate activity levels, beyond which, however, the risk again increased sharply. Men with asymptomatic ischaemic heart disease showed a greater risk of heart attack with higher levels of activity, but they experienced, if stricken, a progressive decrease in case-fatality according to increasing activity class. To test the claim of Morris that only vigorous activity is associated with lower CHD risk, all those who participated in regular sports at least once a month were eliminated from analysis; the association persisted. Shaper and Wannamethee [16] concluded that "the overall level of physical activity is an important independent predictive factor in CHD and

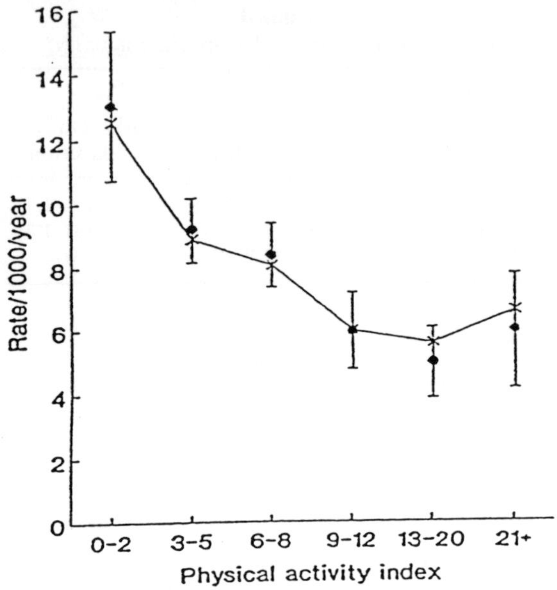

Fig. 1. Heart attack rates (per 1000/year) according to physical activity index. Crude rates (●) with 95% confidence intervals and age-adjusted rates (×). Reproduced from Shaper and Wannamethee [16] with permission.

that vigorous sporting-type exercise, although beneficial in its own right, is not essential in order to obtain such an effect."

Women

In Table 5, modified from Douglas *et al.* [17] and representing five studies from the analysis of Powell *et al.* [12], the RR for activity and CHD in women is of the same order as in men in three out of the five studies, but there is no statistically significant relationship in two, the Framingham and Gothenberg studies, both of which were population-based. Blair *et al.* [18] found that the overall relationship of mortality to activity (fitness) was stronger in women than in men and surmised that exercise and risk factor modification may therefore be potentially more powerful as a preventative measure in women.

Fitness

Fitness, ascertained by a voluntary maximal exercise test, is an objective measure of work capacity and reflects both constitutional characteristics and habitual activity. Blair and colleagues [18] carried out a major study of treadmill performance and disease risk in substantial cohorts of men and women and also reviewed the world literature on fitness and risk. Table 6, taken

Table 5
Physical activity and CHD risk in women

Study	Event	Risk ratio (confidence interval)	Adjusted for:
Israeli kibbutzim	MI	1.8 (0.6–5.1)	
	CHD death	3.0 (0.3–29.4)	Age
North Karelia	MI	1.8 (0.9–3.5)	Age + risk factors
Framingham	CHD death	NS	Age + risk factors
Gothenburg	MI/sudden death angina	NS	Age + risk factors
Netherlands	Angina	5.3 (2.6–10.0)	Age + risk factors

Source: Douglas *et al.* [17].

from their report, shows the considerably greater RR for fitness and CVD than for physical activity classifications, and comparable or greater RR in women than in men. Not shown is the very high RR (around 8) for CVD death. The excess risk for all-cause deaths was due both to excess CVD and cancer deaths. Fitness was independently associated with risk over a variety of single and combined risk factors. Moreover, the slope of association with lower mortality risk appeared with modest levels of fitness and flattened at 9–10 METs, which they equated to an average training effect of 30–60 minutes brisk walking daily.

Table 6
Age-adjusted all-cause death rates per 10,000 person-years of follow-up (1970–85) by physical fitness groups in men and women in the Aerobic Center Longitudinal Study

Fitness group	Person-years of follow-up	No. of deaths	Age-adjusted rates per 10,000 person-years	Relative risk	95% confidence limits
Men					
1 (low)	14,515	75	64.0	3.44[a]	2.05, 5.77
2	16,898	40	25.5	1.37	0.76, 2.50
3	17,287	47	27.1	1.46	0.81, 2.63
4	18,792	43	21.7	1.17	0.63, 2.17
5 (high)	17,557	35	18.6	1.00	—
Women					
1 (low)	4,916	18	39.5	4.65[a]	2.22, 9.75
2	5,329	11	20.5	2.42	1.09, 5.37
3	5,053	6	12.2	1.43	0.60, 3.44
4	5,522	4	6.5	0.76	0.27, 2.11
5 (high)	4,613	4	8.5	1.00	—

Source: Blair *et al.* [8].
[a] Test for linear trend, slope = −4.5; 95% confidence limits, −7.1, −1.9.
[b] Test for linear trend, slope = −5.5; 95% confidence limits, −9.2, −1.9.

Our analyses of other studies reporting both fitness and physical activity assessments found that fitness explained most of the CHD risk associated with activity class [19].

Population attributable risk

In addition to the current fashion of meta-analysis to study these relations, it has become equally fashionable to compute the population attributable risk (PAR), that is, the excess of CHD events in the population attributable to physical inactivity. Table 7, from Paffenbarger *et al.* [15], is the earliest computation of "community risk" based on the RR and the prevalence of sedentary men among Harvard alumni. This computation has been interpreted widely as physical inactivity being more important than either blood cholesterol, hypertension or smoking, and being responsible for the greatest public health influence of all risk factors. Aside from the fallacy of attributing greater importance to *any* risk factor over another in a complex system of cause and effect that operates with different force in individuals and in populations, these claims are re-examined here. For example, physical activity of work and leisure may be overwhelmed by the widespread elevation of other risk factors, particularly by mass hypercholesterolaemia [3]. Which CHD risk factor is "the most important" depends, therefore, on the setting and on the questions asked about individual and population causation. We propose that there is sufficient evidence, palaeontological, anthropological, epidemiological and physiological, that subsistence activity determined the fundamental metabolic adaptations of *Homo sapiens*, and that regular activity remains essential to optimal function in modern "industrial" humans [1]. However, population risk can be modelled on assumptions about shifts in the distribution of sedentary and active groups

Table 7

Relative and attributable risks of death from cardiovascular disease among 18,936 Harvard alumni, 1962–78, according to selected adverse characteristics[a]

Risk characteristic	Prevalence in % man-years	Relative risk of death	% "Clinical" attributable risk	% Community attributable risk
Sedentary lifestyle	62.0	1.3	23.7	16.1
Hypertension	9.4	2.2	54.0	9.1
Cigarette smoking	38.2	1.8	45.7	24.8
Overweight for height	37.2	1.2	15.5	6.4
Parental coronary heart disease	37.1	1.3	24.7	10.9
One or more of the above	90.5	3.0	67.0	64.7

Source: Adapted from Paffenbarger *et al.* [15].

[a] Adjusted for age and for each other characeristic listed.

Sedentary lifestyle = energy < 2000 kcal/week; clinical attributable risk = estimated potential reduction in individual risk by exchanging the adverse characteristic for a more healthy one.

Table 8
Model of population risk attributable to physical inactivity in men aged 45–74 years[a]

Physical activity class	Actual Minnesota % frequency	Relative risk	Case rate	CHD/ 100	Modelled population shift	CHD/ 100	Estimated change in excess risk (%)
Sedentary, work and leisure	37.1	1.8	18	6.7	25	4.5	
Some activity, none vigorous	41.4	1.3	13	5.4	50	6.5	
Any vigorous work or leisure	21.5	1.0	10	2.1	25	2.5	
	100.0			14.2	100	13.5	−4.9

[a] Maximal attributable (excess) risk (if 100% shift to vigorous) = 29.1.

in the population more likely than the complete elimination of physical inactivity from industrial society.

In Tables 8 and 9, we suggest such alternative assumptions of change in the distribution of physical activity. First, we classified physical activity both at work and at leisure in nine population-based surveys carried out by the same team over a several-year period in the same large and small communities of Minnesota [20]. In Table 8, we lump the finer classes of sedentary, active and vigorously active leisure time and work activity among some 9000 adults, aged 25–74 years, into three main classes: (1) a clearly sedentary class, (2) a class that has some activity, and (3) a class that has vigorous activity at leisure or at work, or both. Thirty-seven percent of middle-aged men and 44% of women in our Minnesota samples would be considered sedentary by most criteria, while

Table 9
Model of population risk attributable to physical inactivity in women aged 45–74 years[a]

Physical activity class	Actual Minnesota % frequency	Relative risk	Case rate	CHD/ 100	Modelled population shift	CHD/ 100	Estimated change in excess risk (%)
Sedentary, work and leisure	43.8	1.8	18	7.8	30	5.4	
Some activity, none vigorous	43.7	1.3	13	5.7	50	6.5	
Any vigorous work or leisure	13.3	1.0	10	1.3	20	2.0	
				14.8	100	13.9	−6.1

[a] Maximal attributable (excess) risk (if 100% shift to vigorous) = 32.2.

around 40% of the men and 44% of the women are moderately active and 20 and 13% vigorously active. Using relative risk ratios for CHD and physical inactivity derived from the major statistical summaries – that is, RR = 1.8 for sedentary and 1.3 for moderately active men, compared to 1.0 for the vigorously active – and using an arbitrary CHD rate to standardize, we achieve an estimated number of CHD cases for each class. We then model a shift in the male population distribution to 25% sedentary, 50% moderately and 25% vigorously active, which we suspect is a more feasible public health goal than conversion of all sedentary and moderately active persons to vigorously active (on which the PAR is estimated). Thus, we estimate a *decrease* of 5% from current levels of community risk due to such a "reasonable" shift in the whole distribution towards greater activity.

In Table 9, the model for women poses a shift to 20% of women in the vigorously active group and 50% in the active, with 30% remaining in the sedentary class. This public health model of substantial change, in the realm of possibility, again estimates something on the order of a 5–6% reduction in excess risk. Such a reduction population-wide in excess CHD risk attributable to enhanced physical activity would seem a reasonable population goal for high-risk Western societies. Blair *et al.* [18] also computed PAR based on a shift of the whole distribution upwards but eliminating only the least active class; their model estimated a 9% lowering of deaths in men and a 15% decrease in women. Reductions on the order of 3–5 milligrams percent of average blood cholesterol level in the population would be expected to achieve a similar fall in PAR. In our view, this puts the relative importance of physical activity for affluent sedentary cultures in appropriate perspective.

Physical activity and atherosclerosis

The evidence of a relationship of physical activity to atherosclerosis has, until recently, been indirect, based on experimental effects on blood lipid and blood pressure levels. RCTs using imaging techniques require a major investment to determine experimentally the effects of activity or rehabilitation programmes on the progression of atheroma. But direct evidence from autopsies is available from the Oslo Study [21], the Honolulu Heart Study [22] and the Puerto Rico Study [23], representing populations at high, medium and low CHD rates. In all these studies, total blood cholesterol and blood pressure levels were associated with coronary and aortic atherosclerosis whereas smoking was inconsistently associated. In contrast, various indices of physical activity showed no association.

Longevity

Longevity is not a sensitive indicator of the effect of any specific preventive measure because it is affected by so many influences and changes so little after survival to middle age. Paffenbarger and colleagues [15], however, estimated the effects of high- *vs.* low-activity levels, adjusted for major risk factors, as a gain in longevity of 1.5 extra hours of life for each 1.0 hour of activity for a 40-year-old man, and 1.9 extra hours for a 70-year-old man.

Conclusions and discussion

The results of these meta-analyses and subsequent studies are consistent with a real and significant association in individuals between lack of physical activity or fitness and increased risk of incident CHD, death post-infarction and all-cause death. The association is generally stronger for a high-activity group than a moderate-activity one compared with a sedentary group, suggesting a dose–response relationship. The data support the view that the lack of CHD association in some studies of activity in affluent societies may be due in part to a relatively low "true activity" in groups labelled "active". The data suggest as well that CHD events are prevented rather than reduced in severity. They also indicate that misclassifications of activity and disease probably contribute to the low RR observed in some studies. Bias in classification of CHD, and confounding of the relationship by activity-related risk factors, are considered unlikely to explain the observations because the RR of inactivity does not increase with increasing objectivity of CHD manifestations (e.g. from angina to CHD death). Moreover, multivariate adjustment of the RR for other risk factors does not significantly decrease the magnitude or the statistical significance of the regression coefficients for physical activity. Systematic bias due to the publication of mainly "popular" results that show a significant relationship would be expected to result in uniform and statistically significant results; in fact, this is not found [12,13]. Moreover, an inverse relationship would be expected between study quality and RR if editors and investigators tended to avoid publishing insignificant results. This, too, is not found. Sub-clinical disease at the time of the entry assessment is also considered unlikely to be the cause of the inverse relationship because of the similar RR for early and late follow-up events. Moreover, the fitness study of Blair *et al.* [18] effectively excludes such states by the graded exercise test response itself.

The issues remaining include whether the benefits of physical activity are largely independent of other risk factors or of constitutional (inherited) factors; whether those at higher risk might experience more "benefit" than those at lower CHD risk; and, finally, what is the amount of activity required for optimal "effect". We will not attempt here to update in detail the many analyses from the literature on the association of duration, frequency and intensity of physical activity with CHD. Recent studies of good quality suggest, however, that regular energy expenditure of 300 kcal or more daily, in moderate activities such as walking or working around the house, is associated with significantly lower risk, as is a moderate amount of more vigorous physical activity [24,25]. There may be relatively little added benefit of physical activity levels above an average of 2000 kcal activity weekly, and some potential harm in very vigorous activities ($\geq$3000 kcal) in the setting of sedentary industrial society.

From all these observations taken together, we conclude that physical activity and fitness in middle-aged men and women is associated inversely with, and may protect against, coronary death, sudden death and all-causes death. Uncertainty remains, nevertheless, whether the effect is due mainly to physical activity or to "genes and constitution". People tend to exercise if they "feel good" when doing it. Not everyone does. Fitness may be a major contributor to the apparent "protective effect" of physical activity and fitness has a strong constitutional component variously estimated at 30–90%. It is possible that this component determines both who will be active and who will be protected from clinical CHD events. Several pieces of evidence related to this question, however, suggest otherwise: any protective effect of having once been a college athlete and presumably constitutionally "superior", disappears by time since graduation, while current level of physical activity remains an effective predictor [15]; constitutional "superiority" is likely to be less critical to participants in moderate exercise than in vigorous exercise programmes and associations with lowered CHD risk are found for moderate physical activity and fitness levels [16,24]. All these findings suggest that constitution is not the major factor. From this evidence we are left, none the less, with the lesson that humankind departs at considerable risk from its evolutionary adaptations to regular physical activity!

In the final analysis, safety is foremost in prescribing exercise for the individual as well as in policy recommendations for the public health. Siskovic and colleagues [26] used an innovative approach to estimate the risk of cardiac arrest during exercise by interviewing the families of victims and of a population-based sample of healthy persons. The RR of cardiac arrest during exercise was 56 in habitually sedentary men and 5 in vigorously active men! However, the overall risk of cardiac arrest in habitually active men during and not during actual activity was only 40% of that in sedentary men. This suggests that the reduced risk overall of sudden death due to regular exercise is greater than the excess risk of death during or due to vigorous activities.

Finally, we support strongly the general call to increased habitual physical activity in affluent societies through national policy and preventive practice. In the Minnesota Heart Health Programme, we have over the last decade designed and carried out a community-based approach to the promotion of physical activity using multiple strategies of community organization, promotional campaigns, adult and youth direct education and mass communications [20]. We report elsewhere the encouraging results of this campaign: greater exposure and awareness, greater prevalence of regular physical activity, and increased levels of self-reported LTPA among educated communities [20,27].

References

1. Blackburn H. Physical activity and coronary heart disease: A brief update and population view. *J Cardiac Rehab* 1983; **3:** 101–174.

2. Rose G. Individuals and populations in preventive cardiology: Ancel Keys Lecture. *Circulation* 1991; **84:** 1405–1409.
3. Keys A (ed.) Seven Countries. *A Multivariate Analysis of Death and Coronary Heart Disease.* Harvard University Press: Cambridge, MA, 1980.
4. Naughton J. Role of physical activity as a secondary intervention for healed myocardial infarction. *Am J Cardiol* 1985; **55:** 21D–26D.
5. Haskell WL, Leon AS, Caspersen CJ, Froelicher VF, Hagberg JM, Harlan W, Holloszy JO, Regensteiner JG, Thompson PD, Washburn RA, Wilson PWF. Cardiovascular benefits and assessment of physical activity and physical fitness in adults. *Med Sci Sports Exercise* 1992; **24:** S201–S220.
6. Froelicher V, Battler A, McKirnan MD. Physical activity and coronary heart disease. *Cardiology* 1980; **65:** 153–190.
7. Report of the International Society and Federation of Cardiology. *Physical Inactivity: A Risk Factor for Coronary Heart Disease.* Edited by the Netherlands Heart Foundation, 20 February 1992.
8. Collins R, Yusuf S, Peto R. Exercise after myocardial infarction reduces mortality: Evidence from randomized clinical trials. *J Am Coll Cardiol* (Abstr.) 1984; **2:** 622.
9. WHO Working Group on Rehabilitation Programs for Patients with Myocardial Infarction: Prague, 4–7 October, 1971. EURO 8206(6), WHO Regional Office for Europe, Copenhagen.
10. Oldridge NB, Guyett GH, Fischer ME, Rimm AA. Cardiac rehabilitation after myocardial infarction. *JAMA* 1988; **260:** 945–950.
11. O'Connor GT, Buring JE, Yusuf S, Golbarger RS, Hennekens C. An overview of randomized trials of rehabilitation with exercise after myocardial infarction. *Circulation* 1989; **80:** 234–244.
12. Powell KE, Thompson PD, Caspersen CJ, Kendrick JS. Physical activity and the incidence of coronary heart disease. *Ann Rev Public Health* 1987; **8:** 253–287.
13. Berlin JA, Colditz GA. A meta-analysis of physical activity in the prevention of coronary heart disease. *Am J Epidemiol* 1990; **132:** 612–628.
14. Powell KE, Caspersen CJ, Koplan JP, Ford ES. Physical activity and chronic diseases. *Am J Clin Nutr* 1989; **49:** 999–1006.
15. Paffenbarger RS, Hyde RT, Wing AL, Hsieh CC. Physical activity, all-cause mortality, and longevity of college alumni. *N Engl J Med* 1986; **314:** 605–613.
16. Shaper AG, Wannamethee G. Physical activity and ischaemic heart disease in middle-aged British men. *Br Med J* 1991; **66:** 384–394.
17. Douglas PS, Clarkson TB, Flowers NC, Hajjar KA, Horton E, Klocke KJ, LaRosa J, Shively C. Exercise and atherosclerotic heart disease in women. *Med Sci Sports Exercise* 1992; **24:** S266–S276.
18. Blair SN, Kohl W III, Paffenbarger RS, Clark DG, Cooper KH, Gibbons LW. Physical fitness and all-cause mortality: A prospective study of healthy men and women. *JAMA* 1989; **262:** 2395–2401.
19. Blackburn H, Jacobs David R Jr. Physical activity and the risk of coronary heart disease (editorial). *N Engl J Med* 1988; **319:** 1217–1219.
20. Crow R, Blackburn H, Jacobs D, Hannan P, Pirie P, Mittelmark M, Murray D, Luepker R. Population strategies to enhance physical activity: The Minnesota Heart Health Program. *Acta Med Scand* (Suppl.) 1986; **711:** 93–112.
21. Solberg LA, Enger SC, Hjermann I *et al.* Risk factors for coronary and cerebral atherosclerosis in the Oslo Study. In: Gotto AJ Jr, Smith LC, Allen B (eds) *Atherosclerosis V.* Springer-Verlag: New York, 1980, pp.57–62.
22. Reed DM, MacLean CJ, Hayashi T. Predictors of atherosclerosis in the Honolulu Heart Program. I. Biologic, dietary and lifestyle characteristics. *Am J Epidemiol* 1987; **126:** 214–225.

23. Garcia-Palmieri MI, Costas R, Cruz-Vidal M, Sorlie P, Havel RJ. Increased physical activity: A protective factor against heart disease in Puerto Rico. *Am J Cardiol* 1982; **50:** 749–755.
24. Leon AS, Connett J, Jacobs DR Jr, Rauramaa R. Leisure-time physical activity levels and risk of coronary hearts disease and death. *JAMA* 1987; **253:** 2388–2395.
25. Leon AS, Connett J. Physical activity and 10.5 year mortality in the Multiple Risk Factor Intervention Trial (MRFIT). *Int J Epidemiol* 1991; **20:** 690–697.
26. Siscovick DS, Weiss NS, Fletcher RH, Lasky T. The incidence of primary cardiac arrest during vigorous exercise. *N Engl J Med* 1984; **311:** 874–877.
27. Report of the Minnesota Heart Health Program. Community education for cardiovascular disease prevention: Population risk factor results (in press).

47 Primary Prevention of Coronary Artery Disease by Drugs. Why Calcium Entry Blockers?

Paul R. Lichtlen and the INTACT Study Group

Department of Internal Medicine, Division of Cardiology, Hannover Medical School, Konstanty-Gutschow-Str. 8, D-3000 Hannover 61, Germany

Definition of prevention

Today, the success of preventive measures against coronary artery disease (CAD) can be assessed in humans quite accurately both at the clinical as well as at the angiographic level. Clinically, prevention of CAD is expressed as a reduction in fatal and non-fatal myocardial infarctions and sudden coronary death [1]. Whereas the clinical events are well defined, our knowledge of the underlying processes is still limited, both with regard to the anatomical as well as the functional changes taking place in the arterial wall during prevention of atherosclerosis. Discussion concerning regression of old plaques, i.e. a reduction in volume [2–4] eventually leading to stabilization against rupture, inhibition of the development of new plaques, especially of fatty streaks [5, 6] and restoration of the abnormal endothelial function, i.e. normalization of the elevated vasomotor tone (VMT) [7]. Indeed, severe endothelial dysfunction, i.e. vasoconstriction, was found to be one of the earliest signs of atherosclerosis, especially of elevated cholesterol levels [8, 9] (Table 2). The most probable mechanism is oxidative inactivation of EDRF-NO in the presence of increased free oxygen radicals generated from oxidized LDL particles and free fatty acids [10, 11]. Accordingly, in animals made hypercholesterolaemic, subsequent lowering of serum cholesterol was followed by a significant improvement in endothelial function, restoration of EDRF-NO and normalization of the increased VMT [7] (Table 3). Hence, to what extent in humans with CAD

Proceedings of the Vth World Congress on Cardiac Rehabilitation

undergoing lipid-lowering regimens the angiographically observed mild widening of the coronary lumen (2–3% of diameter stenosis) [3, 4, 12] is due to improved endothelial function (vasodilation) or plaque regression or both cannot be answered to date. There is no technique as yet to assess accurately plaque volume in humans, neither by angiography [13] nor by intravascular ultrasound [14]. Also, the role of new plaques is not yet well defined. It is still not known whether the reduction in acute myocardial infarction is due to stabilization of old plaques or to an inhibition of growth of new plaques, i.e. of fatty streaks [15]. Finally, problems in clinical studies also arise from the usually slow evolution of CAD and the paucity of events per patient (one or two myocardial infarctions per lifetime in the majority of cases) [5]; this often necessitates a long follow-up period (10 or more years) and the inclusion of large numbers of patients [1]. Hence, clinical tests of new drugs in this field become costly and time-consuming.

For all these reasons, several groups recently chose the angiographic approach to test the efficacy of preventive measures in patients undergoing repeated coronary angiograms at fixed intervals, usually 2–3 years [2, 3, 6, 12, 16–18]. In these studies, computer-assisted analysis systems [5, 13] automatically assess minimal stenotic and normal coronary artery diameters and calculate percent diameter stenosis (%*D*). In addition, they search for new stenoses, new isolated narrowings in previously angiographically "normal" segments [5, 6] (Table 1).

Although quantitative, computer-assisted measurements of arterial wall changes are more accurate than qualitative estimates, there also remain a number of limitations for this new technique [5, 13]. Accordingly, very early lesions, especially fatty streaks, protruding only minimally into the vessel lumen (<0.1 mm) or lesions growing initially within the vessel wall [19, 20] are missed by angiography due to its rather low sensitivity. In addition, both the definition of new as well as of old progressing and regressing lesions has to take into account the considerable system variabilities [5, 13].

Mechanisms involved in primary prevention of CAD by drugs

As discussed above, primary prevention of CAD has two targets: to inhibit the formation of new plaques and to induce regression and/or stabilization of existing ones.

Lipid-lowering drugs

The important role of lipids, especially of LDL cholesterol, in the generation of atherosclerotic plaques (fatty streaks) is generally accepted today [1, 15]. Several carefully performed epidemiological studies demonstrated a close, although not linear correlation between total and LDL cholesterol levels and the incidence of coronary events [1, 21]. However, to what extent a reduction in total and LDL cholesterol reduces the production of new plaques is still not known. So

Table 1
Human studies on reduced vascular reactivity due to atherosclerosis

Authors	Results
Bossaller *et al.* [31]	Impaired muscarinic endothelium-dependent relaxation and cGMP formation in atherosclerotic human coronary arteries from explanted hearts
Förstermann *et al.* [8]	Atherosclerosis attenuates EDRF-mediated vasodilation in epicardial human coronary arteries from explanted hearts
Ludmer *et al.* [32]	Vasoconstriction induced by acetylcholine in atherosclerotic coronary arteries
Cox *et al.* [33]	Atherosclerosis impairs flow-mediated dilation of coronary arteries in humans
Yasue *et al.* [34]	Angiographically normal coronary arteries change reactivity on acetylcholine depending on age
Vita *et al.* [35]	Coronary vasomotor response to acetylcholine relates to risk factors for CAD
Zeiher *et al.* [9]	Selective endothelial dysfunction in patients with hypercholesterolaemia and angiographically normal and diseased coronary arteries

far, only a few angiographic studies have analysed the influence of lipid-lowering measures on the formation of new lesions; two of these claimed both regression of old and reduction of new stenoses when compared to placebo [2, 22]. However, due to subjective estimates and retrospective analysis [22] of the %D of new stenoses, they meet with considerable methodological criticism. A third, computer-assisted study applying a reductase inhibitor and initially planned for an interval of 2 years (MAAS), had to be prolonged for another 2 years due to inadequate results [23]. Hence, the mechanisms by which lipid-lowering measures in humans influence the production of new plaques and the regression of old ones (see above) are still unclear and need further evaluation. This is also true for the clinical results of such studies, where for example the lack of suppression of total mortality is so far unexplained [1].

Calcium entry blockers

During the last decade, preventive effects against atherosclerosis have also been demonstrated for calcium entry blockers [24]. These studies, initially performed in cholesterol-fed rabbits, showed a dose-dependent 30–60% reduction in the plaque area of the aorta and of the coronary arteries when calcium entry blockers were added to the diet [25]. The preventive effect was, however, absent when the drug was administered *after* cholesterol feeding. From various animal models and cell cultures, it became evident that calcium entry blockers act on various processes involved in the build-up of plaques:

1. They exert a moderate anti-oxidative effect, i.e. protect membrane phospholipids against oxidative degradation [26].
2. They suppress the accumulation of intracellular lipids by promoting the efflux of free cholesterol from macrophages [27].

Table 2
Evidence for improvement or normalization of endothelial dysfunction in atherosclerosis by reduction of lipid levels

Authors	Animal model	Results
Armstrong *et al.* [36]	monkey	Reversal of impaired dilator capacity after regression of atherosclerosis
Harrison *et al.* [7]	monkey	The attenuated relaxation to acetylcholine in atherosclerotic arteries was normalized in arteries from regressing animals (functional regression)
Heistad *et al.* [37]	monkey	Serotonin-induced increase in segmental pressure (resistance) in atherosclerosis is reversed or normalized after diet

Table 3
Prevention of progression of coronary artery disease, angiographic approach

Underlying anatomical and molecular changes	Changes in repeated angiograms
At the site of pre-existing plaques	
Regression: Reductions in plaque volume (?) Luminal widening by improvement in endothelial function and decrease in vasomotor tone	Increase in minimal stenotic diameter Decrease in percent diameter stenosis (%D)
Stabilization of plaques against fissuring (?)	Fewer progressing stenoses (increase in minimal stenotic diameter (D_{min}), decrease in %D, fewer new occlusions)
At the site of new plaques	
Inhibition of formation of new plaques Reduction of early lesions (fatty streaks) Fewer early lesions "growing" into primary plaques	Fewer new stenoses (primary plaques) in previously "normal" coronary segments
	Limitations: early lesions (fatty streaks) are too small to be visualized by angiography; primary plaques initially often develop intramurally

3. They lower intracellular cholesterol in aortic smooth muscle cells by stimulating acid cholesterol ester hydrolysis activity, an effect also confirmed in human aortic smooth muscle cells obtained during bypass surgery from patients pretreated with nifedipine or diltiazem [28].
4. Most importantly, calcium antagonists exert a strong inhibitory effect on smooth muscle cell proliferation [29].

All of these effects, especially the suppression of various growth factors [30], result in a reduced production of matrix proteins and thus inhibit the build-up of new plaques [24].

Clinical studies with calcium entry blockers: the INTACT study

Four prospective studies [6, 16–18], each applying dihydropyridine-type calcium entry blockers and analysing progression of CAD by repeated quantitated coronary angiograms, are known in humans (Table 4). One of them, the INTACT study [6], will be discussed in more detail here. It included 425 patients, 348 of whom (82%) were undergoing two angiograms at an interval of exactly 3 years, 173 on placebo and 175 on 80 mg nifedipine per day. (For details of the angiographic procedure, and the computerized analysis and assessment of various parameters, see Lichtlen *et al.* [5, 6] and Reiber *et al.* [13].)

Inclusion was limited to patients with moderate CAD: occlusion of no more than one vessel, focal disease only and large segments still angiographically normal. Altogether, 30% of the patients had successfully undergone single-vessel percutaneous transluminal coronary angioplasty (PTCA) prior to inclusion and approximately 30% had previous myocardial infarctions [6].

Angiographic results

At entrance, 1255 lesions with a percent diameter stenosis ($\%D$) $>20\%$ were observed. The placebo group presented 657 lesions, (stenoses and occlusions 3.79 per patient), the nifedipine group 598 lesions (3.42 per patient) (NS). Most of the stenoses were mild, with a $\%D$ averaging $38.9 \pm 10.9\%$ (range 8–78%) and a minimal stenotic diameter (D_{min}) of 1.65 ± 0.52 mm. Accordingly, more than 80% of these stenoses were clinically silent.

Second angiography: Behaviour of pre-existing stenoses

To be classified as progression or regression, the stenoses had to change their $\%D$ by $\geq 20\%$ (for a definition, see [6, 13]). Progression was observed in 118 (11%) of the 1063 pre-existing stenoses recovered from the first angio-

Table 4
Angiographically controlled prevention studies with calcium entry blockers

Study	Medication	Number of patients with two angiograms			Cut-off point for increase in % stenosis	Number of new lesions		% reduction
		Total	PL	Ca-Bl.		PL	Ca-Bl.	
Gottlieb *et al.* [17] 1 year, CABG	3 × 20 mg nifedipine	64	37	27	—	65/37 (1.75/pat.) 48% diseased CABG	31/27 (1.15/pat.) 33%	−34% $P < 0.04$
Loaldi *et al.* [16] 2 years	4 × 20 mg nifedipine *vs* Prop/ISDN	113	74	39	≥20%	23 (0.311 new lesion/pat.)	4 (0.102 new lesions/pat.)	−67% $P < 0.05$
Waters *et al.* [18][a] 2 years	3 × 30 mg nicardipine	217	118	99	≥10%	38 (0.32/pat.)	16 (0.16/pat.)	−50% $P < 0.046$
Lichtlen *et al.* [6] 3 years	4 × 20 mg nifedipine	348	175	173	≥20%	114 (0.82 new lesions/pat.)	103 (0.59 new lesions/pat.)	−28% $P < 0.034$

Abbreviations: PL, placebo; Ca-Bl., calcium entry blocker; Prop, propranol (320 mg); ISDN, isosorbide dinitrate (80 mg) pat., patient.
[a] New Lesions = minimal lesions, degree <20%.

gram, 20 of them (1.9%) becoming occluded during the 3-years follow-up. Most importantly, there was no difference between groups with regard to the number of progressing or regressing stenoses (progressing: 9% placebo, 12% nifedipine; regressing: 4% placebo, 3% nifedipine; NS). Obviously, in patients without excessive risk factors (average cholesterol in this study 260 mg/dl, 50% of patients cigarette smokers, 34 with mild hypertension), progression of CAD was rather slow; the majority of plaques (>80%) had remained unchanged over the 3-years follow-up. In addition, spontaneous progression occurred approximately three times more often than regression and was not influenced by calcium entry blockers.

Progression of new lesions

Stenoses found in previously "normal" segments and defined as new stenoses were already of a considerable size, their %*D* averaging 39.4 ± 10.2% (range 20–70%) (for a definition, see [5,6]); this size is similar to that of pre-existing lesions (NS). Altogether, 247 new lesions (228 stenoses and 19 occlusions) were observed in 155 patients (85 on placebo, 70 on nifedipine, 44.5% of all patients; 0.7 new lesions/patient). In accordance with the findings in animal studies, 28% fewer new lesions were observed in patients on nifedipine ($n = 103$ lesions; 0.59/all patients) than on placebo ($n = 144$ lesions; 0.82/all patients) ($P < 0.034$; Cochran's linear trend test, two-sided) (Fig.1). The trend of 17% fewer patients with new lesions on nifedipine ($n = 70$; 40.5%) than on placebo ($n = 85$, 48.6% of patients) was not significant ($P = 0.1$).

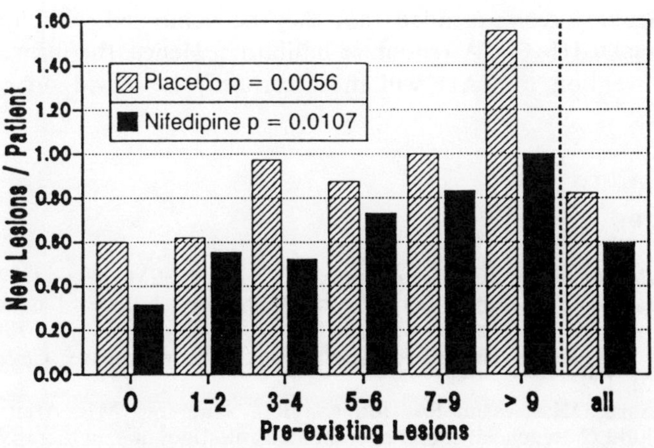

Fig. 1. Influence of nifedipine in patients with low and high progression rate. The number of pre-existing lesions/patient at entrance is compared with the number of newly formed lesions/patient. Note the significant difference on the retardation of new lesions on all levels of progression.

Interestingly, a close correlation was observed between number of preexisting lesions per patient at entrance and number of newly formed lesions after 3 years (Fig.1); the higher the number of pre-existing lesions in the first angiogram, the higher was the number of new lesions after 3 years. This correlation existed both for placebo ($r = 0.192$, $P = 0.0056$) as well as for nifedipine ($r = 0.175$, $P = 0.011$). However, in the latter group, the steepness of the correlation curve was markedly blunted. In summary, nifedipine reduced the number of new lesions at all levels, especially, however, in patients with a high progression rate.

Other studies

The three other human angiographic studies using calcium entry blockers [16–18] all applying computer-assisted analysis systems, confirmed the findings of the INTACT study. They demonstrated significant reductions in the number of new lesions, varying between −34% and −67%, over intervals of 1–2 years (Table 4).

Due to the small number of patients in the four studies (742 altogether) and the short follow-up (maximum 3 years), it is impossible to draw conclusions on the clinical preventive effect of calcium entry blockers. Due to the lack of clinical results, recommendations for the administration of calcium entry blockers in primary prevention of CAD so far remain restricted. Treatment should include only those calcium entry blockers proven to be angiographically effective in humans; it should be limited to patients with an accumulation of risk factors, especially high lipid levels and hypertension, in whom cholesterol and/or high blood pressure cannot otherwise adequately be controlled. As calcium entry blockers have no or only a mild influence on cholesterol levels [6], it is strongly recommended that they be combined with lipid-lowering drugs, especially HMG-CA reductase inhibitors. Hence, the future strategy in primary prevention of CAD will most certainly be based on combination treatment.

References

1. Gotto AM, La Rosa JC, Hunninghake D, Grundy SM, Wilson PW, Clarkson TB, Hay JW, Goodman DS. The task force on cholesterol issues, American Heart Association. The cholesterol facts, a summary of the evidence relating dietary fats, serum cholesterol and coronary heart disease. *Circulation* 1990; **81:** 1721–1723.
2. Blankenhorn DH, Nessim SA, Johnson RL, Sanmarco ME, Azen SP, Cashin-Hemphill LC. Beneficial effects of combined colestipol–niazin therapy on coronary atherosclerosis and coronary venous bypass grafts. *JAMA* 1987; **257:** 3233–3240.
3. Brown G, Albers JJ, Fisher LD, Schaefer SM, Lin JT, Kaplan C, Zhao XQ, Bisson BD, Fitzpatrick VF, Dodge HT. Regression of coronary artery disease as a result of intensive lipid-lowering therapy in men with high levels of apolipoprotein B. *N Engl J Med* 1990; **323:** 1289–1298.

4. Watts GF, Louis B, Brunt JNH, Louis ES, Coltard DJ, Smith LDR, Man JI, Swan AV. Effects on coronary artery disease of lipid lowering diet, or diet plus cholestyramine, in the St. Thomas' atherosclerosis regression study (STARS). *Lancet* 1992; **339:** 563–569.
5. Lichtlen PR, Nikutta P, Jost S, Deckers J, Wiese B, Rafflenbeul W, and the INTACT Study Group. Anatomical progression of coronary artery disease in man, as seen by prospective, repeated, quantitated coronary angiogrpahy; Relation to clinical events and risk factors. *Circulation* 1992; **86**: 828-838.
6. Lichtlen PR, Hugenholtz PG, Rafflenbeul W, Hecker H, Jost S, Deckers JW, and the INTACT Study Group . Retardation of angiographic progression of coronary artery disease by the calcium channel blocker nifedipine – Results of the international nifedipine trial on antiatherosclerotic therapy (INTACT). *Lancet* 1990; **335:** 1109–1113.
7. Harrison DG, Armstrong ML, Freiman PC, Heistad DD. Restoration of endothelium-dependent relaxation by dietary treatment of atherosclerosis. *J Clin Invest* 1987; **80:** 1808–1811.
8. Förstermann U, Mügge A, Alheid U, Haverich A, Frölich AC. Selective attenuation of endothelium-mediated vasodilation in atherosclerotic human coronary arteries. *Circ Res* 1988; **62:** 185–190.
9. Zeiher AM, Drexler H, Wollschläger H, Just H. Modulation of coronary vasomotor tone in humans: Progressive endothelial dysfunction with different early stages of coronary atherosclerosis. *Circulation* 1991; **83:** 391–401.
10. Rubanyi GM, Vanhoutte PM. Superoxide anions and hyperoxia inactivate endothelium-derived relaxing factor. *Am J Physiol* 1986; **250:** H822–827.
11. Jacobs M, Plane F, Bruckdorfer KR. Native and oxidized low density lipoproteins have different inhibitory effects on endothelium-derived relaxing factor in the rabbit aorta. *Br J Pharmacol* 1990; **100:** 21–26.
12. Ornish D, Brown SE, Scherwitz LW, Billings JH, Armstrong WT, Ports TA, McLanahan SM, Kirkeeide RL, Brand RJ, Gould KL. Can lifestyle changes reverse coronary heart disease? *Lancet* 1990; **336:** 129-133.
13. Reiber JHC, Serruys PW, Kooijman CJ, Wijns W, Slager CJ, Gerbrands JJ, Schuurbiers JCH, den Boer A, Hugenholtz PG. Assessment of short-, medium-, and long-term variations in arterial dimensions from computer-assisted quantitation of coronary cineangiograms. *Circulation* 1985; **71:** 280–288.
14. Liebson PR, Klein LW. Intravascular ultrasound in coronary atherosclerosis: A new approach to clinical assessment. *Am Heart J* 1992; **123:** 1643–1660.
15. Fagiotto A, Ross R, Harker L. Studies of hypercholesterolemia in the non-human primate. Part I and part II. *Arteriosclerosis* 1984; **4:** 323–341.
16. Loaldi A, Polese A, Montorsi P, De Cesare N, Fabbiocchi F, Ravagnani P, Guazzi MD. Comparison of nifedipine, propanolol and isosorbide dinitrate on angiographic progression and regression of coronary arterial narrowings in angina pectoris. *Am J Cardiol* 1989; **64:** 433–439.
17. Gottlieb SO, Brinker JA, Mellits ED, Achuff SC, Baughman KL, Traill TA, Weiss JL, Reitz BA, Weisfeldt ML, Gerstenblith G. Effect of nifedipine on the development of coronary bypass graft stenoses in high-risk patients: A randomized, double-blind, placebo-controlled trial. *Circulation* (Suppl. II, abstr.) 1989; **80:** 228.
18. Waters D, Lespérance J, Francetich M, Causey D, Théroux P, Chiang YK, Hudon G, Lemarbre L, Reitman M, Joyal M, Gosselin G, Dyrda I, Macer J, Havel R. A controlled clinical trial to assess the effect of a calcium channel blocker on the progression of coronary atherosclerosis. *Circulation* 1990; **82:** 1940–1953.
19. Glagov S, Weisenberg E, Zarins C, Stankunavicius R, Kolettis GJ. Compensatory enlargement of human atherosclerotic coronary arteries. *N Engl J Med* 1987; **316:** 1371–1375.

20. Freudenberg H, Lichtlen PR. Limitations of intravital coronary angiography: A comparison with postmortem results in 87 cases. *Circulation* (Suppl. IV, abstr.) 1981; **63/64:** 238.
21. Castelli WP, Garrison RJ, Wilson PW, Abbott RD, Kalousdian S, Kannel WB. Incidence of coronary heart disease and lipoprotein cholesterol levels: The Framingham Study. *JAMA* 1986; **256:** 2835–2838.
22. Buchwald H, Varco RL, Matts JP *et al.* Effect of partial ileal bypass surgery on mortality and morbidity from coronary heart disease in patients with hypercholesterolemia: Report of the program on the surgical control of the hyperlipidemias (POSCH). *N Engl J Med* 1990; **323:** 946–955.
23. Oliver M. Coronary atheroma regression trials (Letter to the Editor). *Lancet* 1992; **339:** 1241.
24. Henry PD. Antiatherogenic effects of calcium channel blockers: Possible mechanisms of action. *Cardiovasc Drugs Ther* 1990; **4:** 1015–1020.
25. Nayler WG. *Calcium Antagonists and Atherosclerosis.* Academic Press: London, 1988, pp. 235–247.
26. Janeiro DR, Burghardt B, Lopez R. Protection of cardiac membrane phospholipid against oxidative injury by calcium antagonists. *Biochem Pharmacol* 1988; **37:** 4197–4203.
27. Schmitz G, Robenek H, Beuck M, Krause R, Schurek A, Niemann R. Calcium antagonists and ACAT inhibitors promote cholesterol efflux from macrophages by different mechanisms. I: Characterization of cellular lipid metabolism. *Arteriosclerosis* 1988; **8:** 46–56.
28. Etingin DR, Hajjar DP. Calcium channel blockers enhance cholesterol ester hydrolysis and decrease total cholesterol accumulation in human aortic tissue. *Circ Res* 1990; **66:** 185–190.
29. Nilsson J, Sjolund M, Palmberg L, van Euler AmM, Jonzon B, Thyberg J. The calcium antagonist nifedipine inhibits arterial smooth muscle cell proliferation. *Atherosclerosis* 1985; **58:** 109–122.
30. Nilsson J. Growth factors and the pathogenesis of atherosclerosis. *Atherosclerosis* 1986; **62:** 185–199.
31. Bossaller C, Habib GB, Yamamoto H, Williams C, Wells S, Henry PD. Impaired muscarinic endothelial-dependent relaxation and cyclic guanosine 5-monophosphate formation in atherosclerotic human coronary artery and rabbit aorta. *J. Clin Invest* 1987; **79**: 171–174.
32. Ludmer PL, Selwyn AP, Shook TL, Wayne PR, Mudge GH, Alexander RW, Ganz P. Paradoxical vasoconstriction induced by acetylcholin in atherosclerotic coronary arteries. *N Engl J Med* 1986; **315:** 1046–1051.
33. Cox DA, Vita JA, Treausre CB, Fish MD, Alexander RW, Ganz P, *et al.* Atherosclerosis impairs flow-mediated dilation of coronary arteries in humans. *Circulation* 1989; **80:** 458–465.
34. Yasue H, Matsuyama K, Okumura K, Morikami Y, Ogawa H. Responses of angiographically normal human coronary arteries to intracoronary injection of acetylcholine by age and segment. Possible role of early coronary atherosclerosis. *Circulation* 1990; **81:** 482–490.
35. Vita JA, Treasure CB, Nabel EG, McLennahan JM, Fish RD, Young AC, Vekshtein VI, Selwyn AP, Ganz P. Coronary vasomotor response to acetylcholine relates to risk factors for coronary artery disease. *Circulation* 1990; **81:** 491–497.
36. Armstrong ML, Heistad DD, Marcus ML, Piegors DJ, Abboud FM. Hemodynamic sequelae of regression of experimental atherosclerosis. *J Clin Invest* 1983; **71:** 104–113.
37. Heistadt DD, Marcus ML, Piegors DJ, Armstrong ML. Dietary treatment of atherosclerosis abolishes hyperresponsiveness to serotonine: implications for vasospasm. *Circ Res* 1987; **61:** 346–351.

48 Cellular Interactions and Atherosclerosis Reversal

J. Larrue

Unité de Cardiologie U8 Inserm, Avenue du Haut-Lévêque, 33600 Pessac, France

Introduction

Several hypotheses have been proposed to explain the pathogenesis of atherosclerosis. All of them reflect general disturbances in cellular function that affect the response to various stimuli. Lipid deposition, connective tissue formation, smooth muscle cell proliferation, infiltration of inflammatory cells and endothelial dysfunction are present both at the initiation of the lesion and later (Fig. 1).

In animals, experimentally induced atherosclerosis is achieved either by a dietary-induced hypercholesterolaemia or by producing endothelial denudation and arterial damage by mechanical or toxic injury. So the developing lesions, not surprisingly, appear somewhat different on a morphological basis.

In dietary-induced hypercholesterolaemia models, accumulation of foam cells protruding into the vessel lumen represent the earliest type of atherosclerotic lesion: the fatty streak. Then, proliferating smooth muscle cells (SMCs) give rise to fibrous plaque [1]. In the majority of these models, early lesions develop without any structural signs of endothelial alteration or platelet involvement and, for example, the fatty streaks in swine appear to begin at sites of pre-existing intimal SMC masses. However, recent immunological and morphological evidence suggests functional alteration to the endothelial cells, such as expression of specific endothelial adhesion molecules [2], signs of increased

Proceedings of the Vth World Congress on Cardiac Rehabilitation

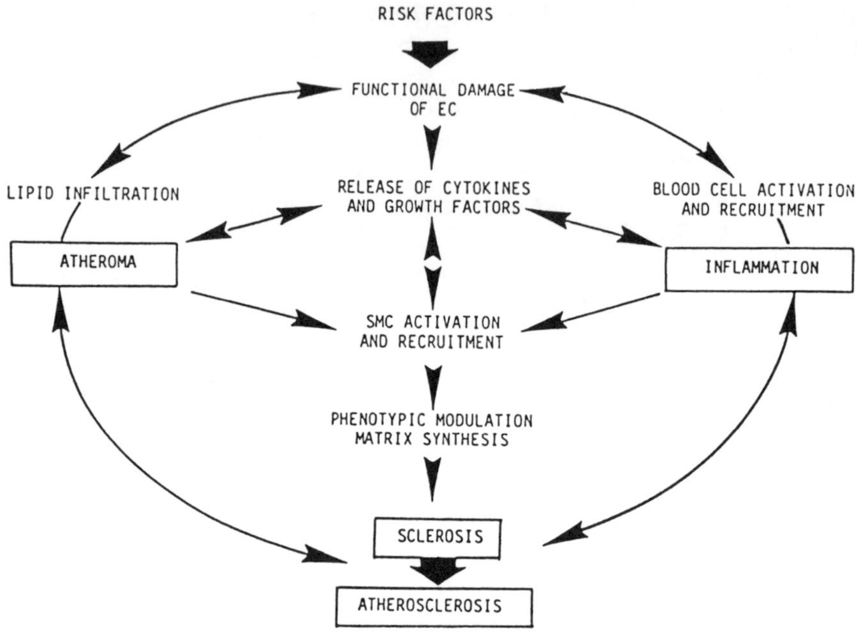

Fig. 1. Schematic diagram of a hypothetical sequence of events and cellular interactions in atherogenesis.

endothelial turnover and the presence of adhering monocytes to the endothelial surface.

Mechanical endothelial injury causes a rapid adherence of platelets to the exposed endothelial tissue [3]. If the wound is deep enough to affect the internal elastic lamina, SMCs start to migrate into the intima where they divide. It is important to note that stretching or dilatation of the media seems to be able to induce first a medial SMC proliferation which is followed by migration and intimal proliferation. However, a superficial injury restricted to the endothelium and devoid of medial stretching does not give rise to SMC proliferation despite platelet adherence [4].

Although there are similarities, atherosclerotic lesions in humans are not necessarily of the same origin and nature as those seen in experimental animals. However, recent immunological evidence has identified the cell composition of fatty streaks or fibrous plaques [5]. Smooth muscle cells in a contractile or synthetic phenotype were found to dominate in the fibrous cap, which also contained many T-cells, whereas macrophage was the most frequent cell type present in the central lipid core, indicating that spontaneous atherosclerotic development in humans or experimentally induced atherosclerosis in animals may be considered essentially a chronic inflammatory response of the arterial wall [6]. The recent development of improved immunological techniques and *in situ* hybridization have largely confirmed this essential feature.

So, the inflammatory nature of atherosclerosis is important in view of atherosclerosis reversal and the major problem remains the modulation or control of wound healing as a reparative response.

Cytokines as potential mediators in atherogenesis

During atherogenesis, vascular cells and infiltrating leukocytes exchange biochemical messengers as information molecules through paracrine pathways. One well-known example is the nitric oxide radical (NO^0, $EDRF_I$) formed by endothelial cells under the influence of various stimuli (neurotransmitters, hormones, drugs), which acts upon smooth muscle cells and induces relaxation and other responses as a function of the phenotypic state [7]. Alternatively, information exchange could involve the autocrine pathway. This seems to be the case for PDGF produced by smooth muscle cells, which amplifies migratory or proliferative signals [8] for many other mediators including inducible NO^0. Among the cytokines, special attention has been given to several monokines which can also be produced by vascular endothelial and smooth muscle cells, at least under culture conditions, and more recently considerable evidence has suggested the expression of several cytokines in arterial tissues *in vivo* when exposed to an inductive stimulus, i.e. a cholesterol diet (see Table 1) [9]. For example, endothelial cells, smooth muscle cells and macrophage-derived cells have been shown to express IL1 genes by *in situ* hybridization or northern blotting experiments monitored in experimental atherosclerotic lesions [10, 11]. In addition, the presence of several cytokines inside the cells of early and complicated lesions in humans has been documented by immunocytochemistry [12].

Therefore, cytokines may provoke local alterations in the functions of intrinsic vascular cells and infiltrating leukocytes during atherogenesis. The cytokines may contribute to the initiation of lesions by inducing the expression of

Table 1
Mediators that can promote atherogenesis and cell origin

	EC	SMC	M	T-cells
IL1	+	+	+++	–
IL2	–	–	–	+++
IL6	+	+++	+++	?
IL8	+	?	++	–
MCP1	+	+	+	–
TNF-α	–	+	+++	+
TNF-β (lymphotoxine)	–	–	–	+++
TGF-α	–	–	++	–
PDGF	++	++	++	–

Abbreviations: EC, endothelial cells; SMC, smooth muscle cells; M, macrophages.

leukocyte adhesion molecules, monocyte chemo-attractant proteins or growth factors involved in monocyte and smooth muscle cell reactivity within the vascular wall during the initial stage of lesion development. Later, the cytokines may trigger the thrombotic events.

In addition to these paracrine or autocrine mechanisms, the storage of soluble informative molecules within the extracellular matrix may represent an important pathway of protection and stabilization of the messengers. Proteoglycans have been found to function as the principal binders of growth factors and cytokines and several enzymatic systems (mainly endoglycosidases) were found to be efficient releasers of active forms from extracellular matrix [13, 14].

Cytokines as negative regulators of atherosclerotic development

Animal models have been used extensively for determining the potential for regression or reversal of atherosclerotic plaques. Regression studies in accelerated and severe lesions in swine have provided evidence of reductions in cellular and extracellular matrix calcium during regression. In a study of swine [15], it was reported that the most important change to the lesions in animals fed a low-fat, low-cholesterol regression diet was the [^{3}H] thymidine labelling index, which returned to normal levels within months. Vascular smooth muscle cells proliferate in response to several peptides (growth factors, cytokines), including PDGF, bFGF, TNF-α and IL1. In healthy adults, the cells of the blood vessel wall normally exhibit a slow turnover rate. The physiological quiescence reflects a balance between the positive and negative factors that influence cell proliferation and activation. So, these results indicate that the cells in the lesion are not in a permanent turned-on state, despite the lesion still containing a great deal of excess lipid as well as necrotic debris and calcium. However, blood lipids returned to normal levels.

These results would seem to imply that a continuing supply of stimulatory factors is necessary for the maintenance of an unbalanced equilibrium leading to excessive replicative activity [16]. These may be growth factors or substances that cause expression of growth factors by the target cells or liberation of factors by the extracellular matrix. In turn, informative molecules participate in the control of smooth muscle cell activation. Possible negative regulators include interferon, nitric oxide radicals, eicosanoids, heparin and heparin sulphate proteoglycans (Table 2) [17].

In addition to interferon-γ coming from activated T-lymphocytes and natural killer cells, the role of interferon-α and -β (INF-α and -β) has been documented [18], indicating that human vascular smooth muscle cells can express INF-β and that INF-α is present in advanced human atherosclerotic lesions. Since INF-β expression is induced in smooth muscle cells under the influence of tumour necrosis factor (TNF-α) which induces SMC growth, this result suggests that SMCs have the capacity to produce a potential autocrine growth regulator

Table 2
Anti-atherosclerotic properties of mediators of vascular origin

	EC	SMC	M	T-cells
TGF-β	++	++	++	–
INF-γ	–	–	–	+++
INF-β	?	+	+	–
$EDRF_I(NO^0)$	++	+/–	–	–
PGI_2, E_2	++	++	+	–
HETEs	+	+	++	+/–
Heparin sulphate	++	+	–	–

Abbreviations: EC, endothelial cells; SMC, smooth muscle cells; M, macrophages.

as it has previously been demonstrated for NO^0 or prostaglandins. Indeed, the production of antiproliferative factors such as heparin, prostaglandins and TGF-β can be achieved by SMCs and also other cells present inside the atherosclerotic plaques. This production can be regulated at several levels as previously indicated for INF-β. This is the case for autocrine stimulators of prostaglandin synthesis by IL1 or PDGF and paracrine stimulation by factors issued from endothelial or macrophage cells.

The link between these multiple interactive factors and cell activation (proliferation) remains difficult to establish even in simplified models. We still know little about the factors involved and the mechanisms of regulation. However, various experimentally and clinically applicable strategies for the inhibition of cytokine effects are under study, including antisense oligonucleotides as inhibitors of intimal SMC accumulation *in vivo*. In turn, stimulation of the endogenous production of protective factors may be proposed. At the moment, these strategies seem unable to protect the vascular wall from accelerated atherosclerosis in humans (i.e. restenosis). However, further understanding of the role of cytokines at various stages of atherogenesis may identify steps susceptible to therapeutic intervention.

References

1. Ross R. The pathogenesis of atherosclerosis: An update. *N Engl J Med* 1986; **314:** 488–500.
2. Cybulsky MI, Gimbrone MAJ. Endothelial expression of mononuclear leucocyte adhesion molecule during atherogenesis. *Sciences* 1991; **251:** 788–791.
3. Ferns GAA, Stewart-Lee AL, Anggård EE. Arterial response to mechanical injury: Balloon catheter de-endothelialisation. *Atherosclerosis* 1992; **92:** 89–104.
4. Fingerle J, Johnson R, Clowes AW, Majesky MW, Reidy MA. Role of platelets in smooth muscle cells proliferation and migration after vascular injury in rat carotid artery. *Proc Nat Acad Sci USA* 1989; **86:** 8412–8416.

5. Jonasson L, Holm J, Skalli O, Bondjers G, Hansson GK. Regional accumulations of T-cells, macrophages and smooth muscle cells in the human atherosclerotic plaque. *Arteriosclerosis* 1986; **6:** 131–138.
6. Munro JM, Cotran RS. The pathology of atherosclerosis: Atherogenesis and inflammation. *Lab Invest* 1988; **58:** 249–261.
7. Moncada S, Palmer RMJ, Higgs EA. Nitric oxide: Physiology, pathophysiology and pharmacology. *Pharm Revs* 1991; **43:** 109–142.
8. Nilsson J. Growth factors and the pathogenesis of atherosclerosis. *Atherosclerosis* 1986; **62:** 185–199.
9. Libby P, Hansson GK. Involvement of the immune system in human atherogenesis: Current knowledge and unanswered questions. *Lab Invest* 1991; **64:** 5–15.
10. Clinton SK, Fleet JC, Loppnow H, Salomon RN, Clark BD, Cannon JG, Shaw AR, Dinarello CA, Libby P. IL1 gene expression in rabbit vascular tissue *in vivo*. *Am J Pathol* 1991; **138:** 1005–1014.
11. Moyer C, Sajuthi D, Tulli H, Williams JK. Synthesis of IL1 α and β in atherosclerosis. *Am J Pathol* 1991; **138:** 951–960.
12. Clinton SK, Underwood R, Hayes C, Sherman ML, Uufe DW, Libby P. Macrophage colony stimulating factor gene expression in vascular cells and in experimental and human atherosclerosis. *Am J Pathol* 1992; **140:** 301–316.
13. Saksela O, Rifkin DB. Release of b FGF-heparan sulfate complexes from endothelial cells by plasminogen activator mediated proteolytic activity. *J Cell Biol* 1990; **110:** 767–775.
14. Vlodavsky I, Folkman J, Sullivan R, Fridman R, Ishai-Michaeli R, Sasse J, Klagsbrun M. Endothelial cells derived basic fibroblast growth factor, synthesis and deposition into subendothelial extracellular matrix. *Proc Nat Acad Sci USA* 1987; **84:** 2292–2296.
15. Kim DN, Schmee J, Ho HT, Thomas WA. The "turning off" of excessive cell replicative activity in advanced atherosclerotic lesions in swine by a regression diet. *Atherosclerosis* 1988; **71:** 131–142.
16. Desgranges C, Larrue J. Smooth muscle cell proliferation and atherosclerosis. *J Nephrol* 1990; **1:** 35–44.
17. Larrue J. Réactivité de la paroie arterielle aux stimuli athérogènes. *Arch Mal Coeur* 1991; **84:** 1635–1643.
18. Palmer H, Libby P. Interferon β: A potential autocrine regulator of human vascular SMC growth. *Lab Invest* 1992; **66:** 715–721.

49 Lipid Management in Secondary Prevention of Coronary Heart Disease

Barry Lewis

University of London, London, UK

Introduction

The justification for intensive management of hyperlipidaemia in secondary prevention is three-fold. Elevated serum cholesterol levels, and also low HDL levels, are powerful predictors of the absolute incidence of recurrent coronary events. Secondary prevention trials have established, particularly in meta-analysis, that measures to lower serum cholesterol levels reduce recurrence rates. And, thirdly, trials employing serial coronary angiography have consistently shown that cholesterol lowering reduces the incidence and extent of progressive coronary atherosclerosis.

Lipids as risk factors for reinfarction

Among 11 longitudinal studies of factors predicting recurrent coronary heart disease in men, 10 showed serum cholesterol to be a predictor of coronary heart disease events [1]. Two studies showed this to be the case in women. Serum cholesterol was not a predictor of total mortality in two studies on men with coronary heart disease, however. The predictive power of cholesterol is shared by other "classical" risk factors: low HDL cholesterol, cigarette smoking, diabetes and hypertension.

Proceedings of the Vth World Congress on Cardiac Rehabilitation

In some studies, the relative risk of recurrent coronary events conferred by elevated serum cholesterol is less than the risk of first events conferred by similar levels in previously healthy subjects; but the reverse has also been observed. However, the absolute number of coronary events attributable to elevated serum cholesterol is several-fold greater in men with pre-existing coronary heart disease than in men free from coronary heart disease [2], and this should guide clinical decisions.

The role of cholesterol is likely to be even greater than is suggested by most epidemiological studies. In most such studies, serum cholesterol was measured only once, at entry; due to regression-dilution bias [3], the predictive power of cholesterol level is substantially attenuated in these studies.

Secondary prevention trials of cholesterol lowering

Interpretation of secondary prevention trials has been constrained by small sample size, inadequate cholesterol lowering, or both. Where sample size has been adequate, as in the Coronary Drug Project [4], or where the decrease in cholesterol has been substantial, as in the Program on Surgical Correction of Hyperlipidemia [5], significant reduction in recurrent coronary heart disease events is often seen. The findings in eight qualifying secondary prevention trials have been subjected to meta-analysis [6]. The number of participants totalled 7837. The combined data show a 25% reduction in non-fatal myocardial infarction and a 22% reduction in all myocardial infarctions ($P < 0.001$). A non-significant 9% decrease in total mortality was seen. In all but one of the eight trials, serum cholesterol reduction was modest, justifying the expectation that more effective lipid lowering would yield better results.

"Regression" trials

Eight trials, employing 10 distinct interventions to lower serum lipids, have utilized coronary angiographic endpoints in randomized controlled designs [7]. A further two were uncontrolled, and another used a non-randomized comparison group. All reported favourable serum cholesterol reductions ranging from 14 to 32%, by use of diet, cholestyramine, lovastatin, drug combinations, multiple changes in lifestyle, or partial ileal bypass. Based on quantitative image analysis, or blinded panels of observers, or both, the trials consistently showed a decreased incidence and/or extent of progression of coronary atherosclerosis. Eight out of 10 intervention groups showed a significant increase in the incidence of regression. Common to all was a reduction in serum cholesterol. Many, but not all, showed a reduction in triglyceride levels and an increase in HDL cholesterol. Progression was directly related to in-trial LDL cholesterol level where this was measured. In most, regression took place in patients in whom LDL cholesterol was reduced to less than 3.5 m mol/l; in one (in which pre-treatment levels were grossly raised due to familial hypercholesterolaemia), the mean LDL cholesterol among those showing regression was 4.5 m mol/l.

In five intervention groups among the randomized controlled regression trials, hard clinical coronary event rates were reduced; angina decreased in a sixth. The regression trials may be considered as a subset of secondary prevention trials.

As an example, the recently reported STARS trial [8] may be summarized. Ninety men with coronary heart disease and serum cholesterol 6–10 (mean 7.2) m mol/l, were randomized to receive usual care (UC), a readily complied with lipid-lowering diet (D), or diet plus cholestyramine 16 g/dose (DC). Serum cholesterol decreased 14% in group D, 26% in DC and 2% in UC. Baseline and 39-month coronary angiograms were compared by quantitative image analysis. The proportion of patients who showed progression of coronary artery disease significantly decreased (46% in UC, 15% in D, 12% in DC), while the proportion showing regression increased significantly (4% in UC, 38% in D, 33% in DC). The mean width of up to 10 proximal coronary segments per patient (total number 489), or MAWS, decreased in UC (−0.201 mm), was little changed in D (+0.003 mm) and increased in DC (+0.103 mm) (P for trend 0.002). Other angiographic indices – minimum width of segment, % diameter stenosis (%D) and edge irregularity – showed congruent changes.

The results were separately analysed for segments showing different degrees of severity of baseline stenoses: <15%, 15–50%, and >50%. All showed progression in UC; in both intervention groups, regression or arrest of progression was seen in mildly, moderately or severely diseased segments. As with other trials, the greatest magnitude of regression was seen in segments bearing >50% stenoses. However, 15–50% stenoses, the range including most precursor lesions for Q-wave myocardial infarction, also showed favourable treatment effects by all four angiographic indices. Hard clinical cardiovascular endpoints were significantly reduced by treatment, occuring in 36% of UC patients at risk, 11% of D ($P < 0.05$) and 4% of DC patients at risk ($P < 0.01$). Progession (decrease in mean width of segments) was directly related to mean in-trial LDL cholesterol ($r = 0.40$), but was not significantly related to HDL cholesterol nor to triglyceride level.

An approach to lipid management in secondary prevention

The following principles are concordant with the 1992 Guidelines of the European Atherosclerosis Society, currently in press. The goals of therapy are, in particular, to lower LDL cholesterol levels to less than 3.0 m mol/l, and also to lower triglyceride to less than 2.3 m mol/l and to ensure that HDL cholesterol is greater than 0.9 m mol/l. The LDL recommendation is based on the linear relation between levels of this lipoprotein and progression of disease in several angiographic trials. The triglyceride target is that currently adopted in primary prevention, but has not been established by trials designed to assess the value of triglyceride lowering. Similarly, there is no definitive evidence as yet of benefit from increasing HDL cholesterol levels, though many believe this to be desirable. In the Leiden Intervention Study [9], progression of coronary narrowing was directly related to in-trial serum cholesterol:HDL cholesterol ratios.

These targets imply that the majority of patients with coronary heart disease require and would benefit from lipid lowering. It should be mentioned that a full lipid profile (cholesterol, triglyceride, HDL cholesterol and LDL cholesterol) should be obtained, in a sample obtained after 14 h fasting, in all patients with coronary heart disease. This should not be carried out during acute illness (or during weight reduction) but reliable measurements may be made within the first 24 h after onset of symptoms of acute myocardial infarction.

Vigorous treatment is not justified in patients with limited life expectation because of myocardial damage, non-cardiovascular disease or very advanced age. A significant reduction in total mortality in the POSCH trial was confined to patients in whom the ejection fraction exceeded 50% [5].

For most hyperlipidaemic persons, carefully supervised dietary management is effective; this is true in secondary as well as in primary prevention. While diet is the preferred management and suffices for many patients, secondary prevention is a clear indication for lipid-lowering drug therapy in patients in whom a 3- to 6-month trial of diet fails to achieve target values. Dietary care includes restriction of energy intake in overweight patients, with a view to reducing weight at the rate of 0.5–1 kg/week. The diet is restricted in total fat to 25–30% of energy intake, and has an increased content of cereal foods, vegetables and fruit with emphasis on those with a high content of soluble fibre [10]. Saturated fat provides 8–10% energy, polyunsaturated fat about 8% and mono-unsaturated fat 10–13% energy. Dietary cholesterol is reduced to 200–250 mg/day. Such a diet will lower serum cholesterol by, on average, 20%, and lowers LDL cholesterol by 20–25% [11, 12]. The physician can do much to provide motivation and enhance compliance, and to assure the patient that the diet does not lessen the pleasures of the table.

For diet-unresponsive patients, several satisfactory lipid-active drugs are available. For reduction of serum cholesterol and LDL cholesterol, the options are a HMG CoA reductase inhibitor, a bile acid sequestrant, or a fibrate such as ciprofibrate or fenofibrate. If serum triglyceride and cholesterol are elevated, a fibrate or a reductase inhibitor is most suitable. Patients with predominant elevation of triglyceride and low levels of HDL cholesterol respond best to a fibrate or nicotinic acid. Severe genetic hyperlipidaemias such as familial hypercholesterolaemia require diet and medication, often with a combination of a reductase inhibitor and a sequestrant; remnant hyperlipidaemia responds well to diet with a fibrate drug. When hyperlipidaemia is accompanied by low levels of HDL cholesterol, a fibrate or nicotinic acid is a suitable choice.

Contribution of lipid lowering to secondary prevention

Trials of lipid lowering in secondary prevention necessarily involve this treatment in a single intervention; but in practice, of course, it is but one component of a regime directed to all cardiovascular risk factors, to anti-platelet therapy and to specific cardio-active drug therapy as indicated. Yet the contribution of lipid lowering is now strongly supported by the evidence summarized, and it deserves a higher priority than is now generally the case. The lipid specialist is all too often referred patients with end-stage coronary heart disease or following an amputation, who have long had florid, hitherto untreated or partly treated hyperlipidaemia.

The absence of clinical trial evidence that total mortality is lessened by lipid lowering is often cited as a reason for this over-conservative attitude. But this absence should not be seen as evidence for or against a favourable effort on longevity: it merely reflects the fact that no trial designed to address this issue has yet been conducted [13]. Until such a trial is completed, policy decisions should be based on three considerations [6]:

1. In patients with coronary heart disease, more than four deaths out of five are from cardiovascular disease.
2. Meta-analysis of *secondary* prevention trials shows a decrease in total mortality.
3. Reduction in coronary heart disease events is in itself a sufficient goal for its role in improving the quality of life.

Finally, the contribution of lipid lowering to secondary prevention is highly cost-effective. In one estimate [12], the cost of extending life by one quality-adjusted life year in men aged 40–69 was £2598 in primary prevention and £223 in secondary prevention: this reflects the far higher incidence of coronary events in the latter category. Comparable costs for detection of breast cancer by mammography are £5500, and for coronary artery bypass grafting £1300 [14].

Secondary prevention is not only good clinical care and good economics; it may also contribute importantly to reduction of the overall rate of CHD in the population, for about one-half of men who have a myocardial infarction have previous manifestations of coronary disease.

References

1. Lewis B. On lowering lipids in the post-infarction patient. *J Int Med* 1991; **229:** 483–488.
2. Pekkanen J, Lin S, Heiss G *et al.* Ten years cardiovascular mortality in relation to cholesterol level among men with and without pre-existing cardiovascular disease. *N Engl J Med* 1990; **322:** 1700–1707.
3. MacMahon S, Peto R, Cutler J *et al.* Blood pressure, strokes, and coronary heart disease. Part I. Prolonged differences in blood pressure: Prospective observational studies corrected for the regression-dilution bias. *Lancet* 1990; **335:** 765–774.

4. Coronary Drug Project Research Group. Clofibrate and niacin in coronary heart disease. *JAMA* 1975; **238:** 360–381.
5. Buchwald M, Varce RL, Matts JP *et al.* Effect of partial ileal bypass on mortality and morbidity from coronary heart disease in patients with hypercholesterolemia. *N Engl J Med* 1990; **323:** 946–955.
6. Rossouw JE, Lewis B, Rifkind BM. The value of lowering cholesterol after myocardial infarction. *N Engl J Med* 1990; **323 :** 1112–1119.
7. Lewis B. Clinical trials of atherosclerosis regression. In: Paoletti R, Gotto AM (eds), *Proceedings of XI International Symposium on Drugs Affecting Lipid Metabolism* (in press).
8. Watts GF, Lewis B, Brent JNH *et al.* Effects on coronary artery disease of lipid-lowering diet, or diet plus cholestyramine, in the St Thomas' Atherosclerosis Degression Study (STARS). *Lancet* 1992; **339:** 563–569.
9. Boutzemius AC, Krombout D, Barth JD *et al.* Diet, lipoproteins, and the progression of coronary atherosclerosis. *N Engl J Med* 1985: **312:** 805–811.
10. Assmann G, Lewis B, Mancini M (Chairman). The recognition and management of hyperlipidaemia in adults: A policy statement of the European Atherosclerosis Society. *Eur Heart J* 1988; **9:** 571–600.
11. Lewis B, Hammett F, Katan MB *et al.* Towards an improved lipid-lowering diet: Additive effects of changes in nutrient intake. *Lancet* 1981; **ii:** 1310–1313.
12. Choudbury S, Jackson P, Katan MB *et al.* A multifactorial diet in the management of hyperlipidaemia. *Atherosclerosis* 1984; **50:** 93–103.
13. Lewis B. Safety aspects of cholesterol lowering: Total mortality, specific side effects, and random associations. *Lipid Review* 1992; **5:** 41–47.
14. Reckless JPD. The cost-effectiveness of clinical care for hyperlipidaemia. In: Lewis B, Assman G (eds), *The Social and Economic Contexts of Coronary Prevention.* Current Medical Literature: London, 1990.

XII Secondary Prevention

50 MULTIFIT: A New System of Coronary Risk Factor Modification After Acute Myocardial Infarction

Robert F. DeBusk,*[1] Nancy Houston Miller,[1] Craig Barr Taylor,[2] Robert H. Superko,[3] Walter E. Berger[4]

[1] Stanford Cardiac Rehabilitation Program, Stanford University School of Medicine, 780 Welch Road, Suite 106, Palo Alto, California 94304-1517, [2] Department of Psychiatry, Stanford University School of Medicine, Stanford, California 94305, [3] Alta Bates–Herrick Hospital, 3030 Telegraph Avenue, Berkeley, California 94705 and *[4] Kaiser Permanente Medical Center, 1150 Veterans Boulevard, Redwood City, California 94063, USA*

A critique of contemporary cardiac rehabilitation

Providing cardiac rehabilitation to patients following acute myocardial infarction (MI) and coronary revascularization procedures entails at least three major problems: (1) there is too little time to initiate intervention during hospitalization, which is increasingly brief; (2) continuity is often lacking between the in-patient and out-patient phases of management, which are often managed by different teams; and (3) too few resources are devoted to risk factor management in both phases of treatment, including not only care-givers, such as nurses, dieticians, psychologists and others, but instructional materials, equipment and facilities.

Comparing the resources devoted to acute care in the in-patient setting with rehabilitation and prevention in the out-patient setting helps to underscore the structural and functional deficiencies in the existing system of disease prevention and rehabilitation. The resources for hospital-based treatment of acute illness during a span of days or weeks are generally adequate: nurses are continuously in attendance, physicians maintain written and verbal communication with nurses and visit patients regularly, and the necessary medical information is available in the medical record. In contrast, nurses and other non-physician

* To whom all correspondence should be addressed.

Proceedings of the Vth World Congress on Cardiac Rehabilitation

health professionals have no continuing contact with patients after hospital discharge. This obliges physicians to carry out the work of gathering and recording medical information and maintaining surveillance of the patient through clinic visits. These clinic visits are not only infrequent, but they are usually devoted to issues of prognosis and symptoms rather than to coronary risk factor modification. Out-patient medical records are often poorly organized, which imposes a further burden on the physician responsible for risk factor modification.

The resources for cardiac rehabilitation are also misallocated. At least in the USA, exercise training remains the primary focus of cardiac rehabilitation, whereas the emerging need is to treat smoking and hypercholesterolaemia. For example, the recent demonstration of regression of coronary atherosclerosis with lipid-lowering drugs will doubtless stimulate the use of these agents. But existing cardiac rehabilitation programmes are not structured to facilitate such use.

Exercise training is no longer an appropriate centerpiece for cardiac rehabilitation, because in the contemporary era of thrombolysis it does not measurably enhance the prognosis of post-MI patients. Equally effective medical therapy such as beta-blocking drugs is much more convenient than exercise training and, unlike exercise training, is covered in the cost of usual care. More effective therapies such as thrombolytic agents and adjunctive medical therapy provided at the very onset of acute MI, have dramatically decreased not only in-hospital but post-hospital mortality, which diminishes the potential of exercise training to lower mortality still further.

In the randomized TIMI IIB study, in which patients receiving thrombolysis for acute MI were randomized to routine or elective balloon angioplasty, the total first-year mortality in both groups *including in-hospital deaths* was 7% [1]. In contrast, the study of cardiac rehabilitation conducted by Kallio *et al.* in the mid-1970s [2] demonstrated an in-hospital mortality of 10% and a first-year post-hospital mortality of 15% among patients receiving usual care and 10% among those receiving cardiac rehabilitation. It is clear that dramatic progress has been made in recent years in reducing the mortality of patients with acute MI.

Today, with optimal thrombolytic and adjunctive medical therapy (beta blocking, antiplatelet and anticoagulant agents) provided at the very onset of myocardial infarction and mechanical revascularization performed as soon as 24 h afterwards, the first-year mortality is so low that many thousands of patients would be required to demonstrate the prognostic value of exercise training. Indeed, the same is true of *any* therapy provided days or weeks rather than hours after acute MI. In the contemporary era of thrombolysis, exercise training also exerts a lesser effect on functional capacity. Thrombolysis, adjunctive medical therapies and revascularization, which decrease early and late mortality, also preserve functional capacity, which reflects the extent of underlying left ventricular dysfunction and myocardial ischaemia. A good prognosis is therefore tantamount to a well-preserved functional capacity. Moreover, the brief duration of contemporary hospitalization for acute MI minimizes physical deconditioning.

MULTIFIT: A new nurse-managed system of coronary risk factor modification

The MULTIFIT programme of medically assisted self-care not only addresses the contemporary need to emphasize smoking cessation and diet–drug management of hypercholesterolaemia, but it does so more efficiently than existing alternatives. Patients' contact with the MULTIFIT nurses occurs primarily by telephone rather than through face-to-face contact in clinics or hospital wards. The nurses communicate with physicians by telephone and through individualized computer-generated reports that characterize patients' current progress in coronary risk factor modification. The relevant medical information is contained in a highly standardized computer format that facilitates assessment of patients' current clinical status and guides nurses' management of coronary risk factors. Finally, patients have access to their individualized medical information through computer-generated reports and other communications initiated by the nurses.

Thus, a single care-giver, the nurse, provides multidisciplinary services in smoking cessation, exercise and the diet–drug management of hypercholesterolaemia. MULTIFIT is not designed to transform nurses into psychologists, exercise physiologists or nutritionists, but rather to enable them to provide patients with the expertise of experts in these areas. In other countries, non-physician health care professionals other than nurses might provide some or all of these services. However, nurses were chosen as the care-givers in this project because they are the most numerous and readily available non-physician professionals, their role is well-integrated into the US medical care system and their training in coronary disease process and medical aspects of coronary care is pertinent to issues of risk assessment and management.

The MULTIFIT system enables a hospital-based nurse to communicate with patients at home through telephone and mail contacts and, where necessary, through visits, which are routinely scheduled at 21 days after acute MI for exercise testing and at 90 days for initiation of lipid-lowering drug therapy for patients who have not achieved goal levels of LDL cholesterol through dietary change. A single additional visit is scheduled for patients relapsing to smoking.

The MULTIFIT system enables nurses to receive appropriate support and telephone consultation from experts including a nurse co-ordinator, lipid specialist, psychiatrist, cardiologist and nutritionist. This mode of consultation augments the decision support provided by computer-based computerized algorithms. This system is also convenient for patients, inasmuch as their visits to the laboratory to provide blood samples for measurement of plasma cholesterol and other chemistry values can be made virtually 24 h per day, at times convenient to them. Once the nurses have obtained the laboratory test results, they initiate and alter lipid-lowering drug therapy by 'phone.

Exercise training in MULTIFIT

Exercise training designed to facilitate weight management and enhance psychological status and physical endurance was provided in a home setting to the following subsets of patients in MULTIFIT:

1. The 70% of patients without significant left ventricular dysfunction or exercise-induced myocardial ischaemia, whose risk is low, initiated exercise training 3 weeks post-MI.
2. The 20% of patients with angina pectoris or exercise-induced myocardial ischaemia, whose risk for subsequent cardiac events was diminished by revascularization, initiated home exercise training 4–5 weeks after coronary artery surgery or 1–2 weeks after percutaneous transluminal coronary angioplasty (PTCA).
3. The 10% of patients with isolated left ventricular dysfunction and other limiting conditions, were considered permanently ineligible for exercise training, although they were encouraged to walk at a comfortable pace for 20–30 min daily. These limiting conditions included chronic obstructive pulmonary disease, peripheral vascular disease, orthopaedic abnormalities and various conditions complicating the prescription of exercise training, including atrial fibrillation and left bundle branch block.

Approximately 70% of MULTIFIT patients underwent symptom-limited treadmill exercise testing 3 weeks after acute MI. Such testing provided the basis for an individualized exercise training programme. The patients were provided with portable heart rate monitors that emitted an audible tone when the heart rate was outside the specified training range. The patients wore these monitors during exercise for the first 2 months to help them to maintain their training intensity within the prescribed range. The exercise training heart rate was set at 60–85% of peak treadmill heart rate. Even such relatively low-intensity exercise training continued over a 6-month period enhances functional capacity [3]. Since the risk of training-induced cardiac arrest is closely related to the intensity of exercise training [4], low-intensity exercise is an important safeguard to home-based exercise training. The prescribed exercise training sessions were of 20–30 min duration, 3–5 times per week.

The actual mean training heart rate was 90–110 beats/min. Walking was elected by 83% of patients, walking/jogging by 12% of patients and cycling by 5%. Self-reported adherence to exercise, verified by exercise logs, exceeded 90% at day 30 and 80% at 6 months. Nurse-initiated telephone contacts were made monthly for the first 5 months and bi-monthly thereafter to help patients assess their progress and address any compliance problems. The patients expressed a high degree of confidence or self-efficacy in their ability to carry out the prescribed exercise training regimen.

Smoking cessation in MULTIFIT

Smoking cessation is an intervention particularly well-suited to the MULTIFIT approach. Patients' greatest likelihood of relapsing to smoking occurs in the first week following hospital discharge, at a time when the vast majority of patients have not yet begun to participate in out-patient cardiac rehabilitation programmes. During the first few days of hospitalization, the MULTIFIT nurses use a 14-item self-efficacy scale to identify the circumstances in which patients state that they are most likely to relapse to smoking. Patients indicate their self-efficacy or confidence in their ability to resist smoking in these individualized high-risk situations. Self-efficacy ratings of less than 70% are the focus of the nurses' counselling sessions prior to hospital discharge. Prior to hospital discharge, the patients are given a workbook to complete at home within the first 2 weeks. They view a videotape portraying successful strategies in smoking cessation and are provided with audiotapes to facilitate relaxation as an adjunct to the smoking cessation intervention.

Within 48 h after hospital discharge, at 7 days, 21 days and monthly thereafter in the first 6 months, the nurses telephone patients to ascertain their success in resisting smoking and to provide additional counselling. Patients who relapse are offered additional counselling in a single out-patient clinic visit with the nurse. Highly addicted patients who relapse to smoking after hospital discharge are provided with a prescription for nicotine gum or patch and detailed instructions for the correct use of these agents. We have not detected significant myocardial ischaemia or ventricular arrhythmias on ambulatory electrocardiograms performed in clinically low-risk patients using these pharmacological agents. The plasma concentration of nicotine associated with use of nicotine replacement strategies is substantially below that noted among smokers. We believe that the short-term risk of these nicotine replacement agents is correspondingly lower than the long-term risk of continued smoking.

Diet–drug therapy for hypercholesterolaemia in MULTIFIT

Diet–drug management for hypercholesterolaemia is perhaps the most demanding of all risk factor interventions, reflecting in part the necessity to evaluate patients' status and provide detailed individualized information and instruction at multiple points in time. To facilitate dietary management, we have created a computer-based expert system called CALS (Computer-Assisted Learning System) that operates very much as an automated bank teller machine (ATM). Patients complete and mail to the nurse a brief *food frequency questionnaire* (FFQ), the analogue to the individualized bank card that provides individualized dietary information. This information is used by the computer to generate individualized *progress reports*, mailed to the patient by the nurse, that summarize the patient's current status. This progress report is the analogue of the individualized account report provided by the ATM. This cycle of FFQ–progress report occurs at baseline and at two subsequent intervals 6 weeks apart. In our experience, this automated system has demonstrated efficacy of the same order of magnitude observed with face-to-face nutritionist counselling. The advantages of the system over nutritionist-mediated counselling include its greater convenience, simplicity and lower cost.

The role of nutritional counselling in the management of hypercholesterolaemia after acute MI has been substantially impacted by the more aggressive treatment goal being advanced by the National Cholesterol Education Program (NCEP) for patients with established ischaemic heart disease. The previous goal of LDL cholesterol of 130 mg/dl is being revised downwards to 100 mg/dl. In MULTIFIT, we have adopted a somewhat more aggressive treatment goal of 95 mg/dl. Inasmuch as the average value of LDL cholesterol at 90 days among MULTIFIT patients was 137 mg/dl, a 10% maximal reduction in this value due to dietary intervention would yield a post-diet value of 123 mg/dl, which is 28 mg/dl above the optimal value of 95 mg/dl. Thus, the magnitude of reduction in LDL cholesterol with drug therapy is twice that of diet therapy: 28 mg/dl compared to 14 mg/dl. In fact, 90 days after acute MI, two-thirds of MULTIFIT patients had values of LDL cholesterol exceeding the present NCEP endpoint of 130 mg/dl and fully 80% were candidates for more aggressive lipid-lowering drug therapy.

Nurse-managed lipid-lowering drug therapy was initiated at 90 days during an out-patient visit and modified as needed by nurse-initiated telephone contacts at 120, 150, 180 and 270 days after acute MI. We used three treatment algorithms for drug therapy, based on combinations of lipoproteins. A total of 79% of patients had isolated hypercholesterolaemia (LDL cholesterol values exceeding 95 mg/dl); they received bile acid binding resin (BABR). A total of 15% had combined hypercholesterolaemia (LDL cholesterol exceeding 95 mg/dl and triglycerides exceeding 250 mg/dl); they received both BABR and nicotinic acid. A total of 6% of patients had isolated hypertriglyceridaemia (triglyceride values greater than 250 mg/dl); they received nicotinic acid. In general, patients in usual care received more lovastatin and less BABR than patients in the intervention group. The average daily dose taken by patients in the intervention group was higher for BABR (32 *vs* 18 g) and for niacin (2000 *vs* 1200 mg) but comparable for gemfibrozil (1200 mg in each group) and lovastatin (25 mg in each group).

The occurrence of self-reported side-effects in the intervention group was 400% overall and was highest for resins and niacin. However, changes in drugs due to side-effects occurred in only 4% of treatment encounters. Unanticipated changes in initial therapy occurred in only 6% of cases overall. In the majority of cases, changes in initial therapy resulted from failure to achieve treatment goals by the second or third step. No serious problems related to lipid-lowering drug therapy were seen in either group.

Results of the MULTIFIT trial

The MULTIFIT trial is an NHLBI-sponsored collaboration between Kaiser Foundation Medical Centers in Redwood City, Santa Clara, Sãn Jose, Hayward and Walnut Creek and the Stanford Cardiac Rehabilitation Program. The primary outcome measures of the trial are smoking cessation rate, functional capacity and plasma LDL cholesterol. The study was designed to evaluate 500 patients receiving a home treatment programme and 500 receiving usual care. To date, a total of 600 patients have been randomized and followed, 300 in each of these assignments.

At 6 months, functional capacity among intervention patients was 9.3 ± 2.4 METs and among usual care patients 8.2 ± 2.0 METs. The smoking cessation rate at 12 months, projected from very early results, was 65% among intervention and 50% among usual care patients. The LDL cholesterol values at 12 months were 110 ± 31 mg/dl in the intervention group and 137 ± 33 mg/dl in the usual care group. A total of 74% of the patients in the intervention group achieved the existing NCEP plasma cholesterol target value of 130 mg/dl or less compared to 21% of the usual care patients.

Conclusions

This highly individualized home-based, nurse-managed system proved superior to usual care for coronary risk factor management and obviated many of the obstacles limiting access to and efficacy of rehabilitative services for post-MI patients.

References

1. The TIMI Study Group. Comparison of invasive and conservative strategies after treatment with intravenous tissue plasminogen activator in acute myocardial infarction – Results of the thrombolysis in myocardial infarction (TIMI) Phase II Trial. *N Engl J Med* 1989; **320:** 618–627.
2. Kallio V, Hämäläinen H, Hakkila J, Luurila OJ. Reduction in sudden deaths by a multifactorial intervention programme after acute myocardial infarction. *Lancet* 1979; **ii:** 1091–1094.
3. King AC, Haskell WL, Taylor CB, Kraemer HC, DeBusk RF. Group- *vs* home-based exercise training in healthy older men and women. *JAMA* 1991; **266:** 1535–1542.
4. Hossack KF, Hartwig R. Cardiac arrest associated with supervised cardiac rehabilitation. *J Cardiac Rehab* 1982; **2:** 402–408.

51 Assisting Coronary Patients with Smoking Cessation

Nancy Houston Miller,*[1] Craig Barr Taylor,[2] Robert F. DeBusk[1]

[1] Stanford Cardiac Rehabilitation Program, Stanford University School of Medicine, 780 Welch Road, Suite 106, Palo Alto, California 94304-1517 and *[2] Department of Psychiatry, Stanford University School of Medicine, Stanford, California 94305, USA*

Patients with ischaemic heart disease who smoke experience an increased rate of morbidity and mortality [1]. For example, both men and women who continue to smoke after a myocardial infarction experience a 50% higher death rate compared to those who stop smoking [2]. Moreover, continued smoking after coronary angioplasty has been reported to be associated with an increased re-stenosis rate [3]. Smoking has been shown to cause silent ischaemia [4], block the increase in coronary blood flow normally associated with exercise [5], reduce the anti-ischaemic effects of both calcium and beta channel blocking agents [6], and trigger coronary spasm and abnormal segmental narrowing of the coronary arteries [7].

Cessation of smoking following a coronary event (acute MI or coronary revascularization procedure) is associated with significant benefits. For example, cessation of cigarette smoking has been shown to reduce the rates of re-infarction and death within 1 year of quitting [8]. In addition, data from the CASS registry indicates total mortality is reduced 25% at 5 years among those who quit smoking. This reduction in risk among patients undergoing coronary artery surgery applies to all patients, even those older than 70 years [9]. Stopping smoking is further associated with a delay in the onset of angina [10] and with an increase in HDL cholesterol levels [11].

* To whom all correspondence should be addressed.

Proceedings of the Vth World Congress on Cardiac Rehabilitation

While the health benefits of smoking cessation continue to be significant, approximately 45–50% of all smokers relapse to smoking within 6–12 months following a myocardial infarction [12]. However, this relapse rate is lower than among the general population of smokers receiving smoking cessation interventions. For example, the 1-year cessation rate in the general US population ranges from as low as 6% following physician advice to as high as 40% following combined behavioural and pharmacological interventions. Because the overall risk of death and myocardial infarction is greater in patients with established ischaemic heart disease, intensive smoking interventions should be provided to these patients.

Most interventions designed to help coronary patients to quit smoking have included physician advice, education or group counselling. Few randomized clinical intervention trials of smoking have been conducted in this population. Most reported studies have used an educational approach stressing the benefits of modifying behavioural risk factors [13] or have attempted to look at the effect of exercise training on the smoking habits of individuals within rehabilitation programmes [14]. Many of these studies are generally limited by small sample size, lack of uniformity regarding the definition of abstinence and reliance upon self-report data for confirmation of non-smoking status [12]. Furthermore, the proportion of "ex-smokers" defined at one point in time ("point prevalence") overestimates the sustained smoking cessation rate because detailed information regarding smoking status over this entire follow-up period is not available. Although approximately 45–50% of all smokers require only minimal intervention, especially after a coronary heart disease event, the remainder require multi-component interventions including physician advice, education and behavioural and pharmacological therapy.

Over the past 7 years, our research programme in smoking cessation has focused on nurse-managed multi-component interventions for patients following acute myocardial infarction. Our smoking cessation programme is based on social learning theory and relapse prevention training. Social learning theory views behaviour as influenced by three interacting systems: behavioural, cognitive and environmental [15]. Social learning theory emphasizes the importance of self-efficacy as a mediator of behaviour change. Self-efficacy is a measure of an individual's confidence in his or her capability to organize and execute a course of action. Self-efficacy measures provide practical information in assessing the effectiveness of programmes or interventions. Such measures have been used extensively in smoking cessation to assess patients' confidence in their capability to resist smoking in a wide variety of situations. In our experience, patients require assistance in undertaking or sustaining a behaviour for which their efficacy ratings are below 70%.

Relapse prevention therapy is a model developed by psychologist Dr Alan Marlatt in his work with addictive behaviours [16]. He notes that the probability of relapse increases when an individual fails to cope with a problem. Most individuals with addictive behaviours such as smoking are in control until the lack of skills to cope with high-risk situations results in decreased self-efficacy and an actual lapse. An increased sense of guilt and conflict associated with failure increases the probability that a lapse will escalate into a full-blown relapse. Years of research have identified the typical situations where smokers are likely to relapse. Self-efficacy scales can help to identify these high-risk situations.

Relapse prevention training helps patients to mobilize their resources for coping with high-risk situations. Such prevention training enables patients to develop cognitive and behavioural strategies to cope with these situations. The coping responses must be rehearsed and practised. Relapse prevention programmes also entail general lifestyle modification. For example, relaxation training provides the patient with a global perception of increased control, which in turn may enhance self-efficacy. Exercise therapy involves replacing a negative addiction with a positive habit. Programming these new activities into the day provides balance and substitutes for activities that may provide immediate gratification such as smoking.

In our original work published in the *Annals of Internal Medicine* in July 1990 [17], 235 of 507 consecutive patients were smoking within the 6 months prior to their acute MI. Of these, 173 were randomly allocated to receive usual care ($n = 87$) or a smoking relapse prevention intervention ($n = 86$). The objectives of the study were to evaluate the efficacy of a nurse-directed smoking cessation programme and to identify the predictors of smoking cessation. Of the 173 smokers, 58 in the usual care group and 72 in the intervention group remained in the study at 1 year. During hospitalization, patients in the intervention group were provided with a strong message about the necessity to quit smoking, an 18-page workbook (*Staying Free*) and audiotape emphasizing how to identify and cope with high-risk situations, and an audiotape to guide relaxation exercises. The workbook was designed to be completed over a 2-week period; the patients completed the first section while in hospital. A 28-item self-efficacy scale was administered during hospitalization to quantify patients' confidence to resist smoking in a variety of situations. The patients were counselled on how to cope with those situations for which they were less than 70% confident. Nurse-initiated telephone contacts were made once per week for the first 2–3 weeks and monthly for the next 4 months to determine if patients had relapsed or lost confidence in their ability to resist smoking and to provide further instruction and support. Those patients who relapsed were asked to meet with the nurse in the out-patient clinic during which nicotine gum was prescribed; only 5 patients received the gum. No further intervention occurred after 6 months. The biochemically confirmed smoking cessation rate at 12 months (6 months post-infarction) was 71% in the intervention group, compared to 45% in usual care ($P < 0.003$). Assuming all patients lost to follow-up or dropping out after randomization were smoking at 12 months, the cessation rate was 61% among the patients receiving the intervention (51/84) and 32% among the patients receiving usual care (26/82) ($P < 0.001$).

What were the important lessons learned from this trial?

1. Timing of the intervention was critical to the success of the intervention. Patients are most likely to relapse during the first week after hospital discharge. In many studies of smoking cessation in patients with coronary heart disease, instruction commences 1 or more weeks after discharge, when many patients have already relapsed. Indeed, of 18 patients who had relapsed by 3 weeks after MI, only 3 were abstinent 1 year later.
2. Patients' stated intention to quit during hospitalization was highly predictive of actual cessation 3 weeks and 1 year after MI. Extra time (an average of 1.5 additional hours) spent with patients expressing little intention of stopping did not enhance the cessation rate. In fact, there was an inverse relationship between time spent in intervention and success in quitting. The cost-effectiveness of the intervention would be enhanced by focusing on the two-thirds of patients expressing an intention to quit who are most likely to benefit from the intervention. However, even a *minimal* intervention may help some patients with low intention to quit to move towards the contemplation stage or at least reduce the number of cigarettes smoked per day.

The success of this study prompted us to incorporate the smoking intervention into a multifactorial intervention trial known as MULTIFIT. This trial evaluated the efficacy of a nurse-managed, home-based programme of exercise training, smoking cessation and diet–drug management of dyslipidaemia. I would like to review the important aspects of the smoking cessation component of the MULTIFIT intervention trial. The hospital provides an ideal setting for a structured individualized approach to smoking cessation following a coronary heart disease event. Patients experience the worst part of withdrawal during the initial 48–72 h after hospitalization, when smoking is forbidden. We initiated the intervention during this period.

A multi-component strategy has been shown in numerous studies to enhance the efficacy of interventions for smoking cessation. We ask physicians to go to the bedside and deliver a strong message to patients about cessation. This is facilitated by a standardized script attached to the patient's chart. In 1–2 min, the physicians are asked to cover four points:

1. To acknowledge that the patient smoked before hospitalization.
2. To provide reinforcement for cessation and indicate that the patient will most likely pass through the worst part of withdrawal during hospitalization.
3. To explain why it is important for the patient to quit smoking and *personalize* the message.
4. To ask if there is anything that can be done to help the patient remain a non-smoker.

A brief smoking history administered by the nurse provides information useful in counselling. Our 20-item history allows our nurses to determine patients' past experiences with quitting, level of addiction, use of alcohol and degree of intention to quit.

Videotapes, audiotapes and other self-help materials not only enhance the health professional's efforts in counselling, but can also save time. We use the videotape on smoking cessation and the smoking cessation workbook from the American Heart Association's Program *An Active Partnership for the Health of Your Heart*. Contracting is useful in enhancing commitment to behavioural change. We have found that contracting with a health care professional, spouse or friend further strengthens patients' commitment and acknowledges the support of another person to facilitate quitting. The *Active Partnership* workbook incorporates a simple contract for smoking cessation.

Our nurses spend approximately 20–30 min working with patients to provide relapse prevention counselling at the bedside. In addition, they cover the aspects of alcohol use, family support, weight gain and loss/deprivation from giving up smoking. Patients are encouraged to develop a specific plan for dealing with slips or a lapse. A lapse is defined as a single event, a re-emergence of a previous habit, which may or may not lead to the state of relapse. In our programme, patients are encouraged to call the nurse if a slip does occur. Nurses then provide additional counselling by telephone to help patients to get back on track. Only a small proportion of smokers telephone, however. A well-developed plan to deal with slips may enable patients to prevent total relapse to smoking.

Appropriate follow-up enhances cessation efforts. In our programmes, structured nurse-initiated telephone interviews at 48 h, 7 days, 21 days and 90 days after hospital discharge provide additional support and reinforcement to patients and facilitate problem-solving in case of relapse. These telephone contacts last approximately 10 min. Patients identified on telephone follow-up as having relapsed are invited to return to the hospital for additional counselling or asked to set another quit date over the telephone. However, further efforts by the nurse after one relapse visit do not appear to be cost-effective.

In our studies, pharmacological therapy is reserved for patients who relapse, or those who are classified as highly addicted during hospitalization. We measure addiction using the Fagerstrom Tolerance Scale. Two items from this scale are highly predictive of addiction in the coronary population: (1) "How soon do you smoke upon arising in the morning?" and, (2) "Do you smoke when you are so ill you are in bed?" Patients who smoke within the first 30 minutes of rising or when they are ill exhibit a high degree of addiction.

To our knowledge, no randomized pharmacological trials have yet been conducted using either nicotine gum or the nicotine patch in the coronary population. This reflects physicians' concern with the risk associated with nicotine replacement therapy in patients with established coronary heart disease. Although nicotine replacement therapy is potentially associated with ventricular arrhythmias and potential myocardial ischaemia, among patients with coronary heart disease we did not document these abnormalities on ambulatory ECG among clinically low-risk post-MI patients. It is important to note that blood nicotine levels average 12 mg/ml with the use of 2 mg nicotine gum, compared to peak levels of 35–54 mg/ml during smoking [18]. We believe that the long-term risks associated with continued smoking far outweigh the short-term risks of nicotine gum or the patch.

Appropriate administration of nicotine replacement therapies requires in-depth written and verbal instruction. A prescribed schedule for administering the gum and caution about the use of acidic agents such as orange juice, coca cola and coffee which may change the pH in the mouth, thus affecting nicotine absorption, is important. A written tapering schedule should be provided. Finally, the hazards of combined use of these agents with smoking must be emphasized. Nurse-initiated follow-up telephone calls provide an opportunity to ensure the proper use of these agents.

It is important to note that although the rates of smoking in the USA have declined to approximately 25.5% of the population as of 1990, among individuals recovering from acute MI the rate continues to be approximately 40–45%. We anticipate the efficacy of MULTIFIT to be similar to that of our original study. In summary, a planned approach to smoking cessation in the coronary population will most certainly lead to enhanced outcomes. Multicomponent strategies combining physician advice, educational aids, behavioural counselling such as contracting and relapse prevention training, and telephone follow-up, as well as pharmacological therapy are useful techniques which can be employed in the hospital and out-patient phases of recovery from a coronary heart disease event.

References

1. Mulcahy R. Influence of cigarette smoking on morbidity and mortality after myocardial infarction. *B Heart J* 1983; **49:** 410–415.
2. Wilhelmsson L, Elmfeldt D, Vedin JA *et al.* Smoking and myocardial infarction. *Lancet* 1975; **i:** 415–420.
3. Galan KM, Deligonul U, Kern MJ *et al.* Increased frequency of restenosis in patients continuing to smoke cigarettes after acute percutaneous transluminal angioplasty. *Am J Cardiol* 1988; **6:** 260–263.
4. Barry J, Mead K, Nabel E *et al.* Effect of smoking on the activity of ischemic heart disease. *JAMA* 1989; **261:** 398–402.
5. Winniford MD, Jansen DE, Reynolds GA *et al.* Cigarette smoking-induced coronary vasoconstriction in atherosclerotic coronary artery disease and prevention by calcium antagonists and nitroglycerin. *Am J Cardiol* 1987; **59:** 203–207.
6. Deanfield J, Wright C, Kirkler S *et al.* Cigarette smoking and treatment of angina with propranolol, atenolol and nifedipine. *N Engl J Med* 1984; **310:** 951–954.
7. Maouad J, Fernandez F, Hebert JL *et al.* Cigarette smoking during coronary angiography: Differences on focal narrowing (spasm) of the coronary arteries in 13 patients with angina at rest and normal coronary angiograms. *Cath Card Diag* 1986; **12:** 366.
8. Sparrow D, Dawber T, Colton T. The influence of cigarette smoking on prognosis after a first myocardial infarction. *J Chron Dis* 1978; **31:** 425–432.

9. Hermanson B, Ȯmenn G, Krommel R *et al.* Beneficial six-year outcome of smoking cessation in older men and women with coronary artery disease: Results from the CASS registry. *N Engl J Med* 1988; **319:** 1365–1368.
10. Daly LE, Graham IM, Hickey N, *et al.* Does stopping smoking delay onset of angina after myocardial infarction? *Br Med J* 1985; **291:** 935–937.
11. Stubbs I, Eskileson J, Nilsson-Ehle P. High-density lipoprotein concentrations increase after stopping smoking. *Br Med J* 1982; **284:** 1511–1513.
12. Burling TA, Singleton EG, Bigelow GE *et al.* Smoking following myocardial infarction: A critical review of the literature. *Health Psychol* 1984; **3:** 83–96.
13. Burt A, Thornley P, Illingsworth D. Stopping smoking after myocardial infarction. *Lancet* 1986; **i:** 304–306.
14. Taylor CB, Miller NH, DeBusk RF. Smoking cessation after acute MI: The effect of exercise training. *Addictive Behav* 1988; **13:** 331–335.
15. Bandura A. *Social Learning Theory*. Prentice-Hall: Englewood Cliffs, NJ, 1977.
16. Marlatt GA, Gordon JR (eds). *Relapse Prevention: Maintenance Strategies in the Treatment of Addiction.* Guilford Press, New York, 1985.
17. Taylor CB, Miller NH, Killen JD, *et al.* Smoking cessation after myocardial infarction: Effects of a nurse-managed intervention. *Ann Int Med* 1990; **113:** 118–123.
18. Benowitz NL. Pharmacologic aspects of cigarette smoking and nicotine addiction. *N Engl J Med* 1988; **319:** 1318–1329.

XIII Return to Work

52 Rehabilitation of Professional Aviators with Potentially Disqualifying Cardiovascular Problems

M. Joy, G. Bennett

Medical Branch, Civil Aviation Authority, Gatwick Airport, South Area, Gatwick, West Sussex RH6 OYR, UK

Introduction

Aviation is the only system of mass transportation regulated by international agreement. The agency involved, the International Civil Aviation Organization, is based in Montreal and all nations are signatories to ICAO, being thus bound by international treaty obligations. ICAO is a safety organization and lays down Internationally Agreed Standards and Recommended Practices known as ISARPs [1]. Aspects of personnel licensing, including medical fitness, are contained in Annex I and are general statements only permitting no degradation of physical fitness. Under ICAO Annex I.2.4.8., the fitness standard may be waivered provided "accredited medical conclusion" indicates that the issuance of the licence for which an application has been made is not likely to jeopardize flight safety. Notwithstanding this waiver clause, failure to meet the promulgated standard may be prejudicial to air transport safety and be prejudical to an applicant's employability. Refusal of medical certification thus represents a personal loss, a loss to an employer who may have invested a significant amount in terms of training and to an industry, in which age and experience have been demonstrated to be associated with a lower accident rate.

The First (1982) and Second (1987) UK and First (1991) European Workshops in Aviation Cardiology [2–4] evolved an approach to licensing based on a predicted probability of event which was not to exceed 1% p.a. for those

Proceedings of the Vth World Congress on Cardiac Rehabilitation

involved in multicrew operations. This is the cardiovascular mortality of a 60–65 year old male in North West Europe and is calculated, making certain assumptions, as follows: there are approximately 10,000 hours in a year (8760) and a 1% event rate is thus equivalent to 1 event per million hours, or one in every 100 years. If it is assumed that 10% of the flight is critical, and an average flight lasts 1 h 40 mins, then 10 min is critical (i.e. during take-off, on the climb out and during the ascent, through the approach to landing). Simulator experience and worldwide incident experience has suggested that in approximately 1% of incapacitating events occurring during this critical period, an accident may not be avoidable. With a cardiovascular event rate of one per million flying hours, it should thus be possible to achieve a medical cause accident rate in multicrew operations of one fatal accident in every 10^{8-9} flying hours (one event in 1×10^6 h with $10^{-1} \times 10^{-2}$ probability of such an event leading to catastrophe).

A 1% event rate cannot be applicable to single crew operations where the serious event rate is likely to equal the accident rate. In that case, there should be no significant degradation of the ICAO minimum standard permitted except that imposed by age. The effect on the identification of patients with cardiovascular conditions satisfying the "1% rule" will now be discussed.

Methods

The Civil Aviation Authority (CAA) is the body responsible in the UK for the implementation of the ICAO ISARPs. Data on loss or non-issuance of professional flying licences has been available since 1972, although it is incomplete for 1988–89 due to computerization difficulties. Figure 1 summarizes the numbers of licences lost over the 16-year period 1972–1989, indicating the predominance of cardiovascular and neuro-psychiatric causes. Other causes include cancer and respiratory illness. Partly due to the age skew of the population – there was a predominance of older pilots flying at the beginning of the period – and no doubt due to increased awareness of the possibility of cardiovascular incapacitation as a cause of accidents, the loss of licences among the 7500 Class I certificate holders at that time was substantial. During the second 5 years of the period, this attrition was reduced somewhat partly due to mandatory flight crew training for the possibility of incapacitation of a colleague and partly to the adoption by the UK CAA of the possibility of the endorsement of a Class I certificate "to fly as/or with co-pilot". This enabled the continuing certification of aircrew with a slightly degraded health standard. To assist with this process, in 1977, the Medical Advisory Panel to the CAA was set up to assist in difficult licensing decisions, i.e. the certification or not of those airmen with potentially disqualifying conditions.

The First UK Workshop in 1982 laid the foundation for the presentation of cardiovascular risk in the same terms as the fatal accident risk to passenger carrying aircraft [2]. Subsequently, as the 1% rule was evolved, it became

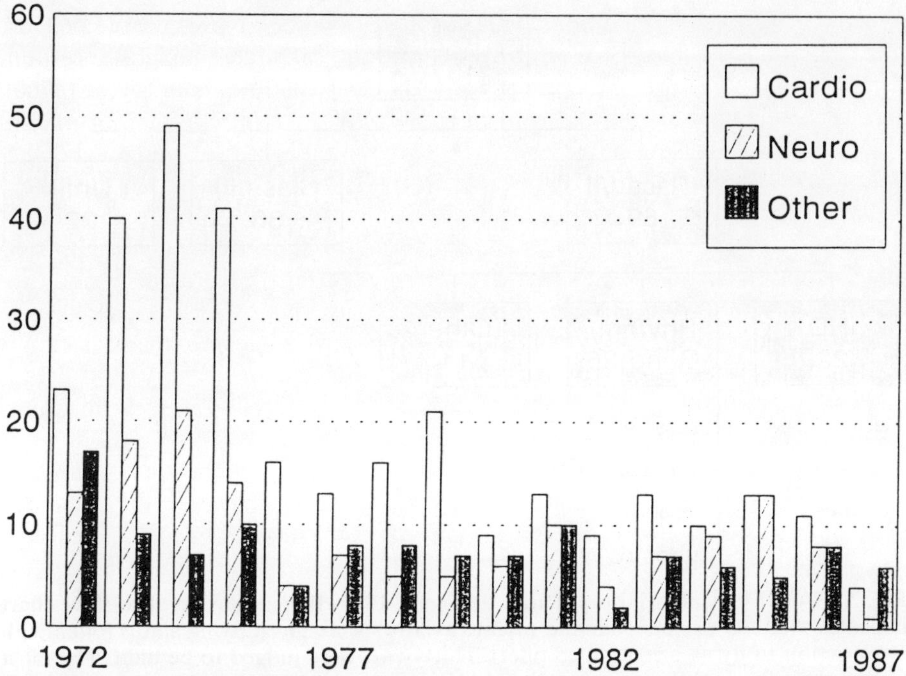

Fig. 1. UK non-loss/non-issuance of professional licences 1972–87. The total number of licences lost each year is indicated on the y-axis. Due to the high mean age of the pilot population in part, significant numbers of licences were lost in the early years of the period (see text).

possible to recertificate, following full evaluation, best risk subjects with a history of conditions previously disqualifying. These included myocardial infarction and coronary artery bypass grafting, for example. The treatment of hypertension also evolved as experience was gained. This initiative was associated with a reduction in the loss of UK professional licences because of cardiovascular problems from 4.1 per 1000 years in 1972–76 to 0.08 per 1000 years in 1986–90.

Results

In the years 1972–82, 61 cases were reviewed by the Medical Advisory Panel – all but 6 of these were for cardiovascular problems. There was a brief pause in activity while the First UK Workshop was published [2], but between 1984 and 1991 inclusive, 142 individual cases were discussed, 5 of which did not involve the speciality of cardiology. The conditions reviewed included myocardial infarction ($n = 30$), coronary artery bypass grafting ($n = 18$), atrial

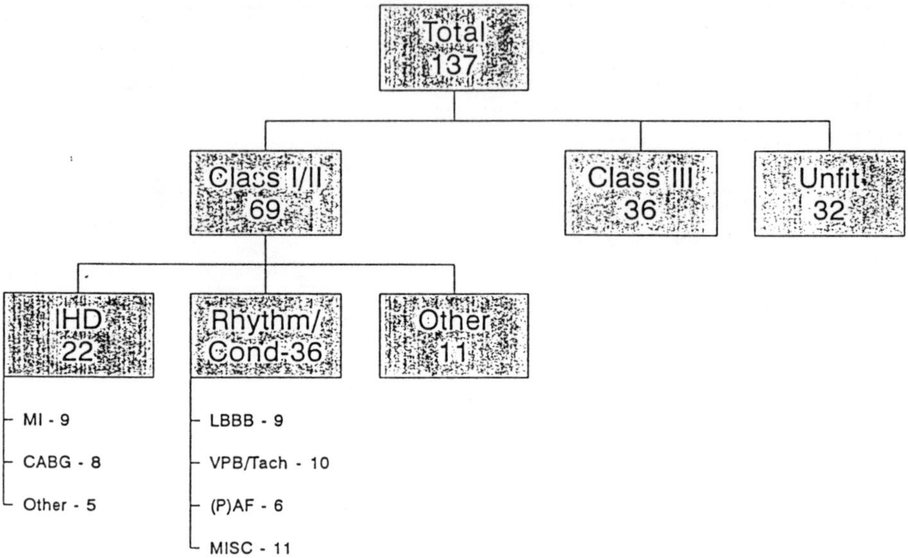

Fig. 2. CAA Medical Advisory Panel decisions 1984–1991 inclusive. The flow chart indicates that 105 professional and private aviators were given flying status (often with a restriction to fly as or with a co-pilot). Thirty-two were judged to be unfit. The most frequently seen conditions are appended below the panels.

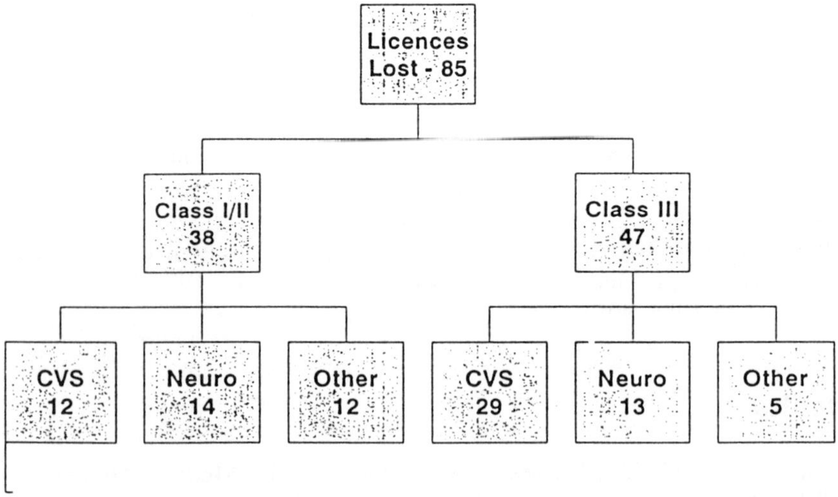

Fig. 3. UK loss/non-issuance of licences 1990–91. Eighty-five licences out of a total pilot population of some 15,000 professionals and 40,000 private certificate holders were refused or withdrawn. The number of certificate holders not renewing their licences for whatever reason is not known. Thirty-eight held Class I certificates, of which 12 were lost because of cardiovascular causes.

fibrillation ($n = 12$), left bundle branch aberration ($n = 8$) and coronary angioplasty ($n = 3$). Six decisions were referred. The outcome is illustrated in Figure 2. Altogether, 69 professional certificate holders were permitted to continue flying, while 36 private certificate holders were also allowed to continue; 32 were judged to be unfit for all forms of certification. The conditions with which certain professional airmen received (usually limited) certification included myocardial infarction ($n = 9$), coronary artery surgery ($n = 8$), left bundle branch aberration ($n = 9$), ventricular premature activity ($n = 10$) and (paroxysmal) atrial fibrillation ($n = 6$). There were 16 miscellaneous problems. Fifteen Class I holders received unrestricted certification to fly, including three with left bundle branch aberration (1 technically only had left anterior hemiblock) and four with AV conduction anomalies of one sort or another. One had suffered a single attack of atrial fibrillation, one had peripheral vascular disease and two were felt to have insignificant abnormality in the coronary circulation.

Licences were also lost or not issued for disqualifying conditions which carry a risk well outside an event rate of 1% p.a. These are not referred to the Medical Advisory Panel. A flow chart totalizing this experience in the years 1990–91 is illustrated in Fig. 3.

Discussion

Professional aircrew are not unique in being required to satisfy certain fitness requirements, but are exceptional in terms of the cost invested in their training. They are also in a high socio-economic group. Until it was suggested that risk of incapacitation could, and should, be expressed in the same terms as the fatal event rate in passenger aircraft operations, decision making in the UK with regard to fitness was at times uneven and inevitably somewhat arbitrary. The adoption of the "1% rule" has identified a target event rate which may permit continued certification, provided sufficient longitudinal data are available in terms of experience of the condition under assessment. This process has led to a fairer and more even standard of certificatory judgement and, furthermore, it has enabled the continued certification of significant numbers of aircrew with potentially disqualifying conditions.

References

1. Personnel licensing. International Standards and Recommended Practices. Annex I to the Convention on International Civil Aviation Medicine. ICAO: Montreal, 1987.
2. Joy M, Bennett G (eds). First UK Workshop in Aviation Cardiology. *Eur Heart J* (Suppl. G) 1984; **5:** 1–179.
3. Joy M, Bennett G (eds). Second UK Workshop in Aviation Cardiology. *Eur Heart J* (Suppl. G) 1988; **9:** 1–179.
4. Joy M (ed.). First European Workshop in Aviation Cardiology. *Eur Heart J* (in press).

53 Results of a Regional Work Aptitude Consultation

C. Blaquière,* E. Mazaudier, H. Douard, M. Koch, J.-P. Broustet

Hôpital Cardiologique du Haut-Lévêque, Avenue de Magellan, 33604 Pessac, France

Introduction

The regional work aptitude consultation was created in 1989 as a combined initiative of the Department of Social Security (DSS) and the Exercise Testing Department at the Hôpital Cardiologique du Haut-Lévêque. It follows a long tradition of cardiac rehabilitation in Aquitaine. The patients in the study were referred by medical officers of the Department of Social Security in the Aquitaine region for half a day, four times a week. They all had problems returning to work because of prolonged sick leave or because of the incompatibility of their cardiovascular condition and their job. Altogether, 231 patients were included between January 1989 and December 1990.

Methods

Every patient underwent an interview and clinical examination, as well as taking part in an adapted exercise test for measuring maximal oxygen consumption ($\dot{V}O_2$ max) and Doppler echocardiography for the evaluation of cardiac function. A Holter electrocardiogram and ambulatory blood pressure were also

* To whom all correspondence should be addressed.

Proceedings of the Vth World Congress on Cardiac Rehabilitation

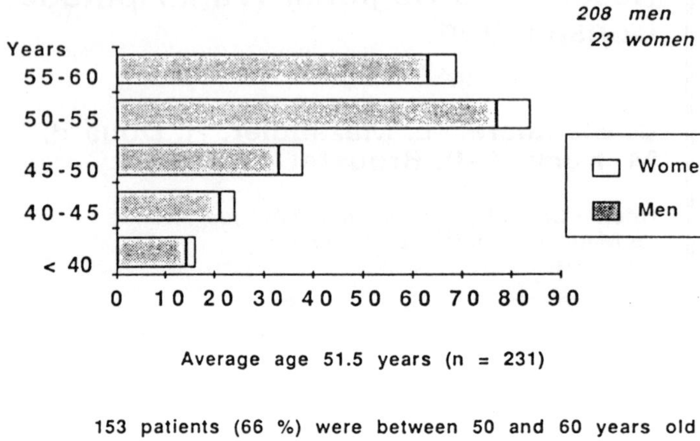

Fig. 1. Age distribution of the patients.

used when necessary, and a questionnaire was sent to both the medical officers and the patients. In total, 231 files were created.

Characteristics of the subjects

There were more men than women in the sample. The average age of the subjects was 51.5 years, which meant that there were an appreciable number of potential

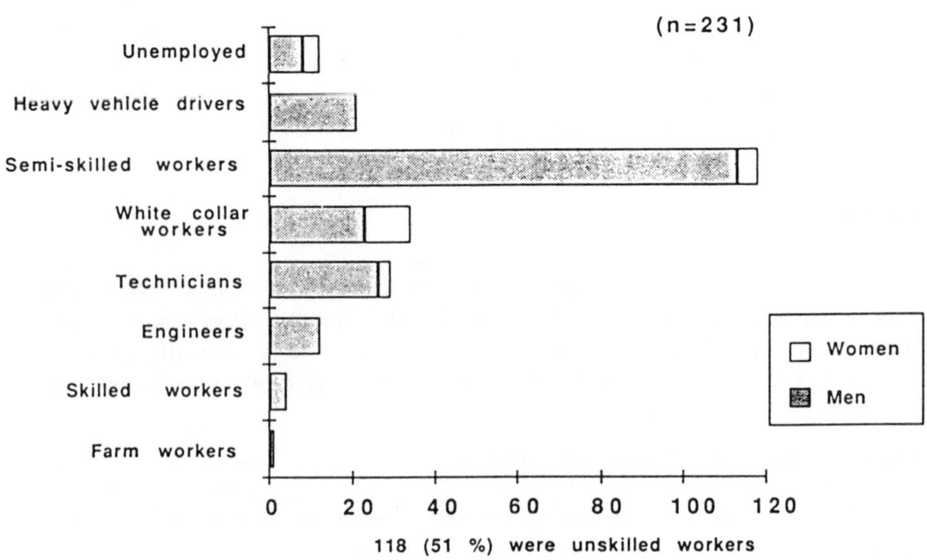

Fig. 2. Patients by profession.

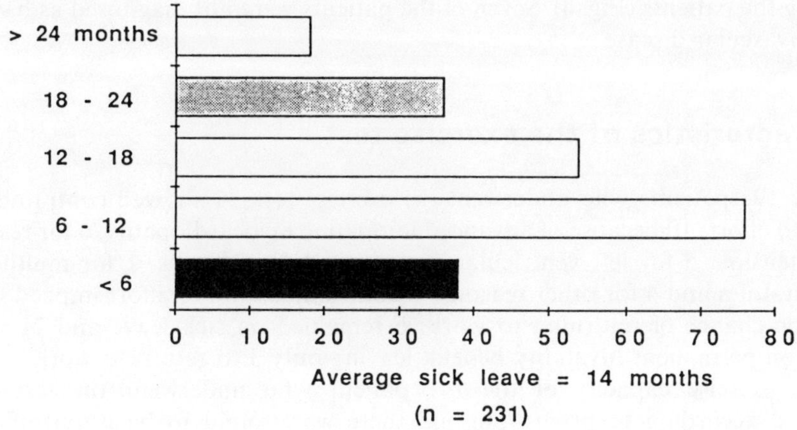

Fig. 3. Duration of sick leave.

active years remaining in their lives (Fig 1). More than half of the men were unskilled or semi-skilled manual workers, which in part explains why they were unable to return to work (Fig. 2). The average time that elapsed between the start of sick leave due to cardiac illness and the time at which we examined the patient was 14 months (Fig 3.). The reasons for this long delay will be commented on in a moment. As was to be expected, the prevalence of coronary heart disease was high; apart from high blood pressure being particularly significant, other diseases were of less importance and were spread evenly

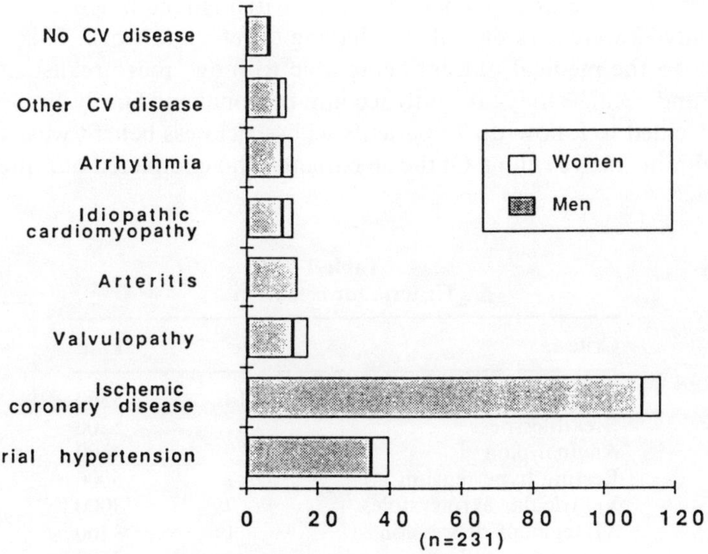

Fig. 4. Distribution of cardiovascular disease.

among the patients (Fig. 4). Seven of the patients were not diagnosed as having cardiovascular disease.

Characteristics of the exercise test

Of the 191 patients who underwent the exercise test, 30 showed contraindications to effort: 10 because of advanced idiopathic myocardiopathy, 6 for resting hypertension, 5 for left ventricular aneurysm, 4 for arteritis, 1 for multifocal extrasystoles and 4 for other reasons. A contraindication to effort implied little realistic chance of returning to work: 6 remained on sick leave and 21 were place on permanent invalidity benefit, leaving only 3 to return to work.

The exercise capacity of the 191 patient who underwent the test was assessed according to profession, and there were found to be no significant differences. Exercise capacity by disease showed no significant differences except for arteritis and hypertrophic myocardiopathy (2000–3000 kpm). The majority of diseases were compatible, with a capacity of 5000 kpm. Of the reasons for cessation, muscular fatigue was the most frequent (Table 1). Six of the nine patients who stopped because of anginal pain had significant ST-segment depression.

We looked at the correlation between the medical advice given and the administrative options, which included remaining on sick leave, stopping benefit because of fitness to work, becoming permanently invalided, premature retirement or adapting the job to the patient (Table 2). In the case of permanent invalidity, the medical recommendations were always followed by the medical officers. However, there were differences of opinion as regards those patients considered fit to return to work; of the 99 patients recommended for return to work, only 72 were actually ruled as having to return to work. This discrepancy was due to the medical officers being able to judge more realistically the job market and because they take into account personal and family circumstances.

We decided to follow-up 72 patients whose sickness benefit was stopped due to an administrative ruling. Of the 56 patients who completed our questionnaire,

Table 1
Criteria for cessation

Criteria	*n*	kpm
Muscle fatigue	114	5300
Breathlessness	37	5200
Anginal pain	9	4600
Resting hypertension	7	5000
Ventricular extrasystoles	7	3000
ST-segment depression	1	3200
Circulatory failure	4	3500

Table 2
Proposals made to medical officers following patient consultation

Proposal	*n*
Remain on sick leave	21
Stop benefit because of fitness to work	99
Permanent invalidity	98
Premature retirement	3
Adapt the job to the patient	10

only 25 in fact returned to work; the other 31 remained on unemployment benefit. The underlying disease did not appear to influence the decision not to return to work. Reasons other than medical ones often prevail – closeness to retirement age, poor job qualifications, being laid off, etc.

Conclusions

All patients who do not return to work within 3 months should be examined thoroughly and assessment should be carried out by a specialized unit. These units should be maintained wherever possible in order to help patients return to as normal a life as possible after a cardiac event and to aid them in finding financial help from Social Security. Unfortunately, at present, most DSS medical officers are unaware of the reasons why patients are placed on sick leave. Such leave can be renewed each month by the family doctor. It is only after 6 months, on average, that medical officers request information pertaining to the patient's disorder and the reason(s) for prolonging sick leave. Doctors are not obliged by law to give reasons for placing a person on sick leave; they are only obliged to reply to requests for information from DSS medical officers.

It was calculated that if the 25 patients who eventually returned to work in 1990 had returned earlier, savings of FF1,476,000 could have been made.

XIV

Implementation of Cardiac Rehabilitation Throughout the World

WHO Working Group

54 Implementation of Cardiac Rehabilitation in Developing Countries*

A. J. Goble

National Heart Foundation Centre for Social and Preventive Research, Suite 1A, 333 Drummond Street, Carlton, Melbourne, Victoria 3053, Australia

Introduction

Many benefits have now been demonstrated from structured cardiac rehabilitation programmes, additional to standard medical care. While most of these benefits have been demonstrated in patients following myocardial infarction, similar benefits have been demonstrated in patients following coronary artery bypass surgery. It is assumed that possibly lesser benefits could be demonstrated among patients with other forms of cardiovascular disease, through improvement in physical, psychological and other functioning.

The initial aims of cardiac rehabilitation programmes after myocardial infarction are to improve psychological, social and physical functioning, to increase return to work and improve occupational adjustments. These benefits have now been demonstrated in randomized controlled clinical trials [1–4], although in some studies the results have proved inconclusive [5, 6].

In addition, risk factor profiles have been shown to be improved [7, 8]. In both meta-analyses of randomized trials [9–11] and in controlled experiment [8], reduced recurrences and complications of cardiac illness, readmissions to hospital and deaths have been reported. Studies have also shown direct savings

*This paper was prepared by A. J. Goble on behalf of the World Health Organisation (WHO) Working Group 1, Expert Committee on Rehabilitation of the Patient with Cardiovascular Disease, whose members were: A. M. A Faruqui, W. F. T Muna, J. Feher, A. J. Goble, I. Gyarfas, and N. K. Wenger.

Proceedings of the Vth World Congress on Cardiac Rehabilitation

for patients, the community, employers, insurers and social security systems [12, 13]. In consequence of these effects, it is now recommended that cardiac rehabilitation programmes should be available to all patients in all countries. This means that they must be at low cost. Low-cost cardiac rehabilitation implies that clinical assessment of the patient and clinical risk stratification can approximate the accuracy of assessment and stratification obtainable through technological investigation [14–16].

High-intensity exercise training requires exercise prescription based upon symptom-limited exercise testing and the training programmes themselves require medical supervision [17]. Light or moderate exercise requires no such prior testing and avoids the need for medical supervision. Some group supervision of activity is required, but, as it would not be at a high level of intensity, the possibility of cardiovascular events arising from the activity is removed. Programmes of supervised group light to moderate intermittent exercises, when coupled with comfortable home walking and resumption of normal home activities, have been demonstrated to induce comparable physical functioning [18, 19] and comparable psychosocial outcomes [20, 21] to programmes of high-intensity exercise three times per week.

Symptomatic progress assessment, though less refined than exercise and other testing, has proved adequate as a means of following the progress of patients and the increase in their physical levels of activity. Group education programmes involve little cost and equipment. Further, they can be undertaken by any health professionals. Resumption of work and re-insertion into normal community and personal activity can be undertaken without significant testing or cost. The challenge, therefore, confronting the working group was to establish the manner in which cardiac rehabilitation programmes could be implemented in developing countries based upon five defined goals.

1. To develop programmes for all patients with cardiovascular disease in all countries.
2. To achieve awareness of this need in all health care professions and all people.
3. To educate all cardiac patients and their families and all health care professionals involved in cardiac rehabilitation.
4. To match the programmes to the needs and resources of each community.
5. To integrate cardiac rehabilitation into existing health care delivery systems.

The achievement of some of these goals may take many years. However, the basic principles whereby such programmes may be developed are presented in this paper, which is a summary of the expert committee report. This report is primarily directed at programmes undertaken during convalescence after acute illness, usually lasting from 4 to 8 weeks (phase 2 programmes).

Entry assessment

Before entry into a rehabilitation programme, it is necessary that there be a formal diagnosis based upon medical examination, with or without an electrocardiogram or other testing. Appropriate medical and surgical treatment should have been delivered to the patient if possible or a plan regarding such treatment should be established. A medical opinion on the prognosis and long-term risk for the patient is required and one needs identification of the rehabilitation requirements and their type. Patients with ischaemic heart disease would require a different form of rehabilitation from that required by those with recent rheumatic fever or chronic rheumatic heart disease who may have presented with a recent episode based upon a complication of that rheumatic heart disease. Similarly, patients with cardiomyopathy or congenital heart disease, with or without overt disability, may require a different pattern of management. Continued evaluation and surveillance of the patients are needed. While some of this surveillance may be through the rehabilitation programme, further medical examination would normally be required.

Programme requirements

The major requirement for a rehabilitation programme is adequately trained personnel. The degree of training and the number of persons would depend upon the level of the rehabilitation programme. A physical facility is required, with the level of equipment and educational materials dependent upon the level of rehabilitation. Financial arrangements need to be understood. The rehabilitation programme itself will be based on exercise and education. There are three types of facilities – basic, intermediate and advanced – each with different requirements.

Basic facility

A basic facility for a cardiac rehabilitation programme would be sited in a village or community and would be integrated into the local community health services. It would usually be conducted by a community health worker trained in cardiac rehabilitation, on a part-time basis. The physical facility could be any community building. There would need to be an exercise or walking area. Equipment could be limited to a sphygmomanometer and stethoscope or there could even be no medical equipment, progress being limited to pulse assessment. Educational materials and charts would be required. The finance would be within the existing health care system and unit. The rehabilitation programme would consist of low or moderate group exercise under the supervision of a health worker, but this supervision could be minimal, requiring no equipment. Basic information would be supplied to the patients using the educational material and charts. Patients and their families would be supported in attempting to achieve long-term compliance with regimens of health care.

Intermediate facility

The site for an intermediate facility would be a local hospital with general medical services. Personnel would usually work part-time and have other responsibilities within the hospital. It is desirable to have the services of a physician with training in cardiology and some knowledge of exercise physiology, cardiac rehabilitation and resuscitation. Nurses and other health professionals are required, also on a part-time basis, with training in exercise supervision, physical therapy, nutrition and patient education.

The physical facilities consist of one office and a multi-purpose exercise room for conducting exercise classes and an area for exercise testing with limited monitoring. Equipment could consist of steps with an electrocardiograph or bicycle ergometer or treadmill with a monitor. An area is required for class group discussions. A small budget is required, taking into account the portion of the time spent in cardiac rehabilitation by the various health professions and a small amount to cover the costs of limited equipment and consumables.

The exercise programme would consist of group low or moderate supervised exercises, conducted with minimal supervision. Patients would receive basic information and long-term compliance support. Exercise or muscle training may be required for some patients dependent upon their specific requirements. These exercises could be undertaken with materials that they would normally handle or some substitute materials.

An intermediate facility, sited in a local hospital, could be used as a centre for support for basic facilities in the surrounding area, for the training of staff, the handling of problems that may arise in the basic facilities and helping to maintain a network throughout the community.

Advanced facility

An advanced facility can be sited in a major medical centre with a significant cardiovascular disease referral base. Such a centre could be developed in a large university teaching hospital or in a sizeable private institution in a major city.

The personnel would probably all work part-time and have other responsibilities. A cardiologist with rehabilitation training may function as a medical director and be the person to whom problems may be referred. A programme co-ordinator would be required, possibly a nurse or a physiotherapist who would have contact with patients while within the hospital. Exercise classes could be under the supervision of a physiotherapist or an exercise specialist depending upon the level of exercise required. Expert nutritional advice, for individual patients and groups, should be available from a dietitian. Occupational therapists, psychologists and/or social workers may also be available. An administrative executive would be required to handle costs and data collection and transmission of information within the hospital. Other staff could include nurses, assistants and trainees.

The physical facilities should include a physician's office, an examination office and an administration office. An exercise testing room is necessary and an exercise room or gymnasium for group activity is required. The equipment includes exercise testing equipment with monitoring, resuscitation equipment and access to imaging techniques in the hospital. A proper classroom and a speciality clinic area are desirable. A budget would need to be worked out as appropriate to the local setting within either a cardiology department, rehabilitation department or a department of medicine.

The exercise programme could be low to moderate intensity with little or no equipment or it could be a high-intensity exercise programme with full equipment. This latter may be desirable for educational and research purposes, recognizing the role of an advanced facility within a community as a core centre, around which expertise may develop and flow to the community. The patient education programme would be similar to that in the other facilities, but additional information may be available, related to the greater expertise of the team available to deliver it.

Special considerations need to be applied to an advanced facility. While the correlation between clinical and technological risk stratification is reasonably close, it is desirable that maintenance of understanding of the association be maintained in at least one centre in any given country or sizeable area. High-intensity exercise programmes may be developed here for their educational content; also, some patients may prefer high-intensity exercise. Further, there could be specific reasons why individuals should receive such training. The level of testing and supervision needs to be viewed in relation to the increasing costs associated with it and the somewhat questionable added benefits.

In an advanced facility, a teaching responsibility must be recognized, the standards should be high and newer methods would be developed. In an advanced facility, there should be sufficient expertise to undertake evaluation and research into rehabilitation programmes and their effects.

Considerations for diagnostic groups

For patients with coronary heart disease, whether it be after myocardial infarction, coronary artery bypass graft surgery, angioplasty or whether patients have stable or unstable angina, one requires an approach based upon risk assessment, exercise prescription and supervision, education directed towards secondary prevention through reduction of risk behaviours and psychological and vocational supports for the patient.

For patients with rheumatic or congenital heart disease, there may be progressive disability. The question of operability or inoperability needs to be reviewed. There are post-operative patients whose requirements are somewhat different from those following coronary artery surgery. Recovery usually is slower and often there is need for anti-coagulant treatment in addition to other medication. For patients with cardiomyopathy, one needs assessment of the rate of progress, which may be slow or rapid, and this progress would determine the pattern and degree of exercise and the direction towards work resumption or resumption of other activities.

Patients with rheumatic heart disease or cardiomyopathy may be pregnant and careful assessment of functional class and associated risk is required.

Exercise: Non-equipment-based programme

Stage 1 design considerations

When contemplating setting up an exercise programme, coupled with an education programme, it is necessary to consider the socio-economic characteristics. These include a view of the occupational, social and financial status of the patients and the structure of the community from which they come. Cultural features of the community, including social structure, beliefs and taboos should be taken into account. The resources of the community in terms of organizational structure, community leadership and finances need to be considered.

Physical characteristics are of considerable importance, particularly the geography, the terrain and the climate. Facilities, activities and timing of activities are dependent on these considerations. Further, one has to consider how best to fit the programme, irrespective of its level, within the health care structure available in the community or hospital in which the programme is to be established.

Stage 2 design considerations

Designing a programme needs consideration of the type of cardiovascular diseases most prevalent in the community. It may be tilted towards coronary heart disease, towards rheumatic heart disease or, in some areas, cardiomyopathic disease. It may be necessary to run two programmes side by side. In some communities, patients do not present with disease until they have significant functional impairment. In others, early presentation may occur. Early presentation would facilitate greater physical activity and risk modification.

Exercise training, both in terms of intensity and duration, could be dictated in part by the levels of activity required by those seeking to resume work or normal activities. Specific muscular training may be required for some subjects, depending on their occupations. The higher the level of activity, the more likely one is to require some monitoring through heart rate or perception of effort. While programmes may be best based on general fitness training, some specific activity training may be required.

Exercise programmes: Content consideration

In general, it is desirable that programmes are adaptable to encompass as many different types of patients as possible. The categorization of risk is to be weighed with the goal of work resumption or community re-insertion. One needs to think about levels of energy expenditure either in terms of METs, watts, or kilocalories per minute. Full recovery of capacity may be achieved by home walking and normal daily activity, facilitated by support through supervised group activity, to assure morale and encouragement through the group. One aims to achieve appropriate functional levels for the individual and for these to be maintained.

The type of exercise programme will depend upon the available personnel, facilities and site of the facility, and be influenced by the geography, climate and the distance the patients have to travel. One needs to develop an accident strategy for handling cardiac events which may occasionally occur in classes or elsewhere and a network of communication for support of those in the programme. The training of staff also depends upon communication with others working at the same level and with others working at a more advanced level. This network is of importance to ensure access to information for all staff.

Assessment for return to work

General factors

The physical demands of work need to be known. Table 1 sets out a general level of the physical demands of work in METs (1 MET represents the oxygen consumption during rest and equals approximately 3.5 ml/O_2/kg/min). It should be noted that in some fields of work there are extreme ranges of effort required. While heavy industry and construction work may be largely undertaken with mechanical handling, occasionally considerable strenuous effort by individual workers is required to move materials. This also applies to mechanized rural work where, although some activity is involved while driving a tractor which is pulling an implement, there may be extremes of effort required or moderate efforts sustained over a period to change implements, unless there are mech-

Table 1
Assessment for return to work

	METs
Office work	1–3
Production line work	2–4
Factory work	3–5
Heavy industry/construction	3–10
Rural work	
Traditional	3–6
Mechanized	2–10
Farm produce handling	3–8

anical aids to achieve that. Farm produce handling may be light and relatively insignificant if one is handling bags or boxes, delivering these to the public or for distribution; however, stacking of such bags or boxes may involve considerable sustained effort. For these reasons, inspection of the type of work undertaken is of importance when in doubt regarding fitness to resume work. However, such information may be simply obtained by asking the individual patient about the nature of the work and which aspects of it would be most difficult. The troublesome aspects are those which may lead to specific muscular training or may lead to the possibility of work modification at the worksite.

The effects of climate influence the speed of work, the time of work and the need for protection against heat or cold, depending upon the circumstances. The site of work also could be important because it may involve significant travel, much of which may be on foot.

Patient factors in work assessment

Individual assessment of the patient's capacity to resume work will depend first upon whether there are any clinical symptoms and, if so, their severity. A clinical examination would be sufficient to reveal residual physical abnormality. The activity level that the patient has achieved is a valuable marker regarding fitness to resume work, provided it is viewed in direct relationship with the particular work. The patient's attitude to work, whether individual or related to community attitudes, should be known. If either the patient or family opposes resumption of work, it is unlikely to be resumed for any length of time. Prior work experience is important and, of course, the availability of suitable work for the patient. The diagnostic group to which the patient belongs is important because it may be, in some instances, inappropriate for the patient to consider resuming work.

Interactive factors in work assessment

While one has the interaction between the patient and his family to consider, it is also important to recognize that one needs a cooperative employer for work to be resumed. If there is uncertainty, work simulation can be undertaken. This may involve such activities as repeated lifting of given weights or stacking of materials or some other repeated simulation of the work which the patient considers potentially most troublesome. When in doubt, it may be possible to return for a trial of work, with the agreement of the employer, to see if the patient can manage the work. Work modification may be required for some. While this may be easy for the self-employed, it may be difficult and require a cooperative employer and a work visit on behalf of those who are employees.

Patient education: Consideration for secondary prevention

For patients with coronary heart disease, it is necessary that the patient and family have an understanding of the nature of the disease. They should know the major risk factors and behaviours which aggravate those risk factors. It is necessary to understand the desirability of compliance and maintenance of behavioural change on a long-term basis. The nature of medications and their purpose should also be understood.

For patients with rheumatic or other forms of heart disease, one again needs understanding of the nature of the disease and its progress and how that may be slowed. The use of prophylactic antibiotics, anticoagulation treatment if necessary, favourable behaviours and compliance with medication need to be understood. Maintenance of satisfactory levels of nutrition for this group of patients is likely to be quite different from the nutritional restrictions likely to be advised for those with coronary heart disease.

Conclusions

The working party considered that low-cost cardiac rehabilitation is possible anywhere. The development of cardiac rehabilitation programmes would be additional to the available medical care. The development of cardiac rehabilitation programmes may start at any level, whether in a village, town or community (a basic facility), a local hospital (an intermediate facility) or a major medical centre (an advanced facility).

Training of local personnel is essential. This training may be obtained at any level, but it is better from the level above. While it may not be possible to establish an advanced facility, intermediate facilities could readily be established in multiple areas and could function as the centres around which training for those who work in basic facilities could be developed. Because of local cultural differences, it is usually desirable that those who conduct basic facilities come from the same culture and geographical area as that in which the basic facility is sited, but they may have to obtain their training elsewhere, in an intermediate facility.

References

1. Stern MJ, Gorman PA, Kaslow L. The group counselling versus exercise therapy study: A controlled intervention with subjects following myocardial infarction. *Arch Intern Med* 1983; **143:** 1719–1725.
2. Taylor CB, Houston-Miller N, Arn DK, Haskell WL, DeBusk RF. The effects of exercise training programmes on psychosocial improvement in uncomplicated postmyocardial infarction patients. *J Psychosom Res* 1986; **30:** 581–587.

3. Erdman RAM, Duivenvoorden HJ, Verhage F, Kazemier M, Hugenholtz PG. Predictability of beneficial effects in cardiac rehabilitation: A randomized clinical trial of psychosocial variables. *J Cardiopulmonary Rehab* 1986; **6:** 206–213.
4. Dennis C, Houston-Miller N, Schwartz RG *et al.* Early return to work after uncomplicated myocardial infarction: Results of a randomized trial. *JAMA* 1988; **260:** 214–220.
5. Sivarajan ES, Newton KM, Almes MJ, Kempf TN, Mansfield LW, Bruce RA. Limited effects of outpatient teaching and counselling after myocardial infarction: A controlled study. *Heart and Lung* 1983; **12:** 65–73.
6. Oldridge N, Guyatt G, Jones N *et al.* Effects on quality of life with comprehensive rehabilitation after acute myocardial infarction. *Am J Cardiol* 1991; **67:** 1084–1089.
7. Kallio V, Hamalainen H, Hakkila J, Luurila OJ. Reduction in sudden deaths by a multifactorial intervention programme after acute myocardial infarction. *Lancet* 1979; **2:** 1091–1094.
8. Hedback B, Perk J. 5-year results of a comprehensive rehabilitation programme after myocardial infarction. *Eur Heart J* 1987; **8:** 234–242.
9. May GS, Eberlein KA, Furberg CD, Passamani ER, DeMets DL. Secondary prevention after myocardial infarction: A review of long-term trials. *Prog Cardiovasc Dis* 1982; **24:** 331–352.
10. O'Connor GT, Buring JE, Yusuf S *et al.* An overview of randomized trials of rehabilitation with exercise after myocardial infarction. *Circulation* 1989; **80:** 234–244.
11. Oldridge NB, Guyatt GH, Fischer ME, Rimm AA. Cardiac rehabilitation after myocardial infarction: Combined experience of randomized clinical trials. *JAMA* 1988; **260:** 945–950.
12. Picard MH, Dennis C, Schwartz RG *et al.* Cost-benefit analysis of early return to work after uncomplicated acute myocardial infarction. *Am J Cardiol* 1989; **63:** 1308–1314.
13. Levin R-A, Perk J, Hedback B. Cardiac rehabilitation: A cost analysis. *J Int Med* 1991; **230:** 427–434.
14. Norris RM, Caughey DE, Deeming LW, Mercer CJ, Scott PJ. Coronary prognostic index for predicting survival after recovery from acute myocardial infarction. *Lancet* 1970; **2:** 485–488.
15. Wolk MJ, Scheidt S, Killip T. Heart failure complicating acute myocardial information. *Circulation* 1972; **45:** 1125–1138.
16. Tibbits PA, Evaul JE, Goldstein RE *et al.* Serial acquisition of data to predict one-year mortality rate after acute myocardial infarction. *Am J Cardiol* 1987; **60:** 451–455.
17. American Heart Association Subcommittee on Rehabilitation. Standards for cardiovascular exercise treatment programs. *Circulation* 1979; **59:** 1084A–1094A.
18. Blumenthal JA, Rejeski J, Walsh-Riddle M *et al.* Comparison of high and low intensity exercise training early after acute myocardial infarction. *Am J Cardiol* 1988; **61:** 26–30.
19. Goble AJ, Hare DL, Macdonald PS, Oliver RG, Reid MA, Worcester MC. Effect of early programmemes of high and low intensity exercise on physical performance after transmural acute myocardial infarction. *Br Heart J* 1991; **66:** 126–131.
20. Blumenthal JA, Emery CF, Rejeski WJ. The effects of exercise training on psychosocial functioning after myocardial infarction. *J Cardiopulmonary Rehab* 1988; **8:** 183–193.
21. Goble AJ, Hare DL, Oliver RG, Reid MA, Macdonald PS, Worcester MC. The effect of exercise training on quality of life after transmural acute myocardial infarction. *J Am Coll Cardiol* 1988; **11:** 189A.

55 Rehabilitation after Cardiovascular Diseases with an Emphasis on Developing Countries: Report of a WHO Expert Committee

Nanette K. Wenger

Department of Medicine, Division of Cardiology, Emory University School of Medicine and Cardiac Clinics, Grady Memorial Hospital, 69 Butler Street, SE, Atlanta, Georgia, 30303 USA

Introduction

Rehabilitative care after cardiovascular disease is designed to improve functional capacity, to alleviate or lessen activity-related symptoms, to decrease unwarranted invalidism, and to enhance return to a useful and personally satisfying role in society.

The prevalence of cardiovascular diseases is increasing in developing countries; coronary heart disease has assumed increased prominence, in addition to rheumatic heart disease, hypertension and cardiomyopathy. Despite differences in the patterns of cardiac disease between and within developing countries, cardiac rehabilitative care can effectively be applied even with modest availability of personnel and equipment. Particularly for societies in transition, with rapid changes in cultures, in foods, in lifestyles and in economics, there is need for guidance to maintain cardiovascular health. The demography of the population and the range of cardiac patients considered eligible for exercise therapy during cardiac rehabilitation has also undergone dramatic change. Among patients with coronary disease, not only individuals recovered from uncomplicated myocardial infarction, but also patients with complications of infarction, those with angina pectoris, and patients recovering from coronary artery bypass surgery and coronary angioplasty are candidates for exercise rehabilitation. Of importance for these diverse patients has been the emergence of varied but

Proceedings of the Vth World Congress on Cardiac Rehabilitation

typically exercise-based test procedures designed to identify both their risk for early recurrent coronary events and their longer-term prognosis. These assessments can concomitantly identify patients able to perform reasonable levels of activity with safety (low-risk patients) and those high-risk patients with a limited exercise capacity and early onset of myocardial ischaemia, ventricular dysfunction or arrhythmias; an intermediate-risk group can also be identified. These delineations can both guide selection of medical and surgical therapies and recommendations for rehabilitative exercise, including the need for and the intensity and duration of professional supervision of exercise; and can comparably guide resumption of pre-illness activities, including return to work. Recently, the data available have expanded the application of exercise rehabilitation.

First is the evidence that low-risk cardiac patients can safely exercise without medical supervision; they can also return promptly to pre-illness activities, including return to work. Equally important is the fact that low- to moderate-intensity exercise training has been demonstrated to improve functional capacity. Lower-intensity exercise is characterized by greater safety, particularly when unsupervised; engenders less discomfort in those unaccustomed to exercise; is more enjoyable; and thereby fosters improved adherence. Also relevant is the safety and value of low-intensity isometric (resistance) exercise in improving the functional status of patients who can safely perform modest levels of dynamic exercise. Next is the evidence of benefit from exercise training for patients receiving all types of anti-anginal drugs. Elderly cardiac patients can participate in exercise rehabilitation with only modest modifications of the usual regimen, with equal improvement of their functional status to their younger counterparts. Further, cardiac enlargement and compensated congestive heart failure do not contraindicate physical activity; exercise rehabilitation can improve functional status without deterioration of ventricular function. Emphasis is warranted regarding the lack of correlation between the severity of ventricular dysfunction and the physical work capacity.

Greater attention in rehabilitative care is currently devoted to education and counselling, with the behavioural approach recommended for coronary risk reduction. This concept involves not simply transmission of cognitive information, but teaching of skills needed to adopt a healthy lifestyle, opportunities to practise these skills, and re-enforcement of successful changes. Active participation of patients is important in the management of their disease; the importance of the family and workplace in coronary risk reduction is also acknowledged. Health professionals at all levels must be trained to be effective teachers of their patients.

Finally, psychological problems, predominantly anxiety and depression, may limit return to work and to pre-illness lifestyles more than decreased physical work capacity. Return to work is often a relevant and desirable outcome of rehabilitation, and is economically, physically and socially appropriate for many cardiac patients. However, resumption of employment in most societies relates poorly to restoration of physical function; hence, attention to psychosocial status warrants attention.

The WHO Expert Committee Charge

The committee was charged with defining the state-of-the-art of rehabilitative care for cardiovascular diseases, and to highlight and interrelate four aspects: (1) implementation of cardiac rehabilitation in developing countries; (2) current and future approaches to the education of patients in cardiac rehabilitation; (3) the use of exercise testing and training in the rehabilitation of cardiac children and young adults; and (4) the rehabilitation of severely disabled, medically complex cardiac patients.

State-of-the-art of rehabilitative care for cardiovascular diseases

Rehabilitation is an integral part of the long-term comprehensive care of cardiac patients. Cardiac rehabilitation includes both an individualized physical activity regimen and the health education and counselling appropriate for an individual patient's needs and specific cardiac problem.

Cardiovascular disease is an increasing problem in developing countries, and includes disease in children and young adults, for whom this will likely be a life-long problem. Adults in developing countries now manifest an increased prevalence of those diseases once considered characteristic of industrialized societies. Further, with increases in the elderly population of developing countries, there will be increased cardiovascular diseases in this group as well.

The benefits of rehabilitative care include improved function and health status, improved quality of life, improved social independence and place in society, and improved work resumption and continuation. This renders efficiently delivered cardiac rehabilitation cost-effective. Both governments and non-governmental organizations can use the training resources available from international and regional agencies to train health providers in cardiac rehabilitation.

Cardiac rehabilitation services can improve recovery from cardiovascular illness by a variety of favourable effects. Rehabilitative services can increase the capability for physical activity, increase the rapidity of physical recovery, and aid in the prevention of cardiac invalidism. They engender improved adherence to treatment recommendations and the adoption of favourable health behaviours. Hospital readmissions have been demonstrated to decrease, as have recurrent episodes of cardiovascular illness. Psychological recovery is faster as well. Cardiac rehabilitation services can increase the rapidity of return to work, the completeness of so doing, as well as adequacy of social reintegration and the maintenance of these important components. There is an enhanced ability to participate in recreational activity. Maintenance of independence for elderly persons is prolonged. Cardiac rehabilitation services can also improve the quality of life and sense of well-being of patients with cardiovascular illness and better their occupational, social, recreational and other adjustments. There is longer maintenance of the physical and social capacities for self-care and self-support.

Because cardiovascular disease will constitute an increasing problem in the workplace, children and young adults with cardiovascular disease require guidance towards appropriate occupations. Adults with cardiovascular disease need guidance regarding their return to work. Most cardiac patients can return to work, and rehabilitative care helps them do so more rapidly and effectively. Therefore, cardiac rehabilitation for employees with cardiovascular disease can engender financial benefit to employers by enabling an earlier return to work; decrease disability; decrease sickness and disability payments; lessen subsequent absenteeism; reduce training costs required to replace personnel; and improve productivity.

Particular benefits to the cardiac child (and that child's family) from rehabilitative care include an enhancement of self-esteem and self-worth in the child. There is a lessening of excessive parental protection, an improvement in the healthy psychological development of the child, and a reduction in unwarranted medical invalidism that may persist to adult life. Healthy childhood development is enhanced. Guidance is provided for family and marital life after childhood. Finally, recurrences and complications of cardiovascular disease are decreased. Most children with cardiovascular disease can safely participate in physical activities, even those of high intensity. Physical activity is a valuable aid in social integration with peers and in the adoption of a healthy lifestyle; it further enhances the quality of life of the cardiac child.

Recommendations of the WHO Expert Committee

Rehabilitation should be a component of long-term comprehensive cardiac care. Therefore, cardiac rehabilitation programmes and services should be available to all children and adults with cardiovascular disease. Cardiac rehabilitation services can and should be provided by any health professional caring for cardiac patients. These services involve participation by the patient and family, and do not necessitate sophisticated equipment or facilities. Cardiac rehabilitation programmes can and should be integrated at low cost into the existing national health care system. These programmes and services require the training of health professionals in exercise recommendations, in health education and in vocational guidance. The implementation of cardiac rehabilitation should be the responsibility of designated trained health professional co-ordinators at a local level. These individuals should be responsible, in turn, to an appropriate department, hospital, physician or health care facility, which may be a governmental or non-governmental organization or agency, varying with the health care system of the country. Evaluation of local efficacy should be included in the rehabilitation plan. School officials should consult with responsible medical personnel about the physical activities that are appropriate for individual children with cardiovascular disease.

The World Health Organization and the International Society and Federation of Cardiology, in collaboration with interested international and national organizations, should be responsible for the transmission of recommendations for cardiac rehabilitation to constituent members, for the provision of international or regional training courses; and for recommendations to governments and professional societies for guidelines on the implementation of cardiac rehabilitation within the existing health care system. International agencies that can and should help with training and with the implementation of cardiovascular rehabilitation include: the International Labour Office; the United Nations educational, scientific and cultural organizations; the World Hypertension League; the International Council of Nurses; the International Telecommunication Union; the International Federation of Sports Medicine; Rehabilitation International; the International Union of School and University Health and Medicine; International Commission on Occupational Health; World Rehabilitation Fund; and World Bank.

Acknowledgements

This chapter forms the recommendations of a WHO Expert Committee whose members included: Drs J.-P. Broustet, France; A.O. Falase, Nigeria; A.M.A. Faruqui, Pakistan (Rapporteur); J. Feher, Brazil; A. Goble, Australia; S. John, India; P. Mathes, Germany (Vice Chairman); W.F.T. Muna, Cameroon; M.M. Al-Nozha, Saudi Arabia; C.H. Oon, Singapore; C. Vongprateep, Thailand; N.K. Wenger, USA (Chairperson). Temporary Advisors included: H. Denolin, Belgium; F.W. James, USA; J.J. Kellermann, Israel; L.F. Nikolaeva, USSR. The secretary was I. Gyarfas (WHO).

References provided for complementary information

1. American Association of Cardiovascular and Pulmonary Rehabilitation. *Guidelines for Cardiac Rehabilitation Programs*. Human Kinetics: Champaign, IL, 1991.
2. American College of Cardiology Position Report on Cardiac Rehabilitation: Recommendations of the American College of Cardiology on Cardiovascular Rehabilitation. *J Am Coll Cardiol* 1986; **7:** 451–453.
3. Blumenthal JA, Rejeski WJ, Walsh-Riddle M *et al.* Comparison of high- and low-intensity exercise training early after acute myocardial infarction. *Am J Cardiol* 1988; **61:** 26–30.
4. Fletcher GF, Frohlicher VF, Hartley LH, Haskell WL, Pollock ML. Exercise Standards: A Statement for Health Professionals from the American Heart Association. *Circulation* 1990; **82:** 2286–2322.
5. Goble AJ, Hare DL, Macdonald PS, Oliver RG, Reid MA, Worchester MC. Effect of early programmes of high and low intensity exercise on physical performance after transmural acute myocardial infarction. *Br Heart J* 1991; **65:** 126–131.
6. Gutgesell HP, Gessner IH, Vetter VL, Yabek SM, Norton JB Jr. American Heart Association: Recreational and Occupational Recommendations for Use by Physicians Counselling Young Patients with Heart Disease. A Statement for Physicians by the Committee on Congenital Cardiac Defects of the Council on Cardiovascular Disease in the Young. *Circulation* 1986; **74:** 1195A–1198A.

7. James FW, Blomqvist CG, Freed MD *et al. Ad hoc* Committee on Exercise Testing: Standards for Exercise Testing in the Pediatric Age Group. American Heart Association Council on Cardiovascular Disease in the Young. *Circulation* 1982; **66:** 1377A–1397A.
8. Kellermann JJ, Shemesh J, Fisman EZ *et al.* Arm exercise training in the rehabilitation of patients with impaired ventricular function and heart failure. *Cardiology* 1990; **77:** 130–138.
9. Schlant RC, Friesinger GC II, Leonard JJ. Position Statement: Clinical Competence in Exercise Testing: A Statement for Physicians from the ACP/ACC/AHA Task Force on Clinical Privileges in Cardiology. *Circulation* 1990; **82:** 1884–1888.
10. Wenger NK, Hellerstein HK (eds). *Rehabilitation of the Coronary Patient*, 3d edn. Churchill Livingstone: New York, 1992.
11. Wenger NK (ed.). *The Education of the Patient with Cardiac Disease in the Twenty-first Century*. LeJacq Publishing: New York, 1986.
12. Wenger NK, Balady GJ, Cohn LH *et al. Ad hoc* Task Force on Cardiac Rehabilitation: Cardiac Rehabilitation Services Following PTCA and Valvular Surgery: Guidelines for Use. *Cardiology* 1990; **19:** 4–5.
13. Wenger NK, Haskell WL, Kanter K, Squires RW, Yusuf S. *Ad hoc* Task Force on Cardiac Rehabilitation: Cardiac Rehabilitation Services After Cardiac Transplantation: Guidelines for Use. *Cardiology* 1991: **20:** 4–5.

56 Current and Future Approaches to the Education in the Rehabilitation of the Patient with Cardiovascular Disease

Oon Chong Hau,* M. M. Al-Nozha, H. Denolin, I. Gyarfas, L. F. Nikolaeva, C. Panchaud, T. Strasser, N. Wenger

World Health Organization, Geneva, Switzerland

Importance of education and counselling in cardiac rehabilitative care

Definition and goals

Patient and family education involves consciously constructed opportunities for learning designed to facilitate changes in behaviour towards a predetermined goal and to enhance their ability to initiate and sustain change in health behaviour over time [1]. Educating the family and the spouse is as important as educating the patient for transforming them into active and informed participants, learning about the disease, the process of rehabilitation, and providing social support to the patient.

Benefits to patients [2]

Acute or episodic care alone is inadequate for most chronic diseases. Hence patients themselves and their families must assume greater responsibility for their care [3]. They must be trained to become active partners in their rehabilitation and to take responsibility for their own health. Information is

* Address all correspondence to Dr Oon Chong Hau, Health Maintenance Centre, Singapore General Hospital, Outram Road, Singapore 0316.

Proceedings of the Vth World Congress on Cardiac Rehabilitation

power, knowledge is strength, and awareness is responsibility. Education can decrease the patient's feelings of hopelessness, increase confidence in a successful outcome, enhance the ability to cope with problems of illness, and increase compliance with recommendations for care. Some of the educational goals under these circumstances are thus short-term and some are long-term. The ultimate aim of patient education is to enable improved cardiovascular "health" plus a good quality of life, and aid in appropriate resumption of family, occupational and social roles and help promote self-responsibility in the family, workplace and community [4, 5].

Benefits to society

Although initially education about cardiac disease may entail an increase in health care costs because of greater use of services, the educated patient may have less disease recurrence, complications or progression, and thereby decrease hospital costs and use of emergency facilities.

Physicians and health professionals should be caring, compassionate and dedicated to patients and to keeping them well and helping them when they are ill. Health professionals should devise a plan of action responsive to the needs of each cardiac patient to impart knowledge, values, skills and attitudes to improve disease outcomes and social integration. In some societies, education is a legal obligation with respect to patients about self-care, and as part of discharge planning after hospitalization, and follow-up care. Health professionals are responsible for the content of the information, the method of communicating the information, and ascertaining patient understanding of the information.

Educational concepts and principles

Overview

In adapting educational programmes, the content may require modification to suit the local language, culture, educational levels, communication media, disease patterns and the target audience. Patient education should be readily applicable by the patient, relatively inexpensive, informative, accurate and attractive. For the patient to form a correct idea about the disease, the subsequent care and needs, a systematic approach and consistent presentation of information is necessary [6]. Motivation must be provided for the patient to continue to participate in an educational programme because knowledge is important for a longer life. Encouraging patients to participate actively in education helps to enhance their motivation.

The factors influencing choice of educational methods are literacy and educational level, multilingual/multi-dialect settings, communication medium and culture. The main principles of education involves presentation of informa-

Table 1
Learning theory emphasizes three components in effecting change [7]

1. Consciousness of need for information
2. Provision of information, which can cause attitude change
3. Implementation of behavioural change based on personal value of the information, with long-term adherence requiring feedback and reinforcement.

tion in a style appropriate to both subject and patient with short words and sentences, important ideas repeated and specific recommendations given. Information should be individualized with questions answered, learning reinforced and corrective feedback provided. Knowledge change should be assessed and education provided at the "teachable" moment when the patient seeks information (see Tables 1–3).

Education of adults [8]

Children learn the domains of knowledge assigned to them while adults learn in order to solve problems. Adults are, therefore, concerned with the immediacy of application. A person learns well those things perceived as involved in the maintenance or enhancement of the structure of self. The atmosphere that promotes learning is one which minimizes threat to the personal perception of the learner and individualized perception of the material as suiting adult needs. Changes in self-concept are reflected in the movement from dependency to increasing "self-efficacy" as an adult learns. Experience causes an adult to learn better, e.g. successfully learning of one aspect facilitates the next. Readiness to learn comes from personal requirements so as to facilitate recovery at home.

Table 2
Relationship between behaviour domains and teaching and learning actions [15]

Domain	Teaching method	Learning outcome
	The teacher will:	*The learner will:*
Cognitive information, knowledge	inform	explain
	instruct	describe
	lecture	discuss
	provide materials	define
Affective attitudes, emotions	counsel	express
	model	affirm
	reinforce	choose
	provide peer exchange	share
Psychomotor skills, performance	demonstrate	perform
	coach	do
	guide	produce
	provide practice	use

Table 3
Checklist for assessing patient readiness to learn [15]

Is the patient ready to learn at this time ?	
Physical ability checkpoints	*Psychological willingness checkpoints*
Stable physical condition (free of pain and complications)	Appropriate emotional state (not too anxious or depressed)
Adequate energy level (not too exhausted or sedated)	Awareness of actual problem (not in total denial)

The behavioural approach

Since lifestyle patterns are complex, long-term behavioural changes made gradually over time are more likely to be successful in the maintenance of a healthy lifestyle [5] (see Table 4).

Education of children with cardiac disease

The objective of the education of the child is to enable optimal intellectual, physical, emotional and social development. This is characterized by the need for long-term lifestyle adherence, and decisions on career options. Education

Table 4
Elements of a successful behaviour change education programme

Building a positive and accurate expectancy about results of knowledge; this involves information
Defining precisely the health behaviour; this involves instruction
Setting realistic short- and long-term goals
Enhancing commitment to behavioural change by contracting with and giving other incentives to participants
Preparing for relapse, if appropriate
Providing a model for the desired behaviour
Promptly practising the desired behaviour
Providing feedback regarding progress in behavioural change
Giving problem-solving advice and identifying difficulties
Rewarding achievements attained by the patient
Enlisting social support as necessary and appropriate.
Thus, treatment plans should be individualized, prioritized and introduced gradually

of girls with cardiac disease about their condition is equally important, even in societies where their general education may be limited. The communication medium and site can vary considerably but important agents of influence are the parents (both mother and father), the teachers and the school, and peers and local role models. Children have a high response to visual, auditory, tactile and kinaesthetic stimuli. The special characteristics which apply to educating children about exercise training for their rehabilitation include the provision of a variety of activities, timed in short bursts and allowing for spontaneous movements, and in a group rather than an individual setting. Parental involvement should be encouraged, since their participation presents the child with a role model. Motivation can involve a system of incentives or rewards. Groups should be separated according to age, up to 8 years, from 8 to 12 years, from 13 to 15 years, 15 and over.

Education of elderly cardiac patients [9]

In planning for educational programmes in an elderly cardiac population, one must be prepared to deal with medical, social and cultural barriers to communication. Impaired vision or hearing are examples of physical handicaps; other obstacles are declining cognitive function, memory and emotional instability. In general, any communication or message to this group must consider the fact that particular subsets of individuals may be fragile and may suffer from concomitant conditions. Educational programming should acknowledge the cultural traditions of the audience, for example, the position of elders in that society. Lifestyle interventions should be made in moderation and at levels compatible with the patient's prior experience and age. They should include the development of social support networks and simplifications of daily activities, and clear written instructions to avoid confusion, especially when multiple drugs or recommendations are made. Educational sites for the elderly can be in the doctor's office, clinic, community centres or retirement homes, where these group settings offer "captive" audiences interested in health issues and supportive of health-related programmes. Home visits do provide important contacts with individual elderly patients. Trans-telephonic monitoring or comparable technology can promote self-care and facilitate surveillance of elderly patients living independently.

Levels of care: Facilities related to educational programmes

Basic, intermediate and advanced

Educational programmes must be provided at three levels of care: *basic*, often far from major medical centres and direct physician supervision; *intermediate*, as in community hospitals; and *advanced*, as in major medical centres. Personnel and resources will vary at the three levels. In developing countries, patients who live in rural areas often have limited transportation or limited access to hospital programmes. The home may therefore serve as a focus for many of the educational efforts. The challenges for effective education include implementation in sites other than the hospital or clinic, including the home, community, school and worksites; greater reliance on non-physician health professionals to implement education; and more effective and creative use of existing basic communication and advanced technology.

Use of technology

Technology has the potential to reduce the workload while increasing the effectiveness of education, as well as helping to initiate behavioural changes at a wide spectrum of educational levels. Printed educational materials should be tailored to a patient's needs and abilities. However, many currently used materials are written at levels above the reading level of the targeted population. The target audience has to be considered in all steps of programme development so that language, illustrations and skills are appropriate. Many of the anticipated sources of information are lacking in the home/community environment of developing societies – books, newspapers and magazines are in short supply, even if the patient can read. The impact of print media in the presence of high levels of illiteracy is less than that of radio or television [10].

Radio, television and video-cassette recorders, which are able to inform, educate and entertain over great distances, are increasingly available in rural villages. However, the cost and storage of batteries, as well as a lack of other power sources, are also important considerations. In developing countries, telephone use has limited potential, and is prohibitively expensive. However, great potential exists in developed societies for telephone education to institute and maintain behaviour change. In the future, the telephone, linked to databases, integrated systems digital networks (ISDNs) and home medical electronics, may become critical educational and behavioural change tools. These are already beginning to be widely applied in business today. Interactive telephonic education systems can be applied in health care settings.

The development of satellite technology (Figs 1 and 2) has made information instantly available globally through television, telephone, faxes and teleconferencing. Technology has become more cost-effective and satellite dishes are getting smaller and more widely available. Rural satellite programmes can carry other forms of information than voice. Pictures, data, text and graphics can be transmitted through microcomputers; printed material through facsimile; and notes, charts and diagrams through telewriters. International education programmes will need to consider cultural characteristics, family values, consumer behaviour, copyright laws and political issues.

In developed societies, increasingly complex medical information will be available in the home through cable television, videotext and optical disc storage. In many countries, hospitals have cable television for patient entertainment and education, as well as medical education. More and better information

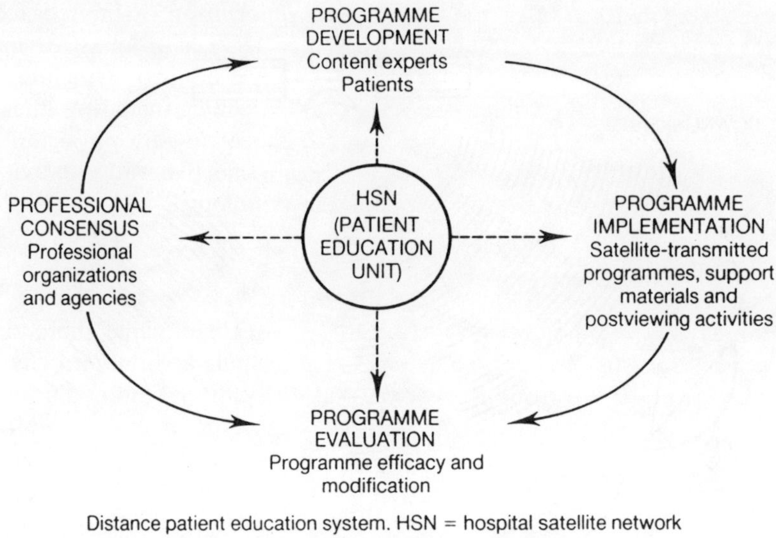

Fig. 1. Hospital-based programmes may require modification to suit local needs. The systems for patient programmes can also be used for professional education systems. Adapted from Wenger [2], with permission.

and assessment will be available in the home through telephone-linked computers, which can transmit ECGs and instruct patients. Educational subscription television with education components is currently available in many countries. Consideration has to be made as to the hardware necessary to display the educational media. Sophisticated, interactive computer programs, which require expensive computers, are unlikely to achieve wide distribution. Other modes of communication, such as audiotapes supplementing simple printed material, may be more useful in developing countries. Computers can help patients assess their knowledge, attitudes, behaviour and skills related to a particular risk factor and then establish specific goals for change. Many computer programs with these characteristics have been developed. New, interactive video, as well as videophones and computer formats, offer even greater potential for more interesting, yet personal instruction.

Despite their potential, computers have achieved little use in most medical practice settings. There are many reasons for this poor utilization: physicians and other health care professionals have limited knowledge about computers; the computers and their programs are expensive; and there is a belief that patients react negatively to the use of computers for education to implement behavioural change. All these factors are rapidly changing as computers are becoming more "user-friendly" and better software programs are being developed. While the cost of developing computer programs is falling, many studies have now shown that patients react favourably to computer education. For

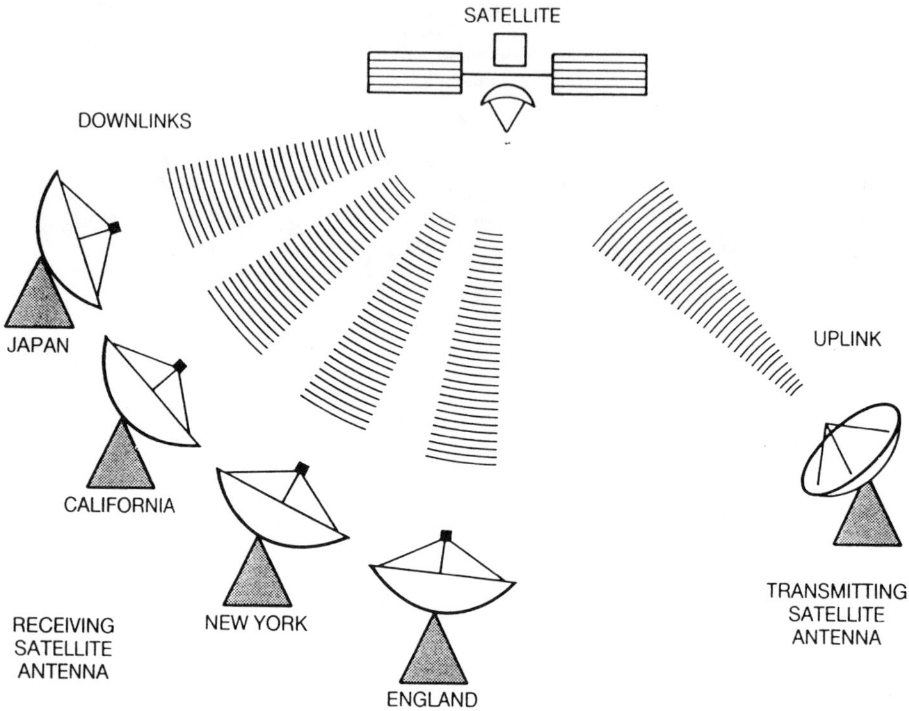

Fig. 2. The satellite link in communication technology. Adapted from Wenger [2], with permission.

instance, interactive computer systems can be developed which function entirely on the basis of symbols. Furthermore, as more people become better educated, they will also become more computer-literate.

Use and availability of personnel

Both physicians and non-physician health professionals can teach. The role of non-physician professionals will assume increasing importance as a cost-effective mode of intervention in patient and family education at community levels, as these people are in close contact with the patients and their families. The following factors should be considered at each level of facility: Who is available to teach? Who can be trained to teach? How should these teachers be trained and what should their educational content be? Furthermore, teachers need to be trained in how to teach, how to interact and what to teach [11, 12]. Non-conventional teachers in rural and village settings include school teachers, religious leaders and model patients.

Levels of care

Basic level of care

The basic level of care may use a community health worker, health visitor or community nurse in the patient's education programme. The community health worker, probably a community nurse, needs training in patient education. Nurses have demonstrated effectiveness in facilitating behavioural change among patients with cardiovascular disease through both individual and group teaching. These people can be trained during basic schooling.

Knowledge requirements for community health worker, health visitor and community nurse (see Table 5)

The community health worker has to develop a line of communication to answer to or refer patients' problems. This worker also has to learn how to establish a network to achieve maximal support and cohesion of activity with neighbouring community health workers.

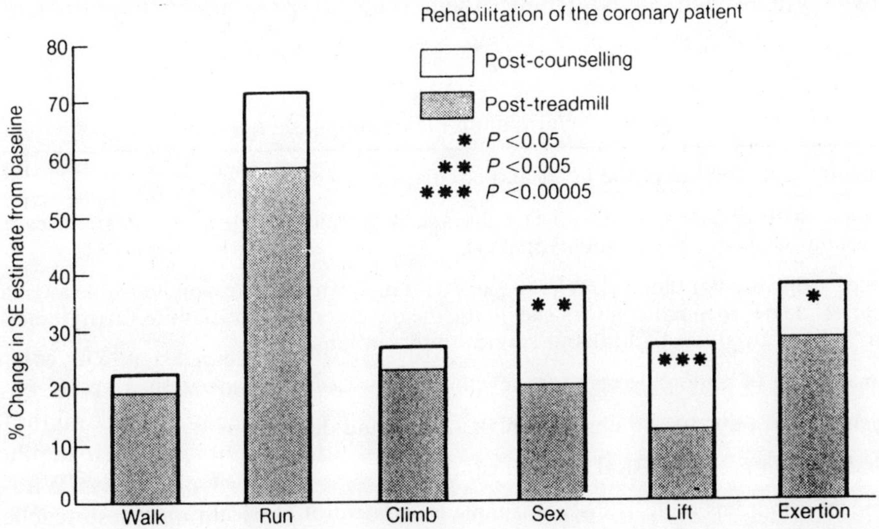

Fig. 3. Increases in self-efficacy (SE) after treadmill exercise and counselling compared with initial values obtained before treadmill exercise and counselling, respectively. Adapted from Nakajima [3], with permission.

Intermediate level of care

Personnel at the intermediate level of care can be trained in a community hospital. Community health workers should learn the requirements for cardiac education appropriate to the rural or village setting where there will be little or no equipment and limited facilities. Physicians can serve as teachers at the intermediate level

Advanced level of care

At the advanced level of care, the areas of expertise will vary and the number and scope of teaching staff will be influenced by the size and complexity of the population to be taught. This group includes primary care physicians, cardiologists, medical specialists, paediatric cardiologists, paediatricians, cardiac surgeons, physicians specializing in rehabilitative medicine, sports medicine and occupational health, as well as general practitioners. They have to learn teaching skills, learn communications skills and be provided with supporting materials to use to teach patients. Nurses, occupational and physical therapists, dietitians, psychologists, health educators and exercise physiologists can also act as trainers of personnel working at the intermediate and basic levels of care as well as teaching patients. Most public health, nursing, nutrition, exercise, medical and even education programmes need improved curricula about patient education for behavioural change. At the advanced level, media experts and specialists in the educational subject matter, teaching methodology and educational systems can all contribute their skills to programme development,

Table 5
Curriculum for training

Structure and function of the heart and circulation
Changes with disease (coronary heart disease, hypertension, rheumatic heart disease, congenital heart disease, cardiomyopathy)
Acute cardiovascular illnesses. What occurs with myocardial infarction, unstable angina pectoris, acute rheumatic fever, rheumatic heart disease, heart failure, arrhythmias (particularly atrial fibrillation) and surgical interventions?
Management of acute illnesses: overview, hospital treatment, medication, surgery
Psychological responses to illness: denial, anxiety and depression
Rehabilitation needs: physical activity, education
Residual symptoms of heart disease; simple assessment of physical capacity
Educational content and methods; group leadership, family education and support; community structure and support
Networks

addressing learning strategies, "testing points" in teaching and optimal modes of presentation for imparting information tailored to specific patient populations. The cost-effectiveness involved in training in developing countries, where one person may be assigned multiple tasks, requires extensive collaboration so that many health professionals can be trained. Hence a potential advantage in using technology for training health professionals is to ensure constancy, quality control and replicability. This is not an unreasonable approach at the intermediate level. Training through an individual teacher or lecturer may lead to considerable variability in message, emphasis, components and the efficacy of transmission of the content. An advantage of videotape, computer-assisted education, or computer-interactive education, would be that the content and emphasis would be uniform and the means of assessment standardized. This is of value in training teachers, and may also be useful in implementing a health curriculum in professional schools.

Educational components for disease categories (see Table 6)

The role of government, voluntary health organizations and international agencies

The government can facilitate cardiac rehabilitation either through legislation or government-sponsored insurance within existing health systems. Rehabilitative services can reduce the burden of cardiovascular disability. Support for and facilitation of such services is a governmental responsibility, including the provision of guidelines for and training of health professionals. Medical professional societies must be strong advocates of cardiac rehabilitation services, including patient education, for which they should develop their own local standards. Voluntary societies and foundations should support cardiac rehabilitation services, develop training systems for patient education, and initiate evaluation research regarding cardiac rehabilitation outcomes.

A challenge for health professionals is to influence governments favourably, so that they adopt a role in patient education, particularly where governments control or influence the media. In the future, governments should provide the educational and communication technology infrastructure characterized by "intelligent" homes with home-based patient monitoring, and facilities for multi-media education. Governments, or private sector educational institutions, should collaborate with universities and colleges to integrate into the current education system for health care professionals (medical schools, nursing schools, health sciences) and specialists (primary, secondary and tertiary), to promote the curricula, teaching skills and information required for patient education.

Curriculum guidelines for non-physician health professionals *are* available through manuals from such bodies as the American College of Sports Medicine and the American Association of Cardiovascular and Pulmonary Rehabilitation and should be incorporated into existing professional education systems [13].

Table 6
Education of the cardiac patient and family [16]

Education component[a]	Coronary heart disease	Systemic arterial hypertension	Rheumatic heart disease	Congenital heart disease	Cardiomyopathy (congestive heart failure)
Medical follow-up	× ×	× ×	× ×	× ×	× ×
Medication taking	× ×	× ×	× ×	× ×	× ×
Rheumatic fever prophylaxis	–	–	× ×	–	–
Endocarditis prophylaxis	+/–	–	× ×	× ×	+/–
Anticoagulant treatment	+/–	–	× ×	+/–	+/–
Response to symptoms of severity	× ×	–	× ×	× ×	× ×
Advice regarding pregnancy	+/–	× ×	× ×	× ×	+/–

Career councelling/ choice	–	–	× ×	× ×	×
Return to work	× ×	× ×	× ×	×	× ×
General nutrition	×	×	× ×	× ×	×
Weight (obesity) control	× ×	× ×	× ×	× ×	× ×
Fat/cholesterol intake	× ×	× ×	×	×	×
Sodium intake	× ×	× ×	×	×	× ×
Blood pressure control	× ×	× ×	+/–	+/–	× ×
Smoking cessation	× ×	× ×	× ×	× ×	× ×
Diabetic education and control	×	× ×	+/–	+/–	×
Physical activity/ exercise	× ×	× ×	× ×	× ×	× ×

[a] Basic educational components, stable phase of disease.
×, routine; × ×, high priority; +/–, if applicable.

It is important for the general practitioner or primary care physician to understand the need to educate their patients, and to acquire the teaching skills to do so. This involves long-term planning for the incorporation of this aspect into the training of medical doctors. Cardiopulmonary resuscitation programmes, basic or advanced, should be taught at the appropriate level of care. Governments, health insurance services and corporations involved in medical cost and payment issues, must be involved in patient education, depending on the country's financial delivery system.

Such agencies as the World Health Organization, the International Society and Federation of Cardiology, the International Telecommunications Union, satellite agencies (INTELSAT), broadcasting unions, the World Federation for Medical Education, international development agencies and banks may support pilot studies to assess the cost-effectiveness of specific, new, educational interventions. Pilot programmes, for example Project SHARE, co-sponsored by INTELSAT and the International Institute of Communications (IIC), may have free satellite time made available for education in developing countries [14].

Acknowledgements

Ms Kelly Kang patiently and painstakingly assisted in the typing and preparation of this manuscript. Permission for submission given by Dr Gyarfas, Chief of Cardiovascular Diseases, World Health Organization. This report is the result of the WHO Expert Committee on Rehabilitation of the Patient with Cardiovascular Disease Working Group 2 chaired by Dr Oon Chong Hau.

References

1. Nutbeam D. Health promotion glossary. *Health Promotion* 1986; **1:** 114.
2. Wenger NK (ed.). *The Education of the Patient with Cardiac Disease in the Twenty-first Century*. Le Jacq: New York, 1986.
3. Nakajima H. The health of nations is changing. *World Health*, 1991; May–June.
4. Wenger NK. Quality of life – issues in chronic cardiovascular illness. *Ann Acad Med* 1992; **21:** 137–140.
5. Taylor CB, Miller NH. Education of the coronary patient and family – the behavioural approach. In: Wenger NK and Hellerstein HK (eds), *Rehabilitation of the Coronary Patient*, 3rd edn. Churchill Livingstone: New York, 1992.
6. Nikolaeva LF, Zaitser WP. School for the Patients after Myocardial Infarction. *Moscow USSR Medicine*, 1989.
7. Evans RI. What can social psychology contribute to increase the probability of adherence on behaviour change through patient-education communication. In: Wenger NK (ed.), *The Education of the Patient with Cardiac Disease in the Twenty-first Century*. Le Jacq: New York, 1986, pp. 46–59.
8. Abadzi H. Cognitive psychology in the seminar room. Economic Development Institute of World Bank, 1990; No. 41.
9. Shephard RJ, Wenger NK, Furberg CD. Education of the aged cardiac patient. In: Wenger NK (ed.), *The Education of the Patient with Cardiac Disease in the Twenty-first Century*. Le Jacq: New York, 1986, pp. 405–410.

10. *Health and Media, Media Technology, Media Asia* 1986; **12:** No. 4.
11. The Patient Education Project (PEP). *A Cross-cultural Project for the Promotion and Evaluation of Health Care in Hypertension.* A Joint WHO/WHL Project Protocol, 1989.
12. Grueninger UJ and Strasser T. Educating the hypertensive patient – teaching the teacher. *J Human Hypertension* (Suppl. 1) 1990; **4:** 3–4.
13. American Association of Cardiovascular and Pulmonary Rehabilitation. *Guidelines for Cardiac Rehabilitation Program.* Human Kinetics: Champaign, IL, 1991.
14. INTELSAT. Bridging the Gap III: A Guide to Telecommunications and Development, 1990.
15. Comoss PM. Education of the coronary patient and family: Principles and practice. In: Wenger NK, Hellerstein HK (eds), *Rehabilitation of the Coronary Patient*, 3rd edn. Churchill Livingstone: New York, 1992, p. 439.
16. Cardiac Rehabilitation Services after PTCA and Valvular Surgery: Guidelines for Use. *Ad Hoc* Task Force on Cardiac Rehabilitation. *Cardiology* 1990; September.

57 The Challenge: Exercise Testing and Training in the Rehabilitation of Children in Developing Countries

Choompol Vongprateep

Children's Hospital, 420/8 Rajvitee Road, Payatai, Bangkok 10400, Thailand

Introduction

Cardiovascular diseases are already the leading cause of morbidity and premature mortality in industrial countries and their emergence as a public health problem in developing countries was already recognized by the WHO Assembly in 1976. Secondary prevention and rehabilitation are part of the WHO strategy to control cardiovascular diseases. Rehabilitation aims not only at training disabled cardiac patients to adapt to their environment, but also at influencing society as a whole in order to facilitate social integration. The goals are to improve functional capacity, decrease unwarranted invalidity, and enable patients to play a useful and personally satisfying role in society. Currently, it is considered an essential part of the care that should be available to all cardiac patients including children, adolescents and young adults. Thus it encompasses the sum of activities required to ensure cardiac patients the best possible physical, mental and social conditions so that they may, by their own efforts, resume and maintain as normal a place as possible in their community.

Exercise testing and training in developing countries

Despite differences in patterns of cardiac disease between and within developing countries, cardiac rehabilitative care as currently conceptualized (low to moder-

Proceedings of the Vth World Congress on Cardiac Rehabilitation

ate intensity exercise with appropriate health education and guidance, as well as vocational counselling) can be applied even in societies with minimal resources. Guidelines are required for so doing. In developing countries, rehabilitative care must be incorporated into the existing health care system, and must conform to cultural traditions and social norms. Although most prominent as a problem in developing countries, such approaches may be applicable to rural areas of industrialized nations as well. Guidance is needed for the maintenance of cardiovascular health, particularly those societies in transition with changes in culture, foods, lifestyle and economy.

The range of cardiac diseases found in children in developing countries such as Thailand are congenital heart disease, rheumatic heart disease (RHD), cardiomyopathy and other aetiologies of ventricular dysfunction (infection, nutrition), and other situations such as mechanical prosthetic valves, chronic anticoagulation, implanted pacemakers and post-cardiac transplantation. Also, those that become inoperable, who have lesions too complex for surgery, who are in post-operative care, with and without residual defect, are especially in need of exercise tests and training in rehabilitation.

While patients with RHD and coronary heart disease may have to be cared for in the same rehabilitation facility as other cardiac patients, it is apparent that groups of children of different ages will need special care and assessment.

The present situation

Exercise testing and training for children in developing countries is not well known nor widely practised, even though it is a very useful non-invasive method for the evaluation of cardiovascular function, since it is a physiological form of stress. Examination of the circulation and cardiac responses to stress is often much more sensitive and informative than evaluation of cardiovascular function at rest. Many subjects with heart disease have abnormal cardiovascular responses to exercise as well as reduced endurance and functional capacity.

Dynamic exercise testing helps in diagnosing and evaluating children and young adults with both cardiac and non-cardiac problems. It provides objective and reliable estimates of physical working capacity, maximal oxygen uptake, and provide clues to mechanisms limiting physical working capacity. In clinical practice, an objective estimate of fitness and information regarding physical activity can be obtained through standard exercise testing, which can be performed with minimal risk. The tests also help in identifying major risk factors which may result in a morbid or fatal event. An abnormal fall or rise in blood pressure, significant ischaemic (e.g. ST-segment and T-wave, rate, rhythm) and conduction abnormalities may occur in the absence of symptoms or a reduction in working capacity.

The guidelines for performing an exercise test are:

1. Evaluate specific symptoms and signs which may be induced or aggravated by exercise.

2. Identify abnormal adaptive responses occurring in subjects with cardiac and other disorders.
3. Assess the effectiveness of specific surgical and medical treatment.
4. Estimate levels of functional capacity for participation in vocational, recreational and athletic activities.
5. Estimate prognosis.

The factors which limit exercise performance and working capacity include: type and severity of heart disease, intolerance to stress, arterial oxygen saturation and acidosis, maximal heart rate, arrhythmia, blood pressure, stroke volume and cardiac output, as well as parental over-protection.

Constraints

Though scientific data have not been compiled, the following conclusion can be drawn from the personal experience of one person involved in the subject over the years, both in the author's own country and through the exchange of information with colleagues in the region.

Exercise testing and training for children in developing countries is not well known nor widely practised, probably because of the following constraints:

1. Lack of trained professional personnel.
2. Lack of facilities, equipment and educational material.
3. Lack of finance and funding.
4. Lack of exercise programmes and patient counselling.
5. Other national priorities.
6. Lack of awareness on the part of both paediatric cardiologists, and patients and their families.

Special considerations in creating exercise testing and training programmes for children in developing countries

Communication, accessibility and socio-cultural elements are limiting factors in most rural communities in developing countries. Significant investment in both financial and trained human resources are frequently the only options available to overcome these obstacles. Simple community-based rehabilitation programmes within the framework of good low-cost medical and community practice are most appropriate for the majority of the population in the developing countries at this stage. Low-intensity exercise programmes are an attractive option because, in most cases, even relatively simple testing may not be required. Thus for the vast majority of patients, sophisticated testing is not required. It could be done within the framework of a basic facility and would consist of:

1. A *facility* (exercise laboratory) to be modified according to sources available and climatic conditions. Any community facility that is available would do.
2. *Personnel*: a trained community health worker, preferably a health professional would need to be available.
3. *Equipment*: step (ergometer) handgrip, sphygnomanometer, stethoscope and also the ability to check pulse rate. Educational material and charts and a suitable area for walking or exercising. Although a multi-stage workload test is preferred, single-stage workload testing, the step test or bending and stretching test is acceptable if resources are limited.
4. *Minimal monitoring and basic measurements* include: general condition of the patient, blood pressure and heart rate before, during and after each workload, and during recovery. Where resources are available, ECG monitoring is required. Some observations are made continuously and others intermittently, depending on the particular protocol.
5. *Protocols*: are available and should be adhered to. The step test and the 9- and 12-min walk/run tests are being investigated further for estimating levels of fitness in the paediatric population.
6. *Normal standards* are available but must be applied appropriately to country and race.

Strategy

The key factor leading to the successful establishment of exercise testing and training for children in developing countries is to inform and convince the clinical community, the health care policy-makers, and the cardiac patients themselves, of the existence and advantages of this service. For the clinical community (physicians and other health professionals), whose initiative the introduction of the programme depends on, it is essential they believe that cardiac rehabilitation is a component of long-term comprehensive cardiac care, which includes exercise testing and training, and that programmes should be available to all patients with cardiovascular diseases, both children and adults. This kind of service can, and should, be provided by any trained health professional caring for cardiac patients. Patients and their families must participate, and sophisticated equipment and facilities are not mandatory. They must also understand that a programme is an individualized regimen of physical activity, health education and counselling, as is appropriate for that specific cardiac problem and that patient's needs. It is also essential that responsibility for implementation should be given to a designated, trained health professional co-ordinator at the local level who is attached to an appropriate health care facility, whether run by a governmental or non-governmental organization. Finally, guidance towards appropriate occupations (for children and young adults) and return to work (for adults) is useful for most cardiac patients.

For health care policy-makers, it is well-known that, in developing countries, policies have to be formulated at the governmental or local level if any health care programme is to be put into effect. This means that not only must the policy-makers themselves recognize the value of this welfare, but they must also be determined to see it through. Every aspect of the programme has to be dealt with: the provision of funds, operational structure, as well as clear instructions to the people involved. They must be persuaded that cardiovascular disease is an increasing problem in developing countries and that it involves children and young adults as well as their elders, and that cardiac rehabilitation is part of the long-term comprehensive care of cardiac patients. These programmes can be integrated at low cost into the existing health care system: the major requirement is the training of health professionals in exercise recommendations, health education and vocational guidance. Training resources are available from international and regional agencies. The programmes are cost-effective because the benefits include improvement in function and health status, quality of life, social independence and place in society, work resumption and continuation.

Both cardiac patients and their families realize the value of rehabilitation as providing a quicker and better chance of a more complete recovery. Even society as a whole can see the benefits that these programmes eventually bring. They in turn will demand that their needs in this respect be provided for.

The benefits to be gained by children and their families from a programme designed to optimize recovery and promote a healthy lifestyle from childhood to adult life, include: improved physical activity capacity and more rapid physical recovery; return to school or work and social re-integration and maintenance there; increased self-esteem and self-worth of the child; a decrease in the risk of excessive parental protection. Such programmes also promote the healthy psychological development of the child, decrease unwarranted invalidity that may persist from childhood into adult life, increase guidance for family and marital life after childhood and decrease recurrent episodes/complications of cardiovascular disease.

Conclusion

Exercise testing and training in the rehabilitation of children can be established in developing countries at low cost. This can be done at a basic level using manual measurements when resources are limited. It can improve quality of health care in general. Cooperation among patients, families, physicians, government and voluntary organizations is needed. The successful rehabilitation of paediatric patients is prudent and will assist them in leading productive lives in the long term. They will benefit medically, socially and psychologically.

References provided for complementay information

1. Adams FJ, Bengtsson E *et al.* The physical working capacity of normal school children. II. Swedish City and Country. *Pediatrics* 1961; **28:** 243–257.
2. Adams FH, Linde IM *et al.* The physical working capacity of normal school children. I California. *Pediatrics* 1961; **28:** 55–64.
3. Alpert BS, Dover E *et al.* Blood pressure response to dynamic exercise in healthy children – black *vs* white. *J Ped* 1981; **99:** 556–560.
4. Alpert BS, Flood NL *et al.* Responses to ergometer exercise in a healthy bi-racial population of children. *J Ped* 1982; **101:** 538–545.
5. American Heart Association. *Standards for Exercise Testing in the Pediatric Age Group.* American Heart Association Council on Cardiovascular Disease in the Young, Vol. 66, 1982.
6. Andersen KL, Seliger V *et al.* Physical performance capacity of children in Norway. *Eur J Appl Physiol* 1974, **33:** 197–206.
7. Bar-Or O. Physical conditioning in children with cardiorespiratory disease. *Exercise Sport Sci Rev* 1985, **13:** 305–334.
8. Beekman RH. Exercise recommendations for adolescents after surgery for congenital heart disease. *Pedatricina* 1986, **13:** 210–219.
9. Cumming GR, Everatt D *et al.* Bruce treadmill test in children: Normal values in a clinic population. *Am J Cardiol* 1978; **41:** 69–75.
10. Garson A, Gillett PC, Gutgesell HP, McNamara DG. Stress induced ventricular arrhythmia after repair of tetralogy of Fallot. *Am J Cardiol* 1980; **46:** 1006.
11. Goldberg B *et al.* Effect of physical training on exercise performance of children following surgical repair of congenital heart disease. *Pediatrics* 1981; **68:** 691–699.
12. James FW, Kaplan S *et al.* Responses of normal children and young adults with cardiovascular disease. *Circulation* 1980; **61:** 902–912.
13. Longmuir PE, Turner JAP, Rowe RD, Olley PM. Postoperative exercise rehabilitation benefits of children with congenital heart disease. *Clin Invest Med* 1985; **8:** 232–238.
14. Muskin CS. Aerobic exercise training in cardiopulmonary disease. In: Weber KT, Janicki JS (eds), *Cardiopulmonary Exercise Testing.* WB Saunders: Philadelphia, PA, 1986.
15. Strong WB, Alpert BS. The Children with Heart Disease: Play, Recreation and Sports. *Current Problems in Cardiology.* Year Book Medical: 1981.
16. Washington RL, Gundy JC *et al.* Normal aerobic and anaerobic exercise data for North American school-age children. *J Ped* 1988; **112:** 223–233.
17. Rheumatic Fever/Rheumatic Heart Disease. Report of a WHO Study Group. *WHO Technical Report* 764, Geneva, 1988.

58 Aspects of Exercise Testing and Training in the Rehabilitation of Children and Young Adults with Cardiovascular Disease

F. W. James*, C. Vongprateep, A. O. Falase, I. Martin, I. Gyarfas, N. Wenger

World Health Organization, Geneva, Switzerland

Introduction

The World Health Organization (WHO) recommends cardiac rehabilitation for all patients with heart disease [1]. Cardiac rehabilitation is less often used in children and young adults than in the adult population. The exercise test is a sensitive and informative method of evaluating cardiovascular function in children. To comply with the WHO recommendations, guidelines are needed which will apply to the young population and the available resources in developing countries.

This chapter briefly discusses certain aspects of exercise testing and training in the rehabilitation of children and adolescents with cardiovascular disease.

Exercise testing

Dynamic exercise testing assists in diagnosing and evaluating young patients with cardiac and non-cardiac problems. Objective and reliable estimates of physical working capacity, maximal oxygen uptake, and clues to mechanisms limiting physical working capacity are feasible through standardized exercise

*Address all correspondence to Frederick W. James, Division of Cardiology, Children's Hospital Medical Center, Cincinatti, Ohio 45229-2899, USA.

testing. The exercise procedure can be performed at minimal risk to patients with conditions of varying severity. The reasons for performing an exercise test are:

1. To assess specific symptoms and signs.
2. To identify adaptive responses.
3. To evaluate medical and surgical treatment.
4. To identify functional capacity levels.
5. To estimate prognosis.

Exercise data combined with other relevant data provide the best information for clinical management. General applications include estimating exercise capacity, directing myocardial ischaemia and rate and rhythm disturbances, and determining the proper type and intensity of exercise training.

The general principles of exercise testing are:

1. Multi-stage workload test is preferred. Single-stage workload test is acceptable in areas where resources are limited.
2. Workload level should begin below the estimated level of impairment.
3. Workload level should be maintained for sufficient time to stabilize the response over 1–2 min.
4. Minimal monitoring requirements are general condition of the patient, blood pressure, heart rate and electrocardiogram where resources are available.
5. Informed consent prior to testing is recommended as appropriate for the medical care setting and culture.
6. Indications to terminate a test and contraindications and special considerations for testing are as outlined by the American Heart Association, Standards for Exercise Testing in Children [2].

Methods of exercise testing

Equipment recommendations for testing at the basic, intermediate and advanced level facilities are listed in Table 1. At the basic and intermediate level facilities, measurements of work, heart rate and ST-segment changes (intermediate only) can be recorded. At the advanced level facilities, recording of multi-lead electrocardiography and estimates of pulmonary ventilation and gas exchange are feasible. Other measurements for assessing cardiovascular function and performance are cardiac output, systolic time intervals, echographic and scintigraphic techniques of function. These techniques are available depending upon the available resources.

Protocols

Normal data are available for several types of cycle or treadmill protocols in young patients. The reader is referred to other published literature for comple-

Table 1
Recommendations for equipment to conduct exercise testing at different treatment facilities [1]

Basic level facilities
Step test, or
Bending and stretching test
Sphygmomanometer
Heart rate by palpitation
Intermediate level facilities
Step test, or
Cycle or treadmill
Bending or stretching test
Single lead electrocardiography
Sphygmomanometer
Advanced level facilties
Cycle and/or treadmill
Multi-lead electrocardiography
Sphygmomanometer
Oxygen uptake and carbon dioxide production system

tion and details [1, 2]. The situations and specific diseases for including exercise testing in the clinical evaluations are: (1) diagnosis of exercise-induced symptoms; (2) evaluation of dysrhythmias; (3) assessment of potential myocardial ischaemia; (4) hypertension; (5) congenital complete A-V block; (6) atrial septal defect; (7) ventricular septal defect; (8) pulmonary stenosis; (9) aortic stenosis; (10) aortic incompetence; (11) coarctation of aorta; (12) tetralogy of Fallot; (13) transposition of the great vessels, post-operatively; (14) Kawasaki disease; and (15) cardiomyopathy.

Exercise training

Increased physical activity, education and counselling of the child and family and reduction of morbidity and mortality are major goals of cardiovascular rehabilitation programmes for your patients. Programmes which involve a variety of fun-related and spontaneous physical activity, group participation including parents for role modelling, use peer-directed approaches and contain an incentive–reward system are more acceptable and successful in the paediatric age group.

Exercise training programmes should have a duration of at least 12 weeks and include activities of flexibility, co-ordination, strength, balance and aerobic training. Also, the programme should be instructional and require goal-setting. High-intensity physical activity at low risk requiring only self-monitoring can be performed by patients with the cardiac conditions listed in Table 2 [1].

Table 2
Cardiac conditions with lowest risk for exercise testing and training [1]

Valvar aortic stenosis (resting gradient <20 mmHg)
Aortic insufficiency (normal heart size and blood pressure)
Atrial septal defect (normal pulmonary artery pressure and conduction)
Coarctation of aorta (normal blood pressure)
Mitral incompetence (normal heart size)
Patent ductus arteriosus (small shunt)
Pulmonic stenosis (resting gradient <50 mmHg)
Ventricular septal defect (small shunt)

Conclusion

Exercise testing and training in the cardiac rehabilitation of children and young adults can be accomplished at low cost in developing countries and can improve the quality of health care with favourable economic benefits to society. In developing countries, the step (ergometer) with manual measurement of pulse rate and blood pressure can be performed at the basic care level. At higher levels of care, more complex measurements are made, depending on the available resources. An exercise procedure used to determine peak working capacity and identify cardiovascular limitations helps to establish the individualized rehabilitation programme. These approaches increase the opportunity for obtaining the best yield, the highest degree of safety of the use of exercise testing and training in young cardiac patients.

References

1. World Health Organization (WHO), Working Group 3, Expert Committee on Rehabilitation of the Patient with Cardiovascular Disease, Geneva, Switzerland, 1991.
2. American Heart Association. Standards for Exercise Testing in the Pediatric Age Group: American Heart Association Council on Cardiovascular Disease in the Young. *Circulation* 1982; **66:** 1387A–1397A.

XV Economics of Cardiac Rehabilitation

59 Economic Evaluation of Cardiac Rehabilitation Soon after Myocardial Infarction

N. Oldridge

Department of Health Sciences, University of Wisconsin, Milwaukee, Wisconsin 53201, USA

Introduction

Choices among alternative health care services have to be made. When health care resources, people, time, facilities, equipment, finances and knowledge are scarce, the answers to the question of choices of alternative services are strongly influenced by estimates of relative merit. One form of evaluation of relative merit is an economic or efficiency evaluation. This is most useful when preceded by assessments of efficacy (randomized clinical trial asking whether the service does more good than harm), effectiveness (whether the service will be accepted in the real world, i.e., whether it will work) and whether it reaches those who need it (whether it is accessible and available to those who can benefit) [1].

The questions of efficacy, effectiveness and availability of cardiac rehabilitation have been extensively examined. The benefits of cardiac rehabilitation include a reduction in cardiovascular risk factors, a decrease in activity-induced symptoms, an improved functional capacity [2] and, possibly, an accelerated early improvement in psychosocial outcomes such as quality of life [3]. In addition, meta-analyses of randomized clinical trials of cardiac rehabilitation [4, 5] have demonstrated a 25% reduction in mortality after myocardial infarction [MI], although, with the impact that routine interventions such as thrombolysis and revascularization have on early reinfarction, the probability of additional improvements in survival with rehabilitation is considerably

Proceedings of the Vth World Congress on Cardiac Rehabilitation

reduced. The overall goals of cardiac rehabilitation, then, clearly should be focused on quality of life as implied in the 1964 WHO definition of rehabilitation: "rehabilitation is the sum of activity required to ensure the best possible physical, mental and social conditions so that patients may by their own efforts regain as normal as possible a place in the community and lead an active productive life" [6].

On the other hand, the economic evaluation of cardiac rehabilitation has not been as rigorously addressed [7–9] as has its efficacy and effectiveness. In the USA alone, it has been estimated that more than 100,000 patients participate in cardiac rehabilitation programmes at a cost exceeding US$108 million per year [10]. Rising health care costs have become a fact of life and efficacy is no longer the only criterion on which to determine whether or not a particular health care service should be used when providing health care for patients. The provision of health care services will increasingly require considerations of costs and, without systematic analysis, including an economic evaluation, it will be increasingly difficult to identify and recommend relevant and efficient health care service alternatives.

Economic evaluation of health care services using cardiac rehabilitation as an example

Economic evaluations help health care policy-makers, health care administrators, physicians and health professionals, as well as patients, compare health care services and technologies in terms of their relative economic efficiencies in providing health benefits. Unless specifically stated, the following comments on economic, or efficiency, evaluation of health care services, specifically cardiac rehabilitation, have been based primarily on the text by Drummond *et al.* [1]. First, economic evaluation deals with both costs (inputs) and consequences (outputs) of the health care service; the linkage between the two factors permits a decision about efficiency to be made. Secondly, economic analysis concerns itself with choices; these choices are made on the basis of explicit, and often implicit, criteria. On the basis of these characteristics, Drummond and colleagues define economic evaluation as "the comparative analysis of alternative courses of action in terms of both their costs and consequences" [1].

We have recently completed a randomized clinical trial (RCT) of cardiac rehabilitation initiated within 6 weeks of myocardial infarction [3]. In this trial 201 patients with mild to moderate anxiety and/or depression while still in hospital were randomized to either 8 weeks of cardiac rehabilitation ($n = 99$) or usual care ($n = 102$) and, for the next year, were followed up with health related quality of life as one of the primary outcomes of interest. The other primary outcome of interest was an economic evaluation of cardiac rehabilitation, considering both the costs and the consequences of cardiac rehabilitation; as examples of an economic evaluation, this presentation utilizes selected preliminary data that will be published in detail elsewhere [11].

Types of costs and consequences

Generally, at least two types of costs and three types of consequences of health care services are considered in an economic evaluation. Using cardiac rehabilitation as an example, these are as follows:

Costs

1. Costs associated with organizing and operating the rehabilitation programme. In the RCT, operating costs per patient amounted to \$670 (to nearest US\$10, 1991); this was made up of space and equipment = \$420, staff (exercise leader, co-ordinator and MD) = \$170 and miscellaneous = \$80.
2. Costs of attending the intervention which are borne by the patient. These direct costs include transportation as well as time spent attending the programme; shoes, clothing and other equipment purchased to participate in the programme or its recommendations; child-care expenses. These patient-borne costs amounted to \$120 per patient in the RCT. There also may be indirect costs associated with cardiac rehabilitation and primarily these include the costs associated with time lost from work (the programme was run in the late afternoon and so these costs were omitted).

The direct costs per patient in the RCT were then the sum of the programme-borne costs (\$670) and patient-borne costs (\$120), amounting to a total direct cost per patient of \$790 or \$50 per session for the 8-week intervention.

Consequences

1. Clinical or therapeutic effects of cardiac rehabilitation can be measured as changes in the physical (e.g. life-years, exercise tolerance), social (e.g. return to work) or emotional (e.g. depression) function of the patient. Survival rates in the two groups during the 12-month follow-up period were not different.

2. There may be changes in resource utilization, often referred to as benefits, as a result of the health care service. In cardiac rehabilitation, these may include direct benefits such as lower utilization of physician services, of emergency visits, of medications, of vocational rehabilitation services; none of these were significantly different in the RCT. A number of usual care patients ($n = 51$) and rehabilitation patients ($n = 33$) were referred by their physicians to community rehabilitation programmes after completion of the experimental intervention, even though the physicians had agreed not to refer their patients to rehabilitation for the first 12 months following discharge from hospital. The mean number of "other cardiac rehabilitation" visits, calculated over the year of follow-up (excluding the 8-week intervention), was significantly greater ($P < 0.0001$) in the control (8.3 visits per patient) than in the experimental group (1.9 visits per

patient). The direct savings, in favour of the rehabilitation patients, associated with these visits to "other cardiac rehabilitation" were $310 per patient.

3. There may be changes in quality of life in both patients and their families. These changes are defined and measured as "utilities" in health care economic evaluation [12]. The conventional utility, or preference valuation of health status, is defined in the interval between 1.00 as the score for perfect health and 0.00 as the score for dead. One example of a "utility" is the time trade-off (TTO) method of estimating health-related quality of life; this approach utilizes a direct preference measure first to estimate utility and then to calculate quality-adjusted life-years (QALY), and was specifically developed for use in health care [13, 14]. In this approach, the patient is given a series of dichotomous choices between the health state being measured for the rest of life as estimated from life-expectancy tables for a person of the same age or a shorter but perfectly healthy life. Dividing the minimum time chosen for perfect health by the time derived from the life tables provides a measure of perceived quality of life, e.g. if life-expectancy is 20 years and the time chosen in full health is 15 years, then TTO = 0.75. The TTO utility scores are then multiplied by duration in years to calculate QALYs. This approach (a) allows patients to consider their present health status so providing an estimation of their quality of life and (b) also permits examination of changes in health-related quality of life.

The differences in mean TTO change scores between the rehabilitation or usual care patients resulted in an estimate of 0.052 QALYs gained per patient in favour of the rehabilitation programme.

Types of economic evaluation

An economic evaluation entails identification, measurement, valuation and comparison of costs and consequences. If only one service is being evaluated, or described, then there is either a cost description (only costs examined), an outcome description (only consequences examined) or a cost–outcome description (both costs and consequences examined). These are each defined as partial economic evaluations. When alternative health care services are being compared but only either costs or consequences are examined, this is defined as either an efficacy or effectiveness evaluation and thus is also considered a partial economic evaluation. Partial economic evaluations do not allow questions of efficiency to be answered. However, when alternative health care services as well as both costs and consequences are examined, this is considered to be a full economic evaluation and efficiency questions can be addressed. There are four types of full economic evaluation. There are cost-minimization and cost–benefit analyses, neither of which was utilized in the present economic evaluation. The remaining two types of full economic evaluation, which were used in the RCT, are cost-utility and cost-effectiveness analyses.

Cost-utility analysis of the randomized clinical trial

In cost-utility analysis, the value of the clinical effects or consequences produced, e.g. life-years gained, is expressed in terms of "utility" (or value) for a specific level of health status or of some improvement in health status. The changes in health-related quality of life with alternative health care services, e.g. cardiac rehabilitation and usual care, can also be considered in a more comprehensive fashion in conjunction with the life-years gained, and quality-adjusted life-years (QALY) can be estimated and costs of the services can then be compared per QALY gained. Cost-utility analysis permits comparison of the efficiency of the health care services under consideration. In the present trial, the TTO technique was used to measure health-related quality of life.

Incremental net direct costs of the RCT were calculated as (direct costs = \$790) – (direct savings = \$310), which amount to a best estimate net direct cost per patient of \$480. The differences in mean TTO change scores between the rehabilitation or usual care patients resulted in an estimate of 0.052 QALYs gained per patient in favour of the rehabilitation programme. As seen in Table 1, using the best estimate of net incremental direct costs (\$480) and 0.052 QALYs gained, the cost (to nearest US\$100, 1991) per QALY per patient with rehabilitation, using TTO scores, was \$9,200. The cost-utility estimate of \$9,200 per QALY for cardiac rehabilitation is considerably lower than that reported for single-vessel bypass surgery in patients with mild angina or for treatment of mild or severe diastolic hypertension in 40-year-old males, but approximately 15% higher than the estimate for bypass surgery in patients with left main vessel disease.

Table 1
Economic evaluation data for cardiac rehabilitation (US\$, 1991)

Incremental costs	
Direct costs	790
Direct savings	310
Net direct costs	480
Cost-utility (year 1 only)	
Net direct costs/QALY[a]	9,200
Cost-effectiveness	
Net direct costs/LYG[b]	21,800
Comprehensive cost-utility	
Net direct costs/QALY gained[c]	6,800

[a] Quality-adjusted life-years from TTO change scores; [b] life-years gained in meta-analysis [5]; [c] quality-adjusted life-years plus quality-adjusted life-years gained.

Cost-effectiveness analysis using meta-analysis

Analyses where costs are related to a single unit of effect are defined as cost-effectiveness analysis. Providing the consequences are measured in common units, i.e. life-years gained (LYG), this approach permits a particular service (e.g. cardiac rehabilitation) to be compared to some other service, either similar (e.g. smoking cessation) or quite different (e.g. rehabilitation following kidney transplantation). Cost-effectiveness analysis also permits comparison of the efficiency of the health care services under consideration.

Estimates of life-years lost over 3 years have been generated from a published meta-analysis of cardiac rehabilitation [5] where mortality with rehabilitation was 10.7%, significantly lower than the 12.9% reported for the control patients; the 0.022 difference between the mortality rates for the groups represents the LYG by patients in the rehabilitation group as compared to the patients in the control group. By the end of year 3, as seen in Table 1 and using net direct costs, the best estimate of the cost per LYG was $21800. At $21800 per LYG, cardiac rehabilitation is not as cost-effective as a brief office visit for smoking cessation, aspirin for all MI or beta-adrenergic antagonist therapy in a 55-year-old male. However, the cost-effectiveness of cardiac rehabilitation per LYG is intermediate to propranolol hydrochloride therapy for diastolic hypertension and Lovastatin (40 mg/day) for hypercholesterolaemia and strikingly more cost-effective than either Lovastatin (80 mg/day), Captopril or Colestipol.

Comprehensive cost-utility

A comprehensive cost-utility measure, or total incremental QALYs gained, associated with rehabilitation, is the sum of the QALY gains attributable to reduced mortality (0.022 incremental LYG) multiplied by the mean TTO score of 0.872 [3] plus the 0.052 QALY gains due to improved health-related quality of life during the first year; this amounts to 0.071 QALYs gained. A comprehensive cost-utility analysis of best estimate costs based on 0.071 incremental QALYs gained over a 3-year horizon results, as seen in Table 1, in a cost per QALY gained due to rehabilitation of $6,800. The costs per QALY gained with early, brief cardiac rehabilitation are similar to the estimated cost of $7,900 (US 1991) per QALY gained reported for bypass surgery for left main vessel disease [15].

Conclusion

These results must be compared to the other interventions when attempting to make decisions about alternative interventions, whether at the individual patient level or the policy level. These economic evaluation data do provide evidence that brief cardiac rehabilitation provided soon after AMI for patients with mild to moderate anxiety and/or depression is an efficient use of health care resources and can be economically justified when compared to published cost-utility and cost-effectiveness results for interventions in coronary heart disease. The RCT does not address the issues of worth or affordability of cardiac rehabilitation. The efficiency of the intervention is enhanced more by the low cost of the rehabilitation services, the subsequent reduction in demand for additional community rehabilitation services and the moderate increase in health-related life quality than by the increased survival among rehabilitation patients. These kinds of data are useful for policy-making decisions, particularly where there is competition for alternative interventions with limited available resources.

References

1. Drummond MF, Stoddart GL, Torrance GW. *Methods for the Economic Evaluation of Health Care Programmes*. Oxford University Press: Oxford, 1987, pp. 1–4.
2. Siegel D, Grady D, Browner WS, Hullet SB. Risk factor modification after myocardial infarction. *Ann Intern Med* 1988; **109:** 213–218.
3. Oldridge NB, Guyatt G, Jones N, Crowe J, Singer J, Feeny D, McKelvie R, Runions J, Streiner D, Torrance G. Effects on quality of life with comprehensive rehabilitation after acute myocardial infarction. *Am J Cardiol* 1991; **67:** 1084–1089.
4. Oldridge NB, Guyatt GH, Fischer M, Rimm A. Cardiac rehabilitation after myocardial infarction: Combining data from randomized clinical trials. *JAMA* 1988; **260:** 945–980.
5. O'Connor GT, Buring JE, Yusuf S, Goldhaber SZ, Olmstaed EM, Paffenbarger RS, Hennekens CH. An overview of randomized trials of rehabilitation with exercise after myocardial infarction. *Circulation* 1989; **80:** 234–244.
6. Rehabilitation of patients with cardiovascular disease: Report of a WHO expert committee. *WHO Tech Rep Ser* 1964: 240.
7. Ades PA, Huang D, Weaver SO. Cardiac rehabilitation participation predicts lower rehospitalization costs. *Am Heart J* 1992; **123:** 916–921.
8. Dennis C. Cost-effectiveness in cardiac rehabilitation. *J Cardiopulmonary Rehab* 1991; **11:** 128–131.
9. Levin LA, Perk J, Hedback B. Cardiac rehabilitation – a cost analysis. *J Intern Med* 1991; **230:** 427–434.
10. Health and Public Policy Committee, American College of Physicians. Cardiac rehabilitation services. *Ann Intern Med* 1988; **258:** 671–673.
11. Oldridge N, Furlong W, Feeny, Torrance G, Guyatt G, Crowe J, Jones NL. Economic evaluation: Cardiac rehabilitation following acute myocardial infarction. *Am J Cardiol*, in press.
12. Torrance GW, Feeny D. Utilities and quality-adjusted life years. *Int J Tech Assess Health Care* 1989; **5:** 559–575.
13. Torrance GW. Social preferences for health states: An empirical evaluation of three measurement techniques. *Socio-Econ Plan Sci* 1976; **10:** 129–136.
14. Torrance GW. Utility, decision, and quality of life. *J Chron Dis* 1987; **40:** 593–600.
15. Weinstein MC. Challenges for cost-effectiveness research. *Med Decision Making* 1986; **6:** 194–198.

Index